Practical Flow Cytometry
in Haematology: 100
Worked Examples

Practical Flow Cytometry in Haematology: 100 Worked Examples

Mike Leach FRCP, FRCPath
Consultant Haematologist and Honorary Senior Lecturer
Haematology Laboratories and West of Scotland Cancer Centre
Gartnavel General Hospital
Glasgow, UK

Mark Drummond PhD, FRCPath
Consultant Haematologist and Honorary Senior Lecturer
Haematology Laboratories and West of Scotland Cancer Centre
Gartnavel General Hospital
Glasgow, UK

Allyson Doig MSc, FIBMS
Haemato-Oncology Laboratory Manager
Haematology Laboratories
Gartnavel General Hospital
Glasgow, UK

Pam McKay
Consultant Haematologist
Haematology Laboratories and West of Scotland Cancer Centre
Gartnavel General Hospital
Glasgow, UK

Bob Jackson
Consultant Pathologist
Department of Pathology
Southern General Hospital
Glasgow, UK

Barbara J. Bain MBBS, FRACP, FRCPath
Professor of Diagnostic Haematology
St Mary's Hospital Campus of Imperial College
Faculty of Medicine, London
and Honorary Consultant Haematologist,
St Mary's Hospital, London, UK

WILEY Blackwell

Library of Congress Cataloging-in-Publication Data

Leach, Richard M. (Haematologist), author.
  Practical flow cytometry in haematology : 100 worked examples / Mike Leach [and 5 others].
    p. ; cm.
  Includes index.
    ISBN 978-1-118-74703-2 (hardback)
  I. Title.
  [DNLM: 1. Hematologic Diseases–diagnosis–Case Reports. 2. Hematologic Neoplasms–diagnosis–Case Reports.
3. Flow Cytometry–methods–Case Reports. 4. Hematology–methods–Case Reports. WH 120]
  RC636
  616.1'5075–dc23
                                                                                            2015007734

A catalogue record for this book is available from the British Library.

Wiley also publishes its books in a variety of electronic formats. Some content that appears in print may not be available in electronic books.

Set in 8.5/11pt, MinionPro by Laserwords Private Limited, Chennai, India

1   2015

Contents

Preface, vii

Acknowledgement, ix

List of Abbreviations, xi

Technical Notes, xv

Laboratory Values, xix

Case 1 1

Case 2 6

Case 3 11

Case 4 15

Case 5 18

Case 6 21

Case 7 24

Case 8 27

Case 9 31

Case 10 35

Case 11 39

Case 12 43

Case 13 46

Case 14 50

Case 15 54

Case 16 59

Case 17 62

Case 18 65

Case 19 68

Case 20 70

Case 21 74

Case 22 77

Case 23 80

Case 24 82

Case 25 87

Case 26 90

Case 27 93

Case 28 95

Case 29 100

Case 30 104

Case 31 106

Case 32 110

Case 33 114

Case 34 117

Case 35 122

Case 36 126

Case 37 129

Case 38 132

Case 39 136

Case 40 140

Case 41 143

Case 42 146

Case 43 151

Case 44 154

Case 45 159

Case 46 163

Case 47 166

Case 48 168

Case 49 172

Case 50 177

Case 51 180
Case 52 183
Case 53 186
Case 54 189
Case 55 193
Case 56 196
Case 57 201
Case 58 206
Case 59 210
Case 60 213
Case 61 216
Case 62 218
Case 63 224
Case 64 227
Case 65 232
Case 66 236
Case 67 240
Case 68 244
Case 69 249
Case 70 253
Case 71 256
Case 72 260
Case 73 266
Case 74 269
Case 75 274
Case 76 276
Case 77 281
Case 78 284

Case 79 289
Case 80 292
Case 81 297
Case 82 300
Case 83 306
Case 84 310
Case 85 315
Case 86 319
Case 87 321
Case 88 325
Case 89 327
Case 90 330
Case 91 334
Case 92 338
Case 93 342
Case 94 347
Case 95 351
Case 96 355
Case 97 359
Case 98 365
Case 99 370
Case 100 375

Antibodies Used in Immunohistochemistry
Studies, 381

Flow Cytometry Antibodies, 386

Molecular Terminology, 389

Classification of Cases According to Diagnosis, 390

Index, 391

Preface

In our first publication 'Practical Flow Cytometry in Haematology Diagnosis' we presented an outline approach to the use and applications of flow cytometric immunophenotyping in the diagnostic haematology laboratory. We showed how this technique could be used to study blood, bone marrow and tissue fluid samples in a variety of clinical scenarios to achieve a diagnosis, taking into account important features from the clinical history and examination alongside haematology, morphology, biochemistry, immunology, cytogenetic, histopathology and molecular data. This text was illustrated with a series of 'worked examples' from real clinical cases presenting to our institution. These cases have proven to be very popular and so a companion publication dedicated to 100 new 'worked examples' seemed justified and is presented here.

The principles used in the approach to each case are exactly the same as used in the first publication and cases are illustrated with tissue pathology and cytogenetic and molecular data, which are integrated to generate, where appropriate, a diagnosis based on the WHO Classification of Tumours of Haematopoietic and Lymphoid Tissues. We present a spectrum of clinical cases encountered in our department from both adult and paediatric patients and of course, if the title is to be justified, flow cytometry plays a role in every case. Furthermore, we present both neoplastic and reactive disorders and the cases appear in no particular order so that the reader should have no pre-conceived idea as to the nature of the diagnosis in any case. May–Grünwald–Giemsa (MGG)-stained films of peripheral blood and bone marrow aspirates are presented with flow cytometry data alongside haematoxylin and eosin (H&E)-stained bone marrow and tissue biopsy sections. Immunohistochemistry is used to further clarify the tissue lineage and cell differentiation. Cytogenetic studies using metaphase preparations are used to identify translocations and chromosome gains and losses whilst interphase fluorescence *in situ* hybridisation (FISH) studies and polymerase chain reaction (PCR) are used to identify gene fusions, break-aparts and deletions. The presentation is brought to a conclusion and the particular features that are important in making a diagnosis are highlighted and discussed. The cases are also listed according to disease classification toward the end (page 390) so that the text can also be used as a reference manual.

The analysis of blood, bone marrow and tissue fluid specimens requires a multi-faceted approach with the integration of scientific data from a number of disciplines. No single discipline can operate in isolation or errors will occur. Flow cytometry technology is in a privileged position in that it can provide rapid analysis of specimens; it is often the first definitive investigation to produce results and help formulate a working diagnosis. The results from flow cytometry can help to structure investigative algorithms to ensure that the appropriate histopathological, cytogenetic and molecular studies are performed in each case. Tissue samples are often limited in volume and difficult to acquire so it is important to stratify investigations accordingly and to get the most from the material available. It is not good scientific or economic practice to run a large series of poorly focussed analyses on every case. Appropriate studies need to be executed in defined circumstances and flow cytometry can guide subsequent investigations in a logical fashion. In some situations a rapid succinct diagnosis can be achieved; immunophenotyping excels in the identification of acute leukaemia. Cytogenetic studies and molecular data give important prognostic information in these patients. But of course the recognised genetic aberrations need to be demonstrated if the diagnosis is to be substantiated. Acute promyelocytic leukaemia can often be confidently diagnosed using morphology alongside immunophenotyping data, but a *PML* translocation to the *RARA* fusion partner, needs to be shown. Flow cytometry cannot operate in isolation; despite having the 'first bite of the cherry' the differential diagnosis can still be wide open. There are a good number of worked examples illustrated here where immunophenotyping was not able to indicate a specific diagnosis. The disease entities with anaplastic or 'minimalistic' phenotypes frequently cause difficulty. Appropriate histopathology and FISH, performed on the basis of flow cytometric findings, highlighting abnormal protein expression and gene rearrangement respectively, can make a major contribution to diagnosis and disease classification. Only when a specific diagnosis is made and prognostic parameters are assessed can the optimal management plan be considered for each individual patient. Finally, the goal posts are constantly moving and developments in the molecular basis of disease, refining disease classification, are evolving rapidly. Whether we are considering eosinophilic proliferations, the myriad of myeloproliferative neoplasms, lymphoproliferative disorders or acute leukaemias we are constantly noting developments and adjusting diagnosis and prognosis accordingly. This is an era of evolving diagnostic challenge and rapid molecular evolution where the practising clinician needs to keep abreast of the significant developments in all areas of haematopathology.

The flow cytometric principles applied to each case have been described in detail in 'Practical Flow Cytometry in Haematology Diagnosis' and some working knowledge is required to interpret the cases described. We also anticipate a reasonable ability in morphological assessment and a capacity to identify morphological variations seen in various disease states. In spite of this we do endeavour to describe the diagnostic logic that we have applied to each worked example and demonstrate how cellular immunophenotypes have helped determine the nature of the disorder.

This text will be of interest to all practicing haematologists and to histopathologists with an interest in haematopathology but it is particularly directed at trainee haematologists and scientists preparing for FRCPath examinations.

Acknowledgement

We are grateful for the substantial assistance of Dr Avril Morris DipRCPath, Principal Clinical Scientist, West of Scotland Genetic Services, Southern General Hospital, Glasgow with regard to the provision of the cytogenetic data and images relevant to the clinical cases presented here.

List of Abbreviations

ADP	adenosine diphosphate
AITL	angioimmunoblastic T-cell lymphoma
AL	acute leukaemia
ALCL	anaplastic large cell lymphoma
ALL	acute lymphoblastic leukaemia
ALP	alkaline phosphatase
ALT	alanine transaminase
AML	acute myeloid leukaemia
AML-MRC	acute myeloid leukaemia with myelodysplasia-related changes
ANA	antinuclear antibody
APC	allophycocyanin
APL	acute promyelocytic leukaemia
APTT	activated partial thromboplastin time
ASM	aggressive systemic mastocytosis
AST	aspartate transaminase
ATLL	adult T-cell leukaemia/lymphoma
ATRA	all-*trans*-retinoic acid
AUL	acute undifferentiated leukaemia
B-ALL	B-lineage acute lymphoblastic leukaemia
BCLU	B-cell lymphoma, unclassifiable, with features intermediate between diffuse large B-cell lymphoma and Burkitt lymphoma
BEAM	carmustine (BCNU), etoposide, cytarabine (cytosine arabinoside) and melphalan
BL	Burkitt lymphoma
BP	blast phase
BPDCN	blastic plasmacytoid dendritic cell neoplasm
c	cytoplasmic
CD	cluster of differentiation
CHOP	cyclophosphamide, doxorubicin, vincristine and prednisolone
CLL	chronic lymphocytic leukaemia
CML	chronic myeloid leukaemia
CMML	chronic myelomonocytic leukaemia
CMV	cytomegalovirus
CNS	central nervous system
CODOX M/IVAC	cyclophosphamide, vincristine, doxorubicin, methotrexate/ ifosphamide, mesna, etoposide, cytarabine
CR	complete remission
CRAB	calcium (elevated), renal failure, anaemia, bone lesions
CSF	cerebrospinal fluid
CT	computed tomography
CTCL	cutaneous T-cell lymphoma
CTD	cyclophosphamide, thalidomide and dexamethasone
CXR	chest X-ray
cyt, cyto	cytoplasmic
DEXA scanning	dual energy X-ray absorptiometry scanning
DIC	disseminated intravascular coagulation
DKC	dyskeratosis congenita
DLBCL	diffuse large B-cell lymphoma
DM	double marking
EBER	EBV-encoded small RNAs
EBV	Epstein-Barr virus
EBV LMP	Epstein-Barr virus latent membrane protein
EDTA	ethylene diamine tetra-acetic acid
eGFR	estimated glomerular filtration rate
EMA	eosin-5-maleimide
EORTC	European Organization for Research and Treatment of Cancer
ESHAP	etoposide, methyl prednisolone, cytarabine, cisplatin
ESR	erythrocyte sedimentation rate

ET	essential thrombocythaemia
ETP-ALL	early T-cell precursor acute lymphoblastic leukaemia
FAB	French–American–British (leukaemia classification)
FBC	full blood count
FDG	fluorodeoxyglucose
FISH	fluorescence in situ hydridisation
FITC	fluorescein isothocyanate
FL	follicular lymphoma
FLAER	fluorescein-conjugated proaereolysin
FLAG	fludarabine, cytarabine, granulocyte colony-stimulating factor
FLAG-IDA	fludarabine, cytarabine, granulocyte colony-stimulating factor, idarubicin
FSC	forward scatter
GGT	gamma glutamyl transferase
GI	gastrointestinal
Gp	glycoprotein
GP	general practitioner
GPI	glycosylphosphatidylinositol
H&E	haematoxylin and eosin
Hb	haemoglobin concentration
HCL	hairy cell leukaemia
HCL-V	hairy cell leukaemia variant
HHV	human herpesvirus
HIV	human immunodeficiency virus
HL	Hodgkin lymphoma
HLA-DR	human leucocyte antigen DR
HS	hereditary spherocytosis
HTLV-1	human T-cell lymphotropic virus-1
ICC	immunocytochemistry
Ig	immunoglobulin
IgA	immunoglobulin A
IgG	immunoglobulin G
IgM	immunoglobulin M
IHC	immunohistochemistry
IPSS	International Prognostic Scoring System
ISCL	International Society for Cutaneous Lymphomas
ISH	in situ hybridisation
ISM	indolent systemic mastocytosis
ITD	internal tandem duplication
ITP	'idiopathic' (autoimmune) thrombocytopenia purpura
IVLBCL	intravascular large B-cell lymphoma
LAP	leukaemia-associated phenotype
LBL	lymphoblastic lymphoma
LDH	lactate dehydrogenase
LFTs	liver function tests
LGL	large granular lymphocyte
LPD	lymphoproliferative disorder
MCH	mean cell haemoglobin
MCL	mantle cell lymphoma
MCV	mean cell volume
MDS	myelodysplastic syndrome/s
MDS/MPN	myelodysplastic/myeloproliferative neoplasm
MF	mycosis fungoides
MGG	May–Grünwald–Giemsa
MGUS	monoclonal gammopathy of undetermined significance
MM	multiple myeloma
mod	moderate fluorescence
MPAL	mixed phenotype acute leukaemia
MPN	myeloproliferative neoplasm
MPO	myeloperoxidase
MRD	minimal residual disease
MRI	magnetic resonance imaging
MZL	marginal zone lymphoma
NLPHL	nodular lymphocyte-predominant Hodgkin lymphoma
NOS	not otherwise specified
NR	normal range
PAS	periodic acid-Schiff
PCR	polymerase chain reaction
PD-1	an antigen, programmed death 1(CD279)
PE	phycoerythrin
PEL	primary effusion lymphoma
PET	positron-emission tomography
Ph	Philadelphia (chromosome)
PMF	primary myelofibrosis
PNET	primitive neuroectodermal tumour
PNH	paroxysmal nocturnal haemoglobinuria
PRCA	pure red cell aplasia
PT	prothrombin time
PTCL-NOS	peripheral T-cell lymphoma, not otherwise specified
PTLD	post-transplant lymphoproliferative disorder
PV	polycythaemia vera
RBC	red blood cell (count)
R-CHOP	rituximab, doxorubicin, vincristine and prednisolone
R-CVP	rituximab, cyclophosphamide, vincristine and prednisolone
RNA	ribonucleic acid
RQ-PCR	real-time quantitative polymerase chain reaction
RS	Reed–Sternberg

RT-PCR	reverse transcriptase polymerase chain reaction	**TdT**	terminal deoxynucleotidyl transferase
SAA	severe aplastic anaemia	**TIA**	T-cell intracellular antigen
Sig	surface membrane immunoglobulin	**TKI**	tyrosine kinase inhibitor
SLE	systemic lupus erythematosus	**T-LBL**	T-lymphoblastic lymphoma
SM	systemic mastocytosis	**t-MDS**	therapy-related myelodysplastic syndrome
SM-AHNMD	systemic mastocytosis with associated clonal haematological non-mast cell disease	**TRAP**	tartrate-resistant acid phosphatase
		TT	thrombin time
SMILE	dexamethasone, methotrexate, ifosfamide, L-asparaginase and etoposide	**TTP**	thrombotic thrombocytopenic purpura
		U&Es	urea, electrolytes and creatinine
		USS	ultrasound
SSC	side scatter	**WAS**	Wiskott–Aldrich syndrome
T-ALL	T-lineage acute lymphoblastic leukaemia	**WASp**	Wiskott–Aldrich syndrome protein
		WBC	white blood cell (count)
TBI	total body irradiation	**WM**	Waldenström macroglobulinaemia

Technical Notes

The patients presented in 100 Worked Examples were all real cases encountered and investigated in a regional flow cytometry laboratory serving a population of approximately 2.5 million over a period of 18 months. These are individually presented with a history that reflects the actual events for each patient, commencing with the presenting clinical features and the initial basic laboratory tests and then proceeding to flow cytometry, bone marrow aspirate morphology, bone marrow trephine biopsy histology with immunohistochemistry studies and other specialised cytogenetic and molecular analyses.

Full blood counts

The full blood counts and marrow counts (for appropriate dilutions in relation to antibody) were performed on a Sysmex XN analyser. The differential leucocyte counts are automated counts from the analyser. It should be noted that sometimes, in an automated count, abnormal cells are misidentified and the leucocyte sub-populations differ from a manual differential performed on a blood film. Such misidentifications are indicated by inverted commas.

Biochemistry and immunology studies

All relevant biochemistry and immunology data is given in relation to the context of each patient presentation and in terms of investigations that were thought to be relevant to the case as the clinical diagnosis evolved. Some retrospectively relevant data may be missing but this reflects the true nature of these actual patient scenarios and the investigations that were considered necessary at that time. Serum calcium values given are all corrected in accordance with serum albumin level.

Flow cytometry analysis

Flow cytometry studies were all performed using a Becton Dickinson FACS Canto II analyser. The findings are presented as a list of positive and negative results in relation to the antigen and target cell population and the gating strategies applied to each case are explained. A series of scatter plots and histograms are presented to illustrate specific informative points. The expression of most membrane antigens is graded as positive when more than 20% of gated events are positive; the exceptions being CD34, CD117 and cytoplasmic antigens where a threshold of 10% has been used. Where the percentage positivity for a given membrane antigen in the gated target population is borderline positive so that some cells appear negative and some positive we have used the term 'partial' to describe antigen expression. Cytoplasmic expression of an antigen is indicated with the prefix 'c' (cytoplasmic expression of CD3 being cCD3) but on some scatter plots 'cyt' or 'cyto' has been used. The intensity of antigen expression in terms of median fluorescence intensity is graded as dim, moderate or bright compared to our laboratory reference ranges for normal cells of each relevant lineage. See Figures 1.1a–g for a schematic representation of these principles.

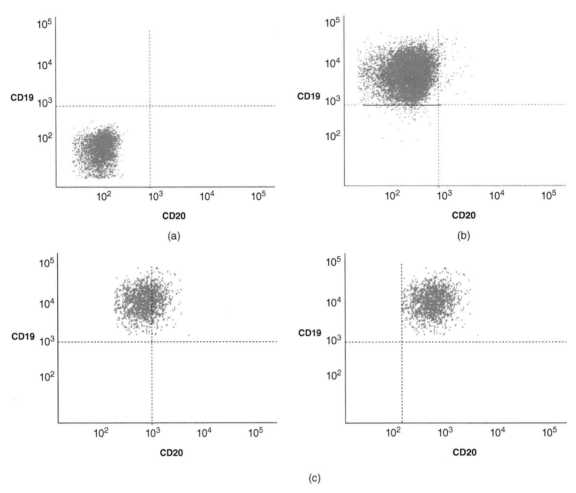

(a)

(b)

(c)

Figure 1.1 Visual representation of strength of fluorescence in flow cytometry (not actual patient specimens), showing an isotype control and eight CD19-positive samples which show fluorescence intensity with CD20 varying from negative to bright. (a) Isotype control, used to set thresholds. (b) Negative (consistent with a CD19-positive, CD20-negative B-cell precursor neoplasm). (c) Partial positive, indicating that CD20 antigen expression varies from negative to positive (consistent with a precursor B-cell neoplasm). (c adjusted) Indicating that the threshold for positivity might be reduced by the cytometrist where a discrete dim positive population is identified. (d) Dim CD20 antigen expression (consistent with chronic lymphocytic leukaemia). (e) Moderate intensity, indicating medium strength of CD20 antigen expression (consistent with B-cell non-Hodgkin lymphoma). (f) bright, indicating strong CD20 antigen expression (consistent with hairy cell leukaemia). (g) Two distinct populations, one partial and dim and one bright (could indicate two unrelated B-lineage neoplasms or transformation of a low grade lymphoma). (h) Contrasting with (g), a heterogeneous single population with fluorescence intensity varying from negative to moderate with a minority being bright.

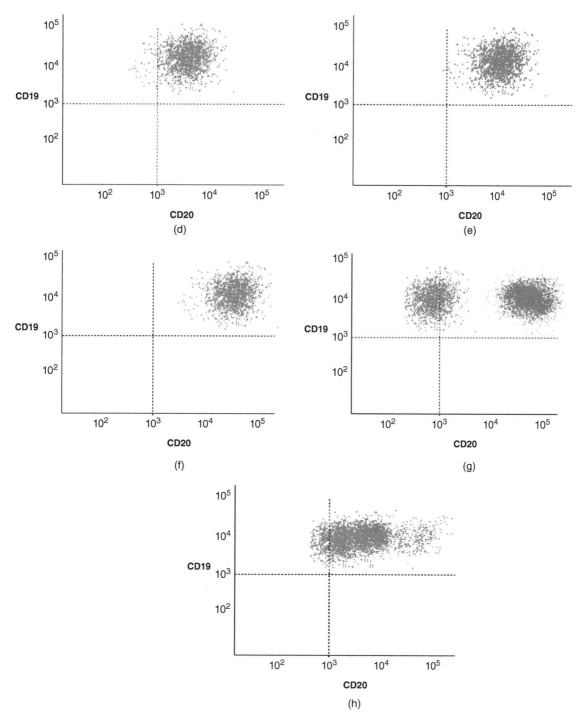

Figure 1.1 (*Continued*)

Immunohistochemistry in paraffin-embedded formalin fixed tissue

In the following section a list is presented of the immunohistochemical reagents used in assessing the paraffin embedded material (bone marrow trephine and lymph node biopsies) in the worked examples described. It should be pointed out that specificities and sensitivities may differ from the antibodies used in flow cytometry due to the effects of formalin fixation and decalcification resulting in antigen loss or masking. For example, CD5 may be detected by flow cytometry in a peripheral blood B cell lymphocytosis but immunocytochemistry may on occasion be negative for the same marker in the trephine specimen. CD56 is aberrantly expressed by plasma cells in myeloma yet immunoreactivity for this antibody within plasma cells in paraffin sections is seen in only a minority of cases. The opposite situation may also occur where an antigen such as TdT is strongly positive by immunohistochemistry on the fixed tissue but is negative on the flow sample. Reticulin fibrosis is reported as per the WHO classification as grade 0, 1, 2 or 3.

These specific features of different techniques need to be appreciated when formulating the combined pathology report and an understanding of the strengths and weaknesses of each approach is essential when establishing a final diagnosis. Cytogenetic and molecular studies have a major influence on disease classification. Specific findings can carry diagnostic significance way in excess of any other single investigative modality e.g. *BCR-ABL1*, *PML-RARA*, *FIP1L1-PDGRFA*. Metaphase cytogenetic studies not infrequently fail, either reflecting the quality of the specimen or the disease entity being studied. Informed FISH and PCR studies can carry great diagnostic importance in certain clinical circumstances and molecular diagnostics will continue to inform disease classification with increasing power and specificity over the decades ahead.

Laboratory Values

Abbreviations and Normal Ranges.

Blood

Haematology

Haemoglobin concentration (Hb)	130–180 g/L (M)
	125–170 g/L (F)
Mean cell volume (MCV)	80–100 fl
Reticulocyte count	$50–100 \times 10^9$/L
White blood cell count (WBC)	$4–11 \times 10^9$/L
Neutrophils	$2–7 \times 10^9$/L
Lymphocytes	$1.5–4 \times 10^9$/L
Monocytes	$0.2–0.8 \times 10^9$/L
Eosinophils	$0.04–0.4 \times 10^9$/L
Basophils	$0.01–0.1 \times 10^9$/L

Haematinics

Serum ferritin	10–275 ng/mL
Serum folate	3.1–20 ng/mL
Serum vitamin B_{12}	200–900 pg/mL

Coagulation

Prothrombin time (PT)	9–13 s
Activated partial thromboplastin time (APTT)	27–38 s
Thrombin time (TT)	11–15 s
Fibrinogen	1.5–4 g/L
D dimer	0–243 ng/mL

Biochemistry

Sodium (Na)	135–145 mmol/L
Potassium (K)	3.5–5.0 mmol/L
Urea	2.5–7.5 mmol/L
Creatinine	40–130 μmol/L
Bicarbonate	20–30 mmol/L

Blood

Urate	0.2–0.43 mmol/L
Lactate	<2.4 mmol/L
Lactate dehydrogenase (LDH)	80–240 U/L
Aspartate transaminase (AST)	<40 U/L
Alanine transaminase (ALT)	<50 U/L
Gamma glutamyl transferase (GGT)	<70 U/L
Alkaline phosphatase (ALP)	40–150 U/L
Calcium adjusted	2.1–2.6 mmol/L
Phosphate	0.7–1.4 mmol/L
C-reactive protein (CRP)	<10 mg/L
Bilirubin	<20 μmol/L
Albumin	32–45 g/L
Globulins	23–38 g/L
Serum osmolality	270–295 mmol/kg
Urine protein/creatinine ratio	0–15 mg/mmol
Immunoglobulin G (IgG)	6–16 g/L
Immunoglobulin A (IgA)	0.8–4.0 g/L
Immunoglobulin M (IgM)	0.5–2.0 g/L

Serum free light chains

Free kappa	3.3–19.4 mg/L
Free lambda	5.7–26.3 mg/L

Cerebrospinal fluid (CSF)

Protein	<0.4 g/L
Cells	$<0.001 \times 10^9$/L (<10 cells/μL)
Glucose	2 mmol/L less than serum glucose

Case 1

An 11-year-old boy was admitted with a short history of fever, sweats, dyspnoea and left chest discomfort. There was no past history of note. Examination identified features of a left pleural effusion. There was also a tender swelling of the left anterior chest in the upper pectoral region and palpable cervical lymphadenopathy. The liver and spleen were not palpable.

Laboratory investigations

FBC and blood film: normal
    U&Es, LFTs: normal. LDH was 1460 U/L.

Imaging

The CXR showed opacification and loss of aeration of the left hemithorax in keeping with a pleural effusion (Figure 1.1).

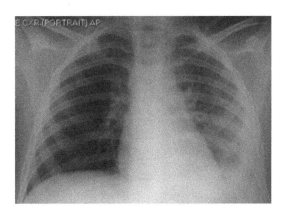

Figure 1.1 CXR.

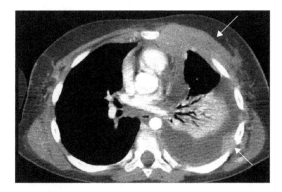

Figure 1.2 CT.

CT imaging confirmed this but in addition identified a left pleural-based mass, abnormal soft tissue in the left pectoral muscles (arrows, Figure 1.2) and cervical lymphadenopathy. In addition, there was collapse/consolidation of the lower left lung, creating the appearance of an air bronchogram. A core biopsy of a cervical node was taken and the pleural effusion was aspirated for analysis.

Flow cytometry

The pleural fluid cell count was 0.98×10^9/L. A cytospin preparation showed three distinct cell types: a small mature lymphoid population in keeping with reactive lymphocytes, an intermediate sized/large sized lymphoid population and a large cell population with pleomorphic morphology and blue cytoplasm (Figures 1.3–1.6). The cells with the abundant cytoplasm (Figures 1.3 and 1.4) and the single binucleate cell (Figure 1.6) are reactive mesothelial cells. The cells with the cytoplasmic blebs (Figures 1.4–1.6) are the disease cells,

Practical Flow Cytometry in Haematology: 100 Worked Examples, First Edition. Mike Leach,
Mark Drummond, Allyson Doig, Pam McKay, Bob Jackson and Barbara J. Bain.
© 2015 John Wiley & Sons, Ltd. Published 2015 by John Wiley & Sons, Ltd.

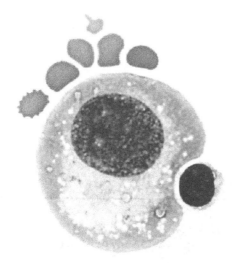

Figure 1.3 MGG, ×500.

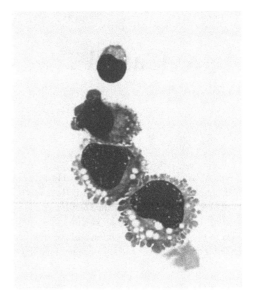

Figure 1.5 MGG, ×500.

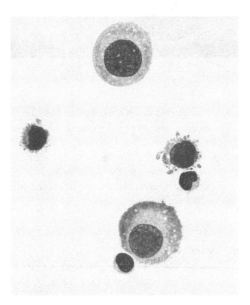

Figure 1.4 MGG, ×500.

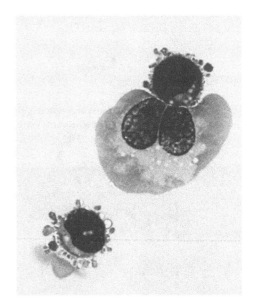

Figure 1.6 MGG, ×500.

which were the subsequent focus for immunophenotyping studies.

By applying a blast gate to the suspected malignant cells in the FSC/SSC analysis (Figure 1.7), they were shown to express CD45^{bright} (Figure 1.8), CD2 (Figure 1.9), cCD3 [whilst surface CD3 was negative apart from a few reactive

T cells (Figure 1.8)], partial CD7 (Figure 1.10) and CD13. Other T-lineage markers were negative.

This is therefore a T-lymphoid neoplasm, indicated by positivity for cCD3 expression, with limited lineage-specific

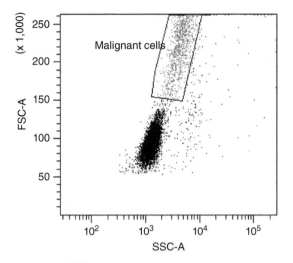

Figure 1.7 FSC/SSC.

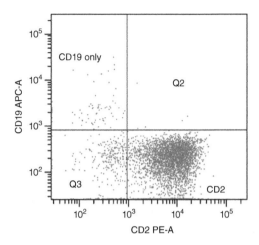

Figure 1.9 CD2/CD19.

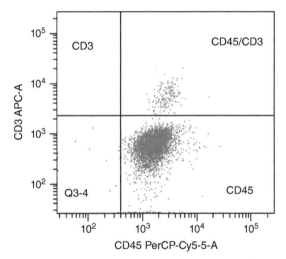

Figure 1.8 CD3/CD45.

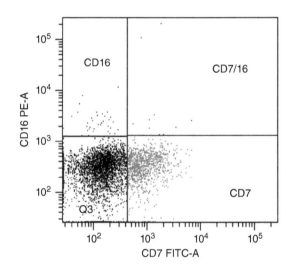

Figure 1.10 CD7/CD16.

markers and an aberrant myeloid marker. The tumour has medium sized/large cell morphology. It was showing aggressive clinical behaviour with extranodal tissue invasion in this 11-year-old patient. An anaplastic large cell lymphoma had to be considered and the medium sized/large cells in the pleural fluid were shown to be strongly expressing CD30 (not shown).

Histopathology

An H&E-stained core biopsy of a cervical node is shown in Figure 1.11. The node is replaced by an infiltrate of undifferentiated pleomorphic large cells with prominent nucleoli.

Immunohistochemistry showed the large cells to express CD45, epithelial membrane antigen (EMA), CD2 focally (Figure 1.12), CD7, granzyme B and CD30 (Figure 1.13). In addition, there was strong nuclear and cytoplasmic staining for anaplastic lymphoma kinase (ALK) protein (Figure 1.14).

The CD30 staining was particularly useful in demonstrating lymphatic invasion within the capsule of the node (Figure 1.15).

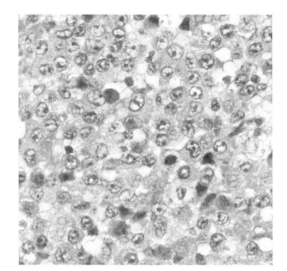

Figure 1.11 H&E, ×400.

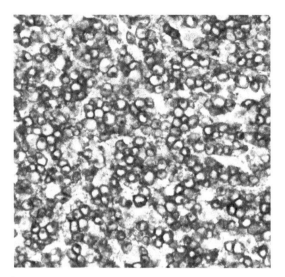

Figure 1.13 CD30, ×400.

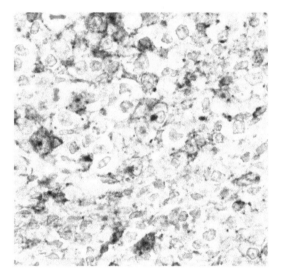

Figure 1.12 CD2, ×400.

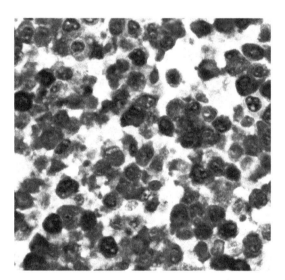

Figure 1.14 ALK, ×400.

FISH studies

A t(2;5)(p23;q35) translocation, rearranging the *ALK* and *NPM1* (nucleophosmin) genes, was shown by FISH studies on paraffin-embedded lymph node tissue. The presence of this specific translocation is highly associated with both nuclear and cytoplasmic positivity for ALK.

Discussion

Anaplastic large cell lymphoma (ALCL) is an aggressive mature T-cell neoplasm with pleomorphic, often large cell, morphology. It frequently fails to show surface expression of T-lineage-specific markers and to potentially further mislead may express aberrant myeloid antigens. This is an

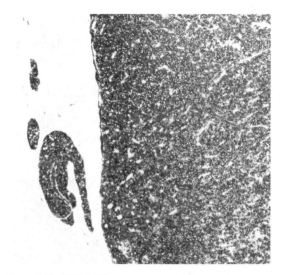

Figure 1.15 CD30, ×100.

important condition to recognise; it frequently shows rapid progression with extranodal tissue involvement and it can rarely appear in the blood. Treatment of ALK$^+$ ALCL is usually rewarding, particularly in paediatric patients, with prompt response to chemotherapy and frequent durable remissions.

Final diagnosis

Anaplastic large cell lymphoma (ALK$^+$)

Case 2

A 72-year-old woman presented with a few months' history of fatigue and the more recent onset of breathlessness and night sweats. On clinical examination she had a large right-sided pleural effusion but no palpable lymph-adenopathy.

Laboratory results

FBC: Hb 158 g/L, WBC 16.6 × 10^9/L (neutrophilia and monocytosis) and platelets 502 × 10^9/L.

U&Es: normal. LFTs were mildly deranged (ALT 52 U/L, alkaline phosphatase 173 U/L). Albumin was low at 29 g/L and serum LDH was raised at 584 U/L.

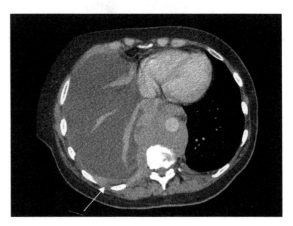

Figure 2.1 CT.

Imaging

A CT scan demonstrated a large right-sided pleural effusion with collapse of the right middle and lower lobes and partial collapse of the upper lobe (Figure 2.1). In addition, there were large volume, confluent, necrotic nodal masses in the right hilar, mediastinal, retrocrural, paracardiac and para-aortic areas (not shown) as well as pleural deposits (arrow, Figure 2.1).

Pleural fluid biochemistry and cytology

The pleural fluid LDH was markedly elevated at 2171 U/L with relatively low glucose at 7.2 mmol/L (patient diabetic) and protein of 43 g/L.

Microscopy of the pleural fluid showed lymphoid cells admixed with neutrophils, histiocytes and mesothelial cells. Most of the lymphoid cells were small but an admixed population of medium-sized cells with slightly irregular nuclei was also present. On morphology alone, the lymphoid cells were thought likely to be reactive but the reporting pathologist suggested that a fresh pleural fluid specimen should be assessed using flow cytometry.

Morphology (pleural fluid)

A specimen of pleural fluid was received by our laboratory. The WBC was found to be 6.3 × 10^9/L. A cytospin preparation showed a cellular specimen with notable macrophages, neutrophils and small lymphocytes. In addition, some large blastoid lymphoid cells were seen (Figures 2.2–2.5).

Practical Flow Cytometry in Haematology: 100 Worked Examples, First Edition. Mike Leach, Mark Drummond, Allyson Doig, Pam McKay, Bob Jackson and Barbara J. Bain.
© 2015 John Wiley & Sons, Ltd. Published 2015 by John Wiley & Sons, Ltd.

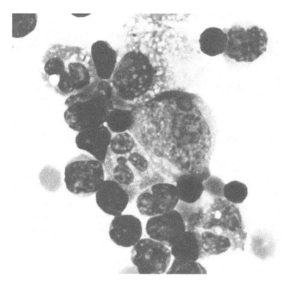

Figure 2.2 MGG, ×500.

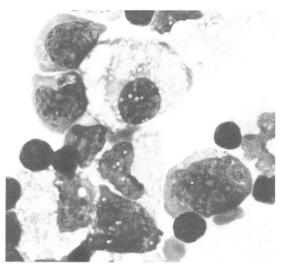

Figure 2.4 MGG, ×500.

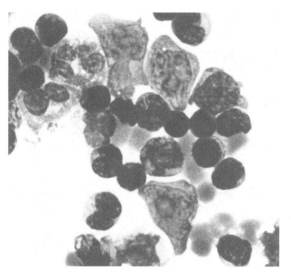

Figure 2.3 MGG, ×500.

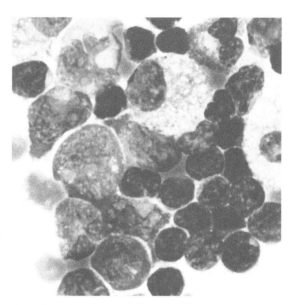

Figure 2.5 MGG, ×500.

Flow cytometry (pleural fluid)

The FSC/SSC plot shows the orientation of the different populations of cells described above. The small lymphoid population (Figure 2.6) comprised mainly reactive T cells (black events with mixture of CD4$^+$ and CD8$^+$ cells) and normal B cells (blue events). Seventeen per cent of all leucocytes were CD19$^+$ B cells (Figure 2.7) showing a mature pan-B phenotype with CD20 positivity and a hint of monoclonality (kappa 73%, lambda 18%). The SSC analysis in Figure 2.7, however, defines 2 B-cell populations with different scatter characteristics, populations P1 and P2.

By gating on the higher SSC profile B cells (P2 red events, Figure 2.7, which are larger indicated by high FSC in Figure 2.6), a clear clonal population was demonstrated showing strong CD20 positivity, expression of CD10/HLA-DR (Figure 2.8), CD38, FMC7, CD79b and CD22 with kappa light chain restriction (Figure 2.9).

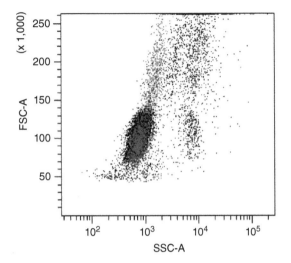

Figure 2.6 FSC/SSC.

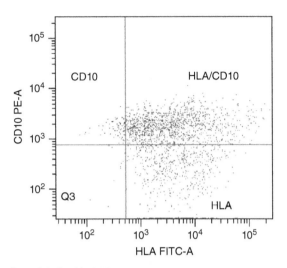

Figure 2.8 CD10/HLA-DR.

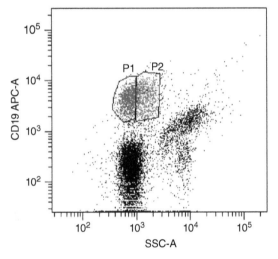

Figure 2.7 CD19/SSC.

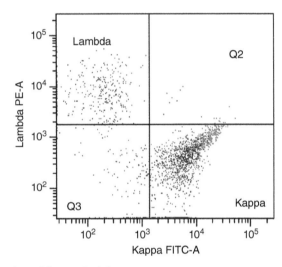

Figure 2.9 Kappa/lambda.

Note the phenotype of the blue events, population P1, representing residual small polyclonal reactive B cells.

Lymph node biopsy

A CT-guided core biopsy of a paravertebral node showed lymphoid infiltration by predominantly small centrocytic cells with occasional larger centroblasts. The cells were positive for CD20, CD10, BCL6 and BCL2 and negative for CD3, CD5, cyclin D1, CD23, CD43 and CD21. The proliferation fraction was low (~10%). The histological and immunohistochemical appearances were in keeping with follicular lymphoma, grade 2, with no evidence of high-grade

transformation. FISH for the t(14;18) translocation was positive.

Bone marrow aspirate and trephine biopsy

These were both normal.

Discussion

The clinical presentation, imaging, pleural fluid morphology and flow cytometry were most in keeping with a diagnosis of an aggressive, mature CD10⁺ B-cell neoplasm. Diffuse large

B-cell lymphoma (DLBCL) would be the favoured diagnosis but a node or tissue biopsy is preferred for confirmation. The percutaneous paravertebral node biopsy showed the typical features of follicular lymphoma (FL). It is highly likely that the diagnosis is DLBCL transformed from a previously undiagnosed FL and that the high-grade transformation has occurred in the mediastinal nodes with subsequent involvement of the pleura. It is not uncommon to see discrepancies in grade of lymphoma when tissue biopsies are taken from different anatomical sites.

This case also illustrates the ability of flow cytometry to detect a small population of neoplastic B lymphocytes within a reactive pleural effusion containing normal lymphocytes, histiocytes and neutrophils. The morphology here was well preserved and a careful gating strategy to analyse the large B cells allowed the confirmation of a neoplastic B-cell clone.

Following three cycles of R-CHOP chemotherapy, a CT scan showed a marked reduction in the lymph node and pleural masses. Despite this encouraging response to treatment, the patient developed increasing breathlessness due to a recurrent pleural effusion. On this occasion the aspirate was chylous (Figure 2.10) with similar protein content to the original serous effusion but normal LDH with a glucose level similar to that of blood (compared with high LDH and low glucose found in the previous effusion). Chyle is a lipid- and protein-rich solution derived from the lymphatic drainage system. It is particularly enriched with fat and proteins absorbed across the small bowel mucosa, delivered to the systemic circulation after drainage of the

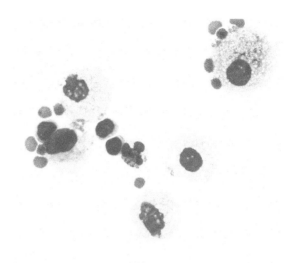

Figure 2.11 MGG, ×500.

Figure 2.12 MGG, ×500.

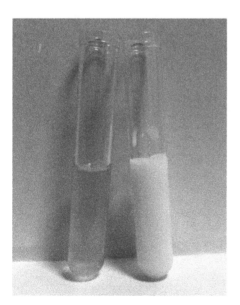

Figure 2.10 Serous (left) and chylous (right) pleural effusions.

thoracic duct into the left subclavian vein. It appears opaque due to the high density of chylomicrons.

The fluid morphology and flow cytometry showed small reactive T cells and foamy macrophages only (Figures 2.11 and 2.12). The large neoplastic B cells were not present.

These results are typical of a chylothorax and this was confirmed by raised triglycerides at 12.3 mmol/L (<2.3) and low cholesterol of 1.8 mmol/L (<5). This case illustrates the different mechanisms by which pleural effusions can develop in patients with lymphoid malignancies. The first effusion developed as a result of direct disease involvement of the pleura with serosal infiltration. Typically, these effusions have a high LDH and low glucose and malignant cells are often identified. The second effusion developed as a result of damage to, or obstruction of, the thoracic duct. In this type of effusion, the LDH is often normal, glucose level is similar to that of blood, triglycerides are high and often no neoplastic cells are seen.

Final diagnosis

1. High grade transformation of follicular lymphoma involving mediastinum and pleura
2. Follicular lymphoma involving paravertebral lymph nodes
3. Chylous pleural effusion, following treatment, from thoracic duct damage by diffuse large B-cell lymphoma

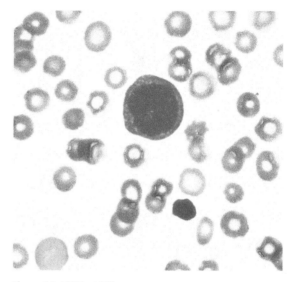

Case 3

A 23-month-old boy presented to the Emergency department of a local children's Hospital, with a 5-day history of pallor and facial swelling. Routine blood test results are shown below. CT imaging of head, neck, thorax and abdomen showed a number of abnormalities including prominent bilateral salivary gland enlargement, moderate bilateral cervical lymphadenopathy and extensive focal low attenuation lesions throughout the liver and both kidneys (not shown).

Laboratory data

FBC: Hb 75 g/L, WBC 6.7×10^9/L (neutrophils 0.2×10^9/L, lymphocytes 5.7×10^9/L) and platelets 321×10^9/L.

Coagulation screen: normal.

U&Es, LFTs: normal. Serum LDH was 1300 U/L.

Marrow aspirate

A cellular sample was difficult to acquire. This hampered the morphological assessment as the smears had scanty cellularity. Small numbers of pathological blast cells were seen, however (Figures 3.1–3.4). These were moderate-to-large in size and had basophilic cytoplasm with occasional fine azurophilic granules. Very occasional vacuolation was seen, but this was not a prominent feature. Occasional fine nuclear folding was seen (Figure 3.4) with nucleoli surprisingly rare.

Flow cytometry (bone marrow aspirate)

Despite low cell numbers, flow cytometry readily identified the pathological population. The immunophenotype of the

Figure 3.1 MGG, ×1000.

blast cells was CD45^{dim}, CD34$^-$, CD117$^+$, CD38$^+$, CD56$^-$, CD15$^+$, CD13$^+$, CD33$^+$, HLA-DR^{++}, CD64$^+$, CD14$^-$ and MPO$^-$. These results were in keeping with acute monoblastic leukaemia.

Cytogenetic analysis

46,XY,t(9;11)(p22;q23) was present in the 10/10 cells examined.

Bone marrow trephine biopsy

This was cellular showing prominent sinusoids (Figure 3.5). The monoblastic infiltrate was negative for CD34 (Figure 3.6,

Practical Flow Cytometry in Haematology: 100 Worked Examples, First Edition. Mike Leach, Mark Drummond, Allyson Doig, Pam McKay, Bob Jackson and Barbara J. Bain.
© 2015 John Wiley & Sons, Ltd. Published 2015 by John Wiley & Sons, Ltd.

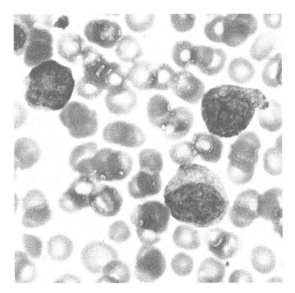

Figure 3.2 MGG, ×1000.

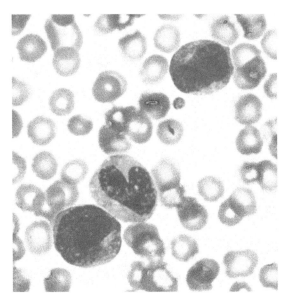

Figure 3.4 MGG, ×1000.

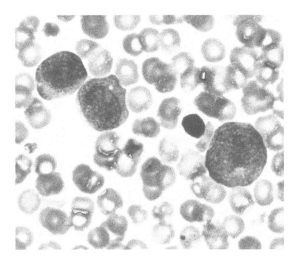

Figure 3.3 MGG, ×1000.

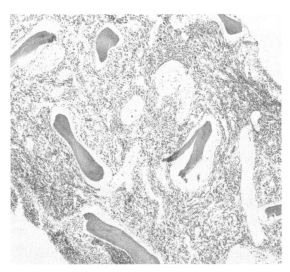

Figure 3.5 H&E, ×40.

noting sinusoidal staining) and MPO (Figure 3.7) but positive for CD4, CD15 (Figure 3.8) and CD68 (Figure 3.9).

Discussion

This case is relatively unusual given the infrequency of circulating leukaemic cells. Monoblastic leukaemias often present with high circulating blast counts and tissue infiltration is very common. The disease burden is therefore often very high at the outset; the risk of tumour-lysis syndrome is significant, which can be further compounded by direct infiltration of kidneys as seen here.

The flow cytometric features of this case were typical of a primitive monoblastic leukaemia: namely, CD34$^-$, CD117$^+$, CD64$^+$ and CD14$^-$. Most cases are CD34$^-$, with CD117 often present on monoblastic rather than the more mature

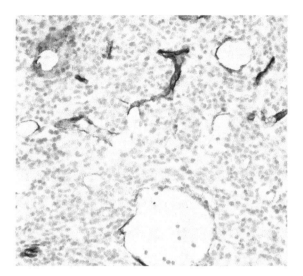

Figure 3.6 CD34, ×200.

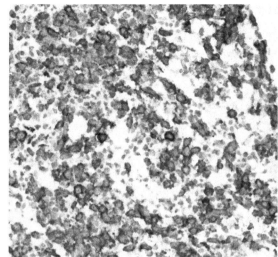

Figure 3.8 CD15, ×200.

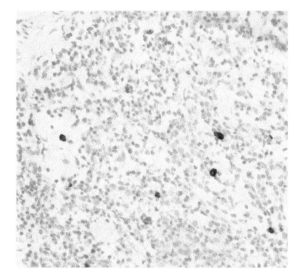

Figure 3.7 MPO, ×200.

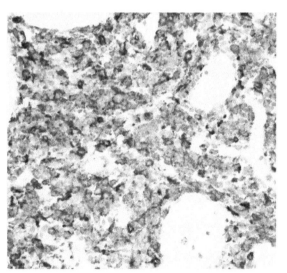

Figure 3.9 CD68, ×200.

monocytic forms. MPO is expressed from the promonocyte stage onwards during normal sequential maturation, so is not infrequently absent in monoblasts. CD14, while specific for the monocyte lineage, is an insensitive marker of monocytic leukaemia due to its frequent absence in primitive cases. CD14 detection may however be epitope dependent, meaning that its apparent expression in these cases may vary according to the antibody clone in laboratory use. CD7 and CD56 are often aberrantly expressed on acute leukaemia of

monocyte lineage (in up to 40% of cases) although neither of these antigens was detected in this case.

The t(9;11)(p22;q23) translocation is one of many reported rearrangements of the mixed lineage leukaemia (*MLL*) gene located on the long arm of chromosome 11. Such rearrangements are commonly found in childhood AML (~20% overall), with a particularly high incidence (50–60%) in those <2 years and are associated with monoblastic/monocytic lineage and extramedullary tissue infiltration. The prognostic implications of *MLL* rearrangements are remarkably heterogeneous, with t(9;11)(p22;q23) in childhood acute monoblastic leukaemia appearing to carry either a favourable (1) or an intermediate (2) prognosis in different studies.

Final diagnosis

Acute monoblastic leukaemia with t(9:11)(p22;q23); *MLLT3-MLL*.

References

1 Rubnitz, J.E., Raimondi, S.C., Tong, X. *et al.* (2002) Favorable impact of the t(9;11) in childhood acute myeloid leukemia. *Journal of Clinical Oncology*, **20**, 2302–2309.
2 Balgobind, B.V., Raimondi, S.C., Harbott, J. *et al.* (2009) Novel prognostic subgroups in childhood 11q23/MLL-rearranged acute myeloid leukemia: results of an international retrospective study. *Blood*, **114**, 2489–2496.

4

Case 4

A 68-year-old woman was brought to the emergency department after her family became concerned with regard to her recent onset of confusion. On admission she appeared pale and was orientated in time and place, but could not answer detailed questions. There was no specific neurological deficit.

Laboratory data

FBC: Hb 88 g/L, WBC 19 × 10^9/L (neutrophils 4.5 × 10^9/L, 'lymphocytes' 5.1 × 10^9/L, 'monocytes' 9.8 × 10^9/L) and platelets 112 × 10^9/L.

U&Es: Na 125 mmol/l, K 4.6 mmol/L, urea 19 mmol/L, creatinine 295 μmol/L.

Bone profile: calcium 3.5 mmol/L, phosphate 1.9 mmol/L, ALP 110 U/L.

LFTs: normal except albumin 26 g/L, total protein 55 g/L.

Immunoglobulins: IgG 2 g/L, IgA not assessable, IgM 0.2 g/L.

Serum electrophoresis: IgA paraprotein quantified at 25 g/L.

Serum-free light chains: kappa 1400 mg/L, lambda 90 mg/L.

Blood film

There was marked rouleaux formation and proteinaceous staining of the plasma (note the pale blue background). In addition, a notable population of plasma cells was evident suggesting a diagnosis of plasma cell leukaemia (Figures 4.1–4.4).

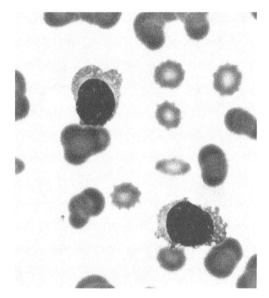

Figure 4.1 MGG, x1000.

Flow cytometry (peripheral blood)

Peripheral blood was examined using a plasma cell panel and a CD138 versus SSC-gating strategy. Plasma cells accounted for 76% of circulating leucocytes and had a neoplastic phenotype expressing CD38 but without CD19, CD45 or CD56 (Figures 4.5–4.7). Cytoplasmic light chain restriction can be used to demonstrate clonality, if there is any doubt, but this is not routinely necessary where the plasma cell phenotype is neoplastic.

Practical Flow Cytometry in Haematology: 100 Worked Examples, First Edition. Mike Leach, Mark Drummond, Allyson Doig, Pam McKay, Bob Jackson and Barbara J. Bain.
© 2015 John Wiley & Sons, Ltd. Published 2015 by John Wiley & Sons, Ltd.

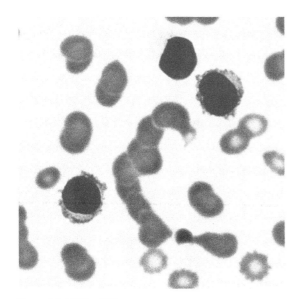

Figure 4.2 MGG, x1000.

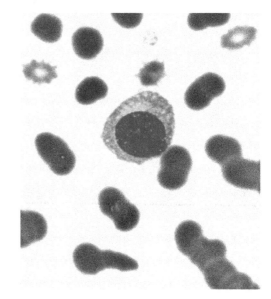

Figure 4.4 MGG, x1000.

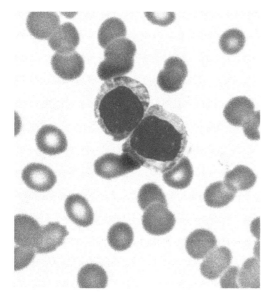

Figure 4.3 MGG, x1000.

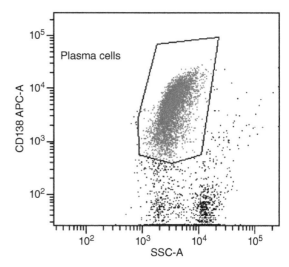

Figure 4.5 CD138/SSC.

CD56 is normally expressed by neoplastic plasma cells in multiple myeloma but it is often not expressed in plasma cell leukaemia. Also known as neural cell adhesion molecule (NCAM), this antigen is involved in tissue homing by plasma cells in multiple myeloma and its absence in plasma cell leukaemia may in part be responsible for the absence of marrow orientation and the release of these cells into the peripheral blood. This hypothesis is supported by the observation that although plasma cell leukaemias usually fail to express CD56, in some cases, examination of bone marrow plasma cells shows CD56 positivity.

Discussion

The clinical presentation here with a recent onset of confusion was due to a combination of hypercalcaemia and

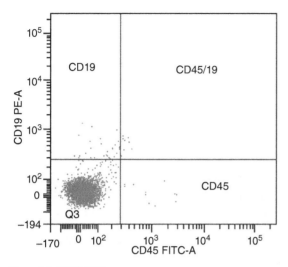

Figure 4.6 CD19/CD45.

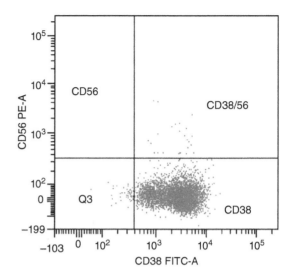

Figure 4.7 CD38/CD56.

acute kidney injury, which were in turn the result of the malignant plasma cell proliferation. The cell morphology in plasma cell leukaemia is extremely variable. Some patients show typical plasma cell morphology, as in this case, making the diagnosis straightforward but others have circulating cells that resemble lymphocytes, monocytes or even hairy cells. Note that in this patient the automated analyser was misidentifying the plasma cells as lymphocytes and monocytes. It is important to consider this diagnosis in any patient presenting with hypercalcaemia or new onset kidney injury where atypical cells are seen in the blood film, particularly when rouleaux and increased background staining

(due to the paraprotein in the plasma) are also present. It will normally take a few days after admission before immunoglobulin quantitation and serum electrophoresis studies become available so the blood film appearances may give the first clear evidence of the underlying diagnosis.

Final diagnosis

De novo plasma cell leukaemia.

5

Case 5

A 32-year-old man presented to the accident and emergency department with acute onset of left upper quadrant pain. He had been complaining of fatigue for 7 days previously. On examination he was haemodynamically stable but had a fever of 38°C and was tender with guarding over his left hypochondrium. He had tender bilateral neck lymphadenopathy.

Laboratory data

FBC: Hb 97 g/L, WBC 25 × 10⁹/L (neutrophils 8.1 × 10⁹/L, lymphocytes 11 × 10⁹/L, 'monocytes' 5.3 × 10⁹/L).

U&Es: normal.

LFTs: AST 95 U/L, ALT 102 U/L, ALP 150 U/L, GGT 50 U/L, albumin 32 g/L, bilirubin 27 μmol/L.

CRP: 35 mg/L.

Imaging

An urgent CT scan confirmed moderate bilateral neck lymphadenopathy but importantly identified the cause of the abdominal pain. The spleen was moderately enlarged but in addition showed a capsular tear (arrow) with an adherent haematoma (Figure 5.1). A core biopsy of a cervical node was taken under ultrasound guidance.

Blood film

The film showed some important features. There was a population of large granular lymphoid cells with a cytotoxic T-cell-type morphology (Figures 5.2–5.5). We initially considered whether this might represent a high-grade hepatosplenic T-cell lymphoma rather than a reactive

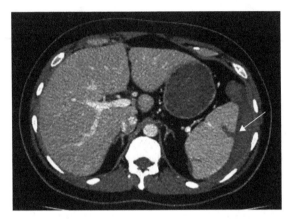

Figure 5.1 CT.

phenomenon. Note that the automated instrument has misidentified abnormal lymphoid cells as monocytes.

Flow cytometry (peripheral blood)

The large lymphoid cells were identified as CD8⁺ T cells with a pan-T phenotype and strong expression of HLA-DR. CD56 and CD57 were not expressed. This is in keeping with an activated, reactive T-cell proliferation typical of that seen as a response to viral infections (Epstein-Barr virus (EBV), in particular). The population was not neoplastic as there was no antigen loss or CD56 expression and there was strong uniform positivity for HLA-DR.

Lymph node core histology

The lymph node showed a degree of architectural effacement but with marked T-zone expansion and an immunoblastic

Practical Flow Cytometry in Haematology: 100 Worked Examples, First Edition. Mike Leach, Mark Drummond, Allyson Doig, Pam McKay, Bob Jackson and Barbara J. Bain.
© 2015 John Wiley & Sons, Ltd. Published 2015 by John Wiley & Sons, Ltd.

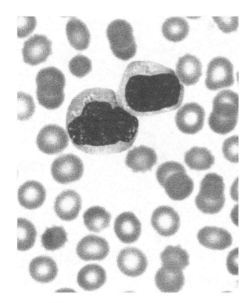

Figure 5.2 MGG, x1000.

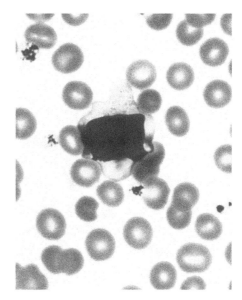

Figure 5.4 MGG, x1000.

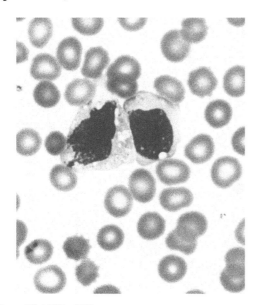

Figure 5.3 MGG, x1000.

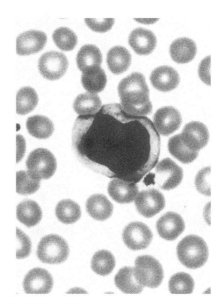

Figure 5.5 MGG, x1000.

reaction (Figures 5.6 (arrows) and 5.7) with areas of necrosis and haemorrhage (Figures 5.6 and 5.8).

The features were of a necrotising lymphadenitis. *In situ* hybridisation for EBER (EBV-encoded RNA) showed positivity within the B cells (Figure 5.9) that are the primary focus for infection. A B-cell immunoblastic response and a T-cell reaction generate the nodal expansion. Peripheral blood PCR for EBV DNA was positive and IgM EBV antibodies were subsequently demonstrated.

The patient was treated supportively and did not require splenectomy. He subsequently made a full recovery.

Discussion

This case illustrates an extreme example of acute EBV infection and its potential sequelae. Epstein-Barr virus is

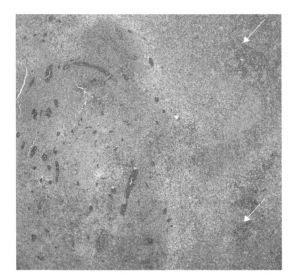

Figure 5.6 H&E, x25.

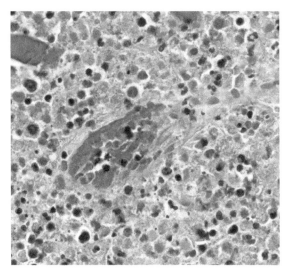

Figure 5.8 H&E, x400.

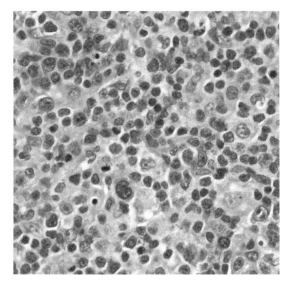

Figure 5.7 H&E, x400.

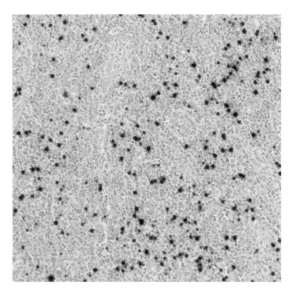

Figure 5.9 EBER ISH, x40.

a ubiquitous DNA virus of the herpes superfamily, which is transmitted by direct person-to-person contact. Primary infection is common in young adults and normally causes a minor illness with fever, sore throat, reactive lymphadenopathy, splenomegaly and mild hepatitis. It commonly causes a reactive CD8$^+$ T-cell lymphocytosis that should not be mistaken for other pathological processes. The T-cell reaction and expansion within the spleen in infectious mononucleosis can cause spontaneous rupture but this is a rare event estimated to occur in less than 0.5% of

cases. The management has traditionally been splenectomy but there is increasing evidence that in patients who are haemodynamically stable a conservative approach is justified.

Final diagnosis

Acute EBV infection with reactive CD8 lymphocytosis, necrotising lymphadenitis and spontaneous rupture of the spleen.

6

Case 6

A 75-year-old man was noted to have a chronic mild pancytopenia. A blood film reported at the referring hospital showed no specific features. The counts had slowly deteriorated and further investigations were therefore warranted. A myelodysplastic syndrome was thought to be the most likely diagnosis by the referring hospital.

Laboratory results

FBC: Hb 101 g/L, WBC 3.2×10^9/L (neutrophils 0.9×10^9/L, lymphocytes 1.9×10^9/L, monocytes 0.3×10^9/L) and platelets 109×10^9/L.

Renal and hepatic function normal.

LDH normal.

Normal immunoglobulins with no paraprotein detected.

Flow cytometry (bone marrow aspirate)

A hypocellular, aparticulate aspirate was received by our laboratory. The aspirate white cell count was 3.3×10^9/L. A good cellular aspirate will have a white cell count approaching 100×10^9/L (in-house observations). Morphological review of the aspirate did not show obvious blasts but a few lymphoid cells were noted; a good morphological assessment was hindered by the hypocellularity. Flow analysis using a FSC versus SSC approach showed an abnormal cell population lying between the lymphoid cells and larger granular myeloid cells (population P1 in Figure 6.1). Monocytes normally occupy this zone.

These cells were found to be CD19, CD20^{bright}, HLA-DR and surface lambda positive. There was insufficient material

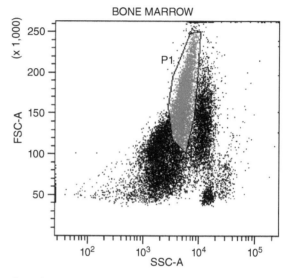

Figure 6.1 FSC/SSC.

for further analysis. On the basis of these findings a peripheral blood sample was requested for morphological review and flow cytometric studies to further define the clonal lymphoproliferative disorder.

Peripheral blood morphology

Careful review of the blood film showed a population of medium/large lymphoid cells with pale blue cytoplasm. The cell margins were indistinct and many cells had bi-lobed nuclei (Figures 6.2–6.4). These findings were highly suggestive of a diagnosis of hairy cell leukaemia.

Practical Flow Cytometry in Haematology: 100 Worked Examples, First Edition. Mike Leach, Mark Drummond, Allyson Doig, Pam McKay, Bob Jackson and Barbara J. Bain.

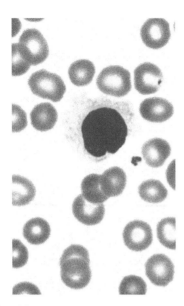

Figure 6.2 MGG, ×1000.

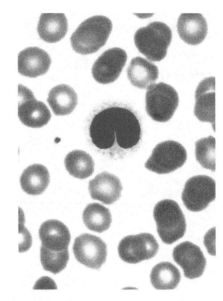

Figure 6.4 MGG, ×1000.

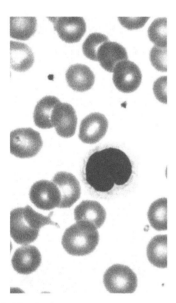

Figure 6.3 MGG, ×1000.

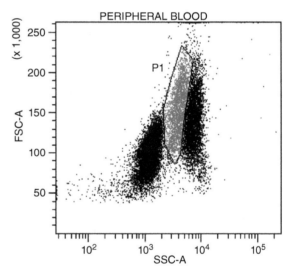

Figure 6.5 Blood, FSC/SSC.

Flow cytometry (peripheral blood)

Peripheral blood was analysed using an extended mature B-lymphoid panel (as the population in the marrow aspirate was expressing surface lambda). Thirteen per cent of cells were B cells that had the same scatter characteristics as noted in marrow (Figure 6.5).

These expressed CD19, CD20[bright], CD79b, CD22, FMC7 and surface lambda. A secondary panel also showed positivity for CD25, CD11c, CD103 and CD123, in keeping with a diagnosis of hairy cell leukaemia.

Histopathology

The bone marrow trephine biopsy sections showed increased cellularity (60%) with a subtle interstitial infiltrate of

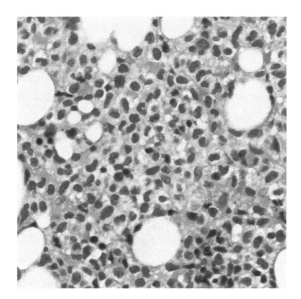

Figure 6.6 H&E, ×400.

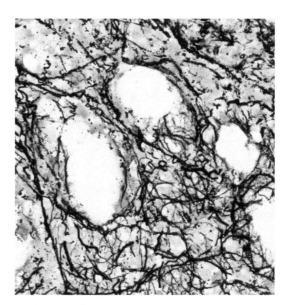

Figure 6.7 Reticulin, ×400.

lymphoid cells with reniform, often bilobed, nuclei and clear cytoplasm with associated grade 2 reticulin fibrosis (Figures 6.6 and 6.7). The lymphoid cells expressed pan-B-cell markers plus CD11c, CD25, CD123, CD72 (DBA-44), TRAP and annexin-1, an immunophenotype that is essentially diagnostic of hairy cell leukaemia (HCL).

Discussion

Hairy cell leukaemia (HCL) is a clonal mature B-cell disorder characterised by peripheral blood cytopenias (particularly neutropenia and monocytopenia) with circulating neoplastic cells, bone marrow infiltration with marrow fibrosis and splenomegaly from diffuse red pulp involvement. The cytopenias are due to bone marrow infiltration and hypersplenism. The condition is rare, being 10 times less frequent than chronic lymphocytic leukaemia. It is important to consider this diagnosis in any patient presenting with cytopenias and splenomegaly and to search the blood film carefully looking for the characteristic cells. A careful manual differential count should also be performed to identify the monocytopenia that is expected and is a useful supplementary aid to the diagnosis of hairy cell leukaemia. It should be noted that the automated monocyte count in this patient is likely to have been wrong, since hairy cells are often misidentified as monocytes by automated counters. Bone marrow aspirates are often hypocellular or dry, so the diagnosis is often not possible on such poor specimens. Flow cytometry studies on peripheral blood should therefore be an early investigation if this diagnosis is considered; hairy cells show a surface light chain-restricted pan-B phenotype, CD20[bright] with a 4/4 hairy cell score (CD11c[+], CD25[+], CD103[+], CD123[+]). Flow cytometry can also help discriminate between hairy cell variant, splenic marginal zone lymphoma and splenic diffuse red pulp lymphoma, unclassifiable. Finally, the bone marrow trephine biopsy is a reliable means of making this diagnosis and makes an important contribution where the diagnosis has not been considered by the haematologist. Marrow infiltration can however be patchy in early stage disease and may potentially be missed, especially if trephine samples are small, fragmented or subcortical in origin. Where other specimens are of poor quality, or not carefully examined, the bone marrow trephine biopsy remains a reliable means of making this diagnosis.

Final diagnosis

Hairy cell leukaemia

Case 7

A 30-year-old man was referred for a haematology assessment by an ear, nose and throat surgeon. He had presented with nasal congestion due to multiple bilateral nasal polyps and a surgical polypectomy was planned. He had no significant bleeding history but he recalled the story of a large scalp haematoma as a child following a fall with a head injury. He was also aware that a number of members of his Iraqi family were known to have low platelet counts though this had never been fully explained. He was otherwise in good health and was taking no regular medication. General physical examination was normal.

Laboratory data

FBC: Hb 151 g/L, WBC 5.8 × 10⁹/L and platelets 7 × 10⁹/L.
 U&Es, LFTs, CRP were normal.
 Coagulation screen and D-dimer were normal.

Blood film

This showed a true thrombocytopenia with prominent large platelets. Some were approaching the size of red cells such that the automated platelet count was likely to be an underestimate and the automated instrument failed to calculate a mean platelet volume (Figures 7.1 and 7.2). The neutrophils did not show inclusions and the film was otherwise unremarkable.

Platelet aggregation studies

In view of the incomplete family history, the presence of a macrothrombocytopenic syndrome and the potential for

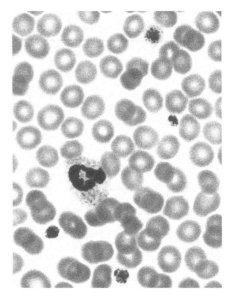

Figure 7.1 MGG, ×500.

a significant surgical challenge, we proceeded to perform platelet aggregation studies. The results are reproduced in Figure 7.3. This illustrates normal aggregation to all agonists except ristocetin. This finding is in keeping with a diagnosis of Bernard–Soulier syndrome (BSS).

Flow cytometry studies

The patient's platelets had markedly reduced expression of CD42 (GpIb-IX-V) with normal expression of CD41 and CD61.

Practical Flow Cytometry in Haematology: 100 Worked Examples, First Edition. Mike Leach, Mark Drummond, Allyson Doig, Pam McKay, Bob Jackson and Barbara J. Bain.
© 2015 John Wiley & Sons, Ltd. Published 2015 by John Wiley & Sons, Ltd.

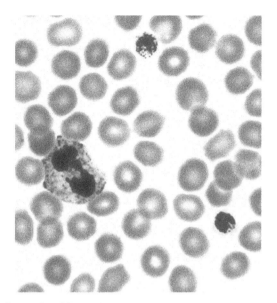

Figure 7.2 MGG, ×1000.

Molecular studies

The patient was found to be homozygous for the C.10 T>G mutation in exon 1 of the *GP1BB* gene.

Management

The patient was counselled with regard to the presence of this inherited platelet disorder and the need for family studies on his siblings in Iraq. The situation was discussed with surgical colleagues and the patient was planned for surgery following a preoperative desmopressin infusion and intravenous tranexamic acid with the latter continued orally for 7 days. Platelets were available for transfusion, if required. The surgical procedure was uncomplicated and there was no excess bleeding.

Discussion

Bernard–Soulier syndrome is an autosomal recessive disorder characterised by the constellation of thrombocytopenia, macro-platelets and abnormal platelet function due to defects in the GpIb-IX-V complex. Typically, platelets fail to aggregate in response to ristocetin and von Willebrand factor (VWF) but show a normal response to other agonists. The GpIb-IX-V complex acts as a receptor for von Willebrand factor exposed following trauma to vascular endothelium. It initiates platelet adhesion at sites of tissue injury but is also involved in complex interactions with the subendothelial matrix in the processes of thrombosis and inflammation.

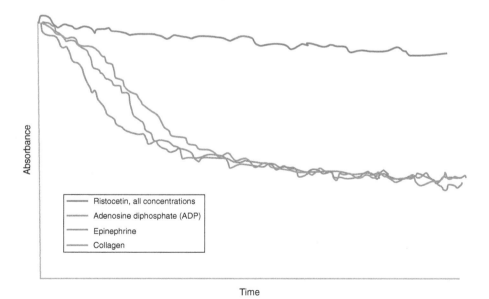

Figure 7.3 Platelet aggregation.

The clinical phenotype is variable but most patients describe mucosal type bleeding with epistaxis, gingival bleeding and bleeding following trauma or surgery. Menorrhagia is common in affected females.

The patient described is unusual in that the bleeding history was mild though he had never been subjected to a surgical challenge. Surgery on nasal polyps can induce significant bleeding and it was this that led to a careful consideration of the nature of the thrombocytopenia. The platelet aggregation studies were strongly suggestive of BSS and sequencing of the *GP1BB* gene identified homozygosity for a recognised mutation.

Macrothrombocytopenia is a generic term that encompasses a number of inherited platelet disorders. The thrombocytopenia is real but automated counts may be disproportionately low due to very large platelets that have the impedance characteristics of small red cells and thus are excluded from the count. In addition to assessment of platelet size and morphology on the blood film, it is important to assess neutrophils for the presence of inclusions. These are present in May–Hegglin anomaly, Sebastian and Fechtner syndromes (*MYH9*-related disorders). They are not present in Bernard–Soulier syndrome and other giant platelet disorders; see Mhawech and Saleem (1) for an excellent concise review .

Final diagnosis

Bernard–Soulier syndrome

Reference

1 Mhawech, P. & Saleem, A. (2000) Inherited giant platelet disorders. Classification and literature review. *American Journal of Clinical Pathology*, **113** (**2**), 176–190. PubMed PMID: 10664620.

Case 8

A 79-year-old man presented with a recent onset of fatigue. There was no past medical history of note and physical examination was unremarkable except for pallor. A full blood count from 9 months earlier was normal.

Laboratory data

FBC: Hb 87 g/L, WBC 36 × 10⁹/L (neutrophils 0.75 × 10⁹/L, monocytes 34 × 10⁹/L) and platelets 140 × 10⁹/L.

U&Es, LFTs, LDH and bone profile were normal.

Blood film

This showed a large population of monocytes with pale blue vacuolated cytoplasm and folded nuclei without obvious nucleoli (Figures 8.1 and 8.2). There was also a population of promonocytes, recognisable from their delicate chromatin pattern (Figure 8.2, lower cell). In small numbers these cells might not have generated much attention as many cells had morphology very similar to normal monocytes. However, their large number and the presence of promonocytes indicated a high likelihood of clonal proliferation and in view of the normal blood count from earlier that year, this was likely to represent an acute monocytic leukaemia rather than chronic myelomonocytic leukaemia (CMML). The neutrophil proliferation typically seen in CMML was also lacking.

Bone marrow aspirate

In view of the patient's age, a decision for supportive care was made. A bone marrow aspirate was therefore not obtained.

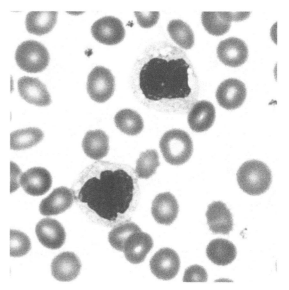

Figure 8.1 MGG, ×1000.

Flow cytometry on peripheral blood

This confirmed a large population of abnormal monocytic lineage cells (CD34⁻, CD117⁻, CD13⁺, CD33⁺, HLA-DR⁺, CD15⁺, CD14⁺, CD64⁺) (73% of all cells) with 15% of these having an immunophenotype suggestive of monoblasts (CD14⁻, CD64⁺) whilst the remainder were consistent with promonocytes (CD14ᵈⁱᵐ, CD64⁺) and monocytes (CD14ᵇʳⁱᵍʰᵗ, CD64⁺). CD56 was expressed, in keeping with a neoplastic proliferation, and this expression was largely confined to the monoblast and promonocyte population (40% of monocyte lineage cells). In addition to the expression of CD56, CD64 was expressed more strongly than on normal cells of monocyte lineage. This abnormal antigen expression is not only useful in diagnosis but is also important in

Practical Flow Cytometry in Haematology: 100 Worked Examples, First Edition. Mike Leach, Mark Drummond, Allyson Doig, Pam McKay, Bob Jackson and Barbara J. Bain.
© 2015 John Wiley & Sons, Ltd. Published 2015 by John Wiley & Sons, Ltd.

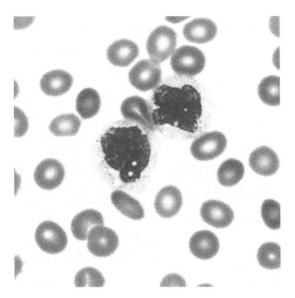

Figure 8.2 MGG, ×1000.

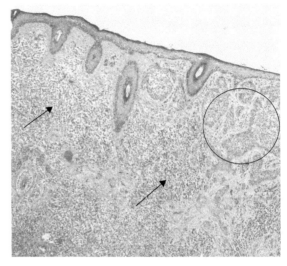

Figure 8.3 H&E, ×40.

defining remission status following chemotherapy for acute monocytic/monoblastic leukaemias as normal monocytes are prominent in remission bone marrows.

Cytogenetic analysis on peripheral blood

Metaphase preparations showed a normal 46,XY karyotype.

Clinical course

In view of the patient's age, preserved platelet count and resolution of all symptoms following blood transfusion, we elected for management with supportive care only.

The patient attended dermatology, unknown to our department, regarding a chronic nodular/ulcerating lesion on his face and this was biopsied. This showed two features. Firstly there was a basal cell carcinoma, likely to be the pathology responsible for the symptomatic skin lesion (circled, Figure 8.3) but in addition, the dermis was infiltrated by a monotonous population of medium to large cells with plentiful cytoplasm (arrows, Figures 8.3 and 8.4). These cells were negative for CD34, weakly positive for MPO and positive for CD33 and CD15 in keeping with cells of monocytic lineage (Figures 8.5–8.8). CD33 also highlighted normal Langerhans cells within the epidermis.

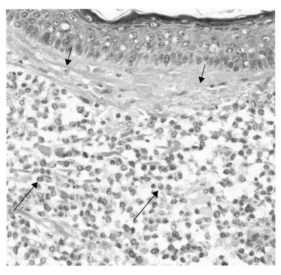

Figure 8.4 H&E, ×200.

Note that the epidermis is not involved by the monocytic infiltrate and this may explain why this component was not causing symptoms. Note the Grenz zone in Figure 8.4 (short arrows); this is a collagenous band between epidermis and dermis that is often not breached by non-T-cell neoplasms. CD34 clearly identifies the endothelium of the blood vessels (Figure 8.5).

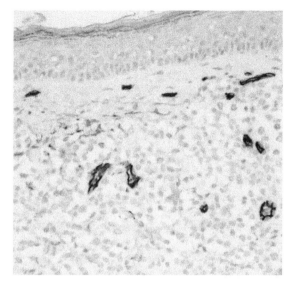

Figure 8.5 CD34, ×200.

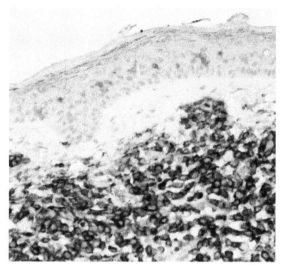

Figure 8.7 CD33, ×200.

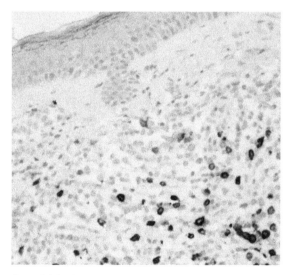

Figure 8.6 MPO, ×200.

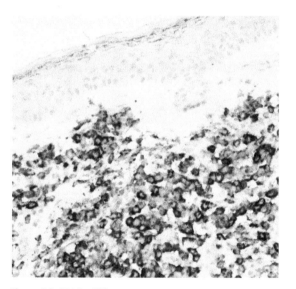

Figure 8.8 CD15, ×200.

Discussion

Acute leukaemia diagnosis is based on the morphological assessment of leukaemic cells and this provides a working template on which to structure subsequent investigations. A primary morphological diagnosis, supported by flow cytometric analysis, can guide appropriate cytogenetic, FISH and molecular studies. These directed investigations can activate requests for necessary follow-on tests so that time

There was no significant bleeding following the procedure but the skin wound did become infected and required intravenous antibiotic therapy.

and money are not wasted and resources are not stretched by 'doing everything in every case'. However, the extent of investigation must also be related to their appropriateness in an individual patient and, as in this case, once a management decision has been made, unnecessary investigations should be avoided.

In this patient, the size of the monocytic clone in the peripheral blood, the reduction of normal granulopoiesis and the normality of blood counts earlier in the same year all suggested an acute process despite the preservation of the platelet count. This diagnostic suspicion was supported by the immature phenotype of many of the leukaemic cells of flow cytometry. When no bone marrow aspirate is available, a suspicion of acute monocytic leukaemia can be based on the recognition of promonocytes as well as monocytes in the blood film. The presence of 20% 'blast equivalents' (monoblasts plus promonocytes) in either the bone marrow or peripheral blood is sufficient for a diagnosis of acute leukaemia. Usually, when there is monocytic differentiation, the cells in the bone marrow are less mature than those in the blood so that sometimes a diagnosis of acute monocytic leukaemia is only possible with marrow examination.

Because of the therapeutic implications, it is important that acute monocytic leukaemia is clearly differentiated from CMML. Both diseases can affect the elderly and both show a tendency for extranodal tissue involvement. In addition to cytology and immunophenotyping, cytogenetic and molecular studies can be informative, although this was not so in this patient. The finding of an *MLL* rearrangement at 11q23, when present, is indicative of acute monocytic leukaemia and is not seen in CMML. Conversely, *TET2* mutations are frequently seen in CMML but are not a feature of *de novo* acute monocytic leukaemia.

This patient was managed supportively for almost a year, spending relatively little time in hospital and precious time with his family and friends.

Final diagnosis

Probable acute monocytic leukaemia with subclinical dermal infiltration.

9

Case 9

A previously well 79-year-old man attended his GP for a routine health check. An FBC was taken. The patient reported 2–3 kg weight loss over the previous 6 months as well as night sweats. Clinical examination revealed 5 cm splenomegaly and a 4 cm liver edge. There was no lymphadenopathy or skin rash and chest examination was normal. An FBC taken 1 year previously had been entirely normal.

Laboratory data

FBC: Hb 147 g/L, WBC 38.3×10^9/L (neutrophils 26.0×10^9/L, monocytes 7.4×10^9/L) and platelets 463×10^9/L.

U&Es, bone profile and LFTs were normal. Serum LDH was 1620 U/L and urate 0.48 mmol/L.

Blood film

This confirmed the marked monocytosis (20% of cells), with dysplastic features evident in both monocyte and neutrophil populations. Monocytes were of mature appearance. Neutrophils were mainly mature but hyposegmented (Figures 9.1–9.4). Some eosinophils were hyposegmented with reduced granules (Figure 9.3). A very occasional nucleated red blood cell was noted, with no teardrop forms and no blast cells. The platelets were generally large, some abnormally so, and well granulated.

Flow cytometry

Flow cytometry on blood confirmed an abnormal monocyte population, with CD64+ and CD14dim, but CD56 negative.

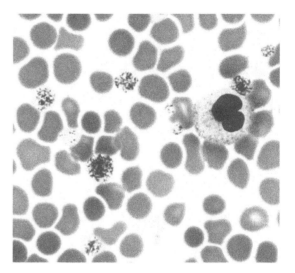

Figure 9.1 MGG, ×1000.

No loss of HLA-DR was noted and circulating CD34+ cells were not detected.

The marrow aspirate was difficult to acquire and was hypocellular but CD34+ cells comprised <1% of events and an abnormal monocyte population, of identical immunophenotype to that present in blood, accounted for 25% of cells.

Bone marrow trephine biopsy

The trephine biopsy sections demonstrated 90% cellularity, with increased granulopoiesis and a striking proliferation of megakaryocytes (Figures 9.5–9.8). These were of varying size, with numerous loose clusters noted and there was abnormal localisation adjacent to the bony trabeculae

Practical Flow Cytometry in Haematology: 100 Worked Examples, First Edition. Mike Leach, Mark Drummond, Allyson Doig, Pam McKay, Bob Jackson and Barbara J. Bain.
© 2015 John Wiley & Sons, Ltd. Published 2015 by John Wiley & Sons, Ltd.

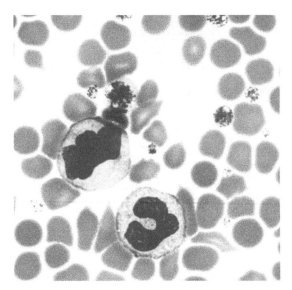

Figure 9.2 MGG, ×1000.

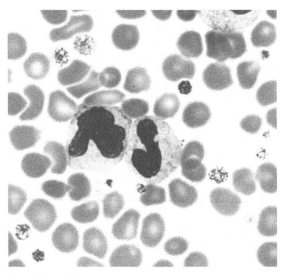

Figure 9.4 MGG, ×1000.

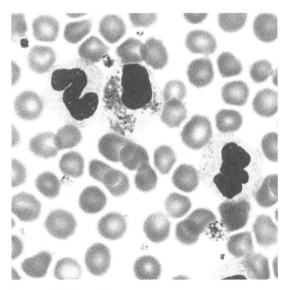

Figure 9.3 MGG, ×1000.

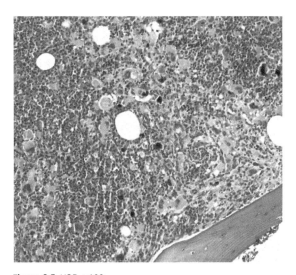

Figure 9.5 H&E, ×100.

(Figure 9.7); some megakaryocytes had hyperchromatic nuclei. The interstitium was expanded further with myeloid precursors and monocytes (Figure 9.9). Reticulin was increased to grade 2. No collagen fibrosis, cell streaming or osteosclerosis was seen.

Cytogenetic analysis

Normal male karyotype, 46,XY, in 20 metaphases.

Molecular studies

Analysis for the *JAK2* V617F mutation in peripheral blood was positive (*BCR-ABL1* was negative).

Discussion

This case presents some diagnostic difficulty. Initial clinical assessment led to the assumption that it was likely to represent primary myelofibrosis (PMF), given the

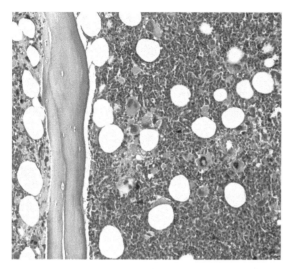

Figure 9.6 H&E, ×100.

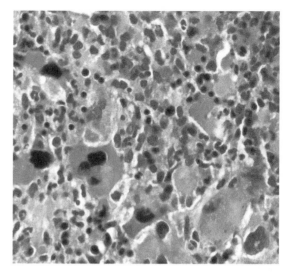

Figure 9.8 H&E, ×400.

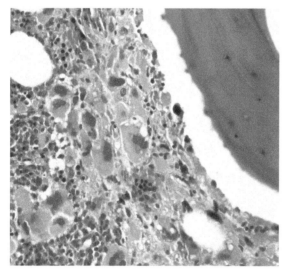

Figure 9.7 H&E, ×200.

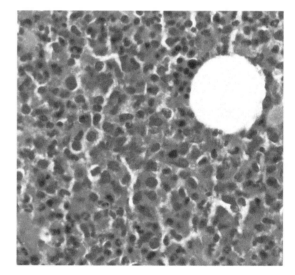

Figure 9.9 H&E, ×100.

hepatosplenomegaly and systemic symptoms. However, the blood film examination was not typical, namely lack of teardrop poikilocytes, <10% myeloid precursor cells, the presence of dysplastic neutrophils and monocytes as well as a marked monocytosis. No reactive process was evident and marrow examination confirmed a primary haematological disorder, *JAK2* +ve. The monocytosis is the key here; PMF and the other *BCR-ABL1*-negative myeloproliferative disorders do not usually exhibit monocytic proliferation. While the monocytic cells were dysplastic, they were towards the mature end of the spectrum by morphology and flow

cytometry (including CD14 positivity). Blast cells in both marrow and blood were infrequent (1% or less). Given the additional presence of neutrophilia and dysplastic changes, with increased bone marrow granulopoiesis, chronic myelomonocytic leukaemia (CMML) is therefore considered a more likely diagnosis, with secondary acquisition of *JAK2* explaining the unusual megakaryocyte proliferation and the degree of reticulin fibrosis. Monocyte infiltration can be difficult to assess on H&E-stained marrow sections and therefore immunohistochemistry or flow cytometry may be required to demonstrate monocyte excess. The monocyte compartment in a normal, steady state marrow is usually between 1% and 8% of cells by flow cytometry (1), and is clearly increased in this case. Identifying an abnormal monocyte immunophenotype is important in supporting a clonal disorder; in this case, the dim CD14 expression and relatively bright CD64 indicated an immature monocytic population. CD56 is the most common aberrant antigen detected in CMML, in approximately 80% of cases (2) although it was not seen in this case.

CMML is characterised by a monocytosis of $>1.0 \times 10^9$/L, usually in conjunction with either a predominantly myeloproliferative phenotype (CMML-MP, 40% of cases) or a predominantly dysplastic phenotype (CMML-MDS, 60% of cases), these exhibiting mainly proliferative features or mainly cytopenias, respectively. Thrombocytosis is occasionally seen in such patients, although thrombocytopenia is much more common. A significant incidence of *JAK2* mutation has been described (~5–10% of cases) in this disorder over recent years (3, 4). It would appear to be associated with a more proliferative phenotype, in particular neutrophilia, thrombocytosis and splenomegaly as well as megakaryocytic clustering in the marrow and reticulin fibrosis. The considerable genetic, clinical and laboratory heterogeneity of CMML is likely to lead to further such genotypic-phenotypic correlative observations in the near future.

Final diagnosis

Chronic myelomonocytic leukaemia with acquisition of the *JAK2* V617F mutation.

References

1 van Lochem, E.G., van der Velden, V.H., Wind, H.K., te Marvelde, J.G., Westerdaal, N.A. & van Dongen, J.J. (2004) Immunophenotypic differentiation patterns of normal hematopoiesis in human bone marrow: reference patterns for age-related changes and disease-induced shifts. *Cytometry Part B, Clinical Cytometry*, **60** (1), 1–13.

2 Kern, W., Bacher, U., Haferlach, C., Schnittger, S. & Haferlach, T. (2011) Acute monoblastic/monocytic leukemia and chronic myelomonocytic leukemia share common immunophenotypic features but differ in the extent of aberrantly expressed antigens and amount of granulocytic cells. *Leukemia & Lymphoma*, **52** (1), 92–100. PubMed PMID: 21219126.

3 Schnittger, S., Bacher, U., Eder, C. *et al.* (2012) Molecular analyses of 15,542 patients with suspected BCR-ABL1-negative myeloproliferative disorders allow to develop a stepwise diagnostic workflow. *Haematologica*, **97** (10), 1582–1585.

4 Pich, A., Riera, L., Sismondi, F. *et al.* (2009) JAK2V617F activating mutation is associated with the myeloproliferative type of chronic myelomonocytic leukaemia. *Journal of Clinical Pathology*, **62** (9), 798–801.

10

Case 10

A previously well 70-year-old man was admitted with a short history of fever, night sweats and general malaise.

Laboratory investigations

FBC: Hb 140 g/L, WBC 31.9 × 10⁹/L (neutrophils 14.7 × 10^9/L, lymphocytes 11.7 × 10^9/L, 'monocytes' 4.8 × 10^9/L) and platelets 132 × 10^9/L.

U&Es: Na 135 mmol/L, K 3.6 mmol/L, urea 9 mmol/L, creatinine 124 µmol/L, eGFR 50 mL/min.

Bone profile: calcium 4.75 mmol/L, phosphate 1.35 mmol/L, ALP 350 U/L, albumin 30 g/L.

Serum LDH 2428 U/L, urate 1.12 mmol/L.

Blood film

This showed a population of large, lymphoid cells with prominent nucleoli and basophilic cytoplasm, sometimes vacuolated (Figures 10.1–10.3). The morphology was 'Burkitt like' but quite pleomorphic with a lot of variation in cell size. Apoptotic cells were easily identified and the cell cytoplasm was fragile and shedding fragments (Figure 10.3).

Flow cytometry (peripheral blood)

The large circulating cells were monoclonal B cells expressing lambda^bright, CD19^dim, CD20^mod, CD10, CD38, FMC7^dim, HLA-DR, CD22 and CD79b. CD5 and CD23 were negative. This phenotype is of a mature B-cell disorder but note the reduced intensity of CD19 and FMC7 expression.

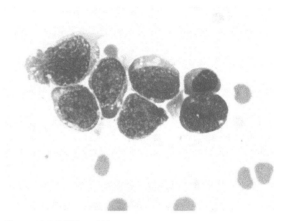

Figure 10.1 MGG, ×1000.

Imaging

A CT scan showed extensive lymphadenopathy from the base of skull to the groins. There was evidence of superior vena cava (SVC) obstruction.

Lymph node core biopsy

A core biopsy from a supraclavicular lymph node showed a diffuse infiltrate of pleomorphic large blast cells. There were numerous tingible body macrophages conferring a 'starry sky' appearance. By immunohistochemistry, the abnormal cells were shown to express CD20, CD10, BCL6, BCL2 and MUM1. They were negative for CD5, CD30 and cyclin D1. The proliferation fraction was 90%.

Practical Flow Cytometry in Haematology: 100 Worked Examples, First Edition. Mike Leach, Mark Drummond, Allyson Doig, Pam McKay, Bob Jackson and Barbara J. Bain.
© 2015 John Wiley & Sons, Ltd. Published 2015 by John Wiley & Sons, Ltd.

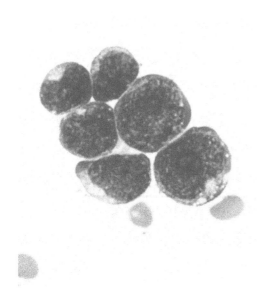

Figure 10.2 MGG, ×1000.

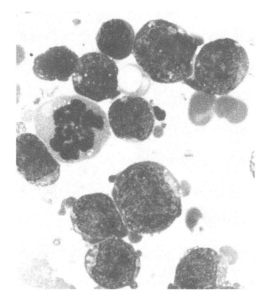

Figure 10.3 MGG, ×1000.

Bone marrow aspirate and trephine biopsy

The aspirate showed identical cells to those seen in blood. Trephine biopsy sections showed cellularity to be increased to 70–80% with a diffuse infiltrate of large blast-like cells

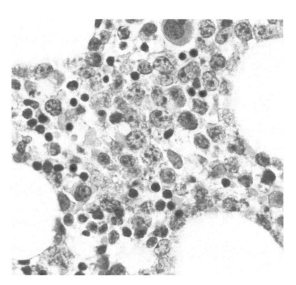

Figure 10.4 H&E, ×500.

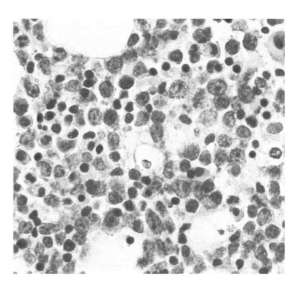

Figure 10.5 H&E, ×500.

(Figures 10.4 and 10.5). The cells had large pleomorphic nuclei with one or more prominent nucleoli. The cytological features were identical to those shown in the lymph node biopsy.

Molecular studies

The lymph node tissue was positive for a translocation involving *MYC* by fluorescence *in situ* hybridisation (FISH).

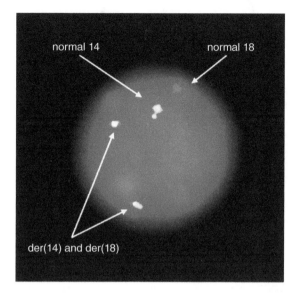

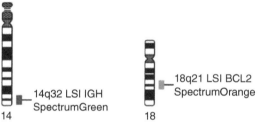

Figure 10.6 Abbott Molecular Vysis LSI IGH/BCL2 Dual-Color, Dual-Fusion Translocation Probe.

In addition, an *IGH/BCL2* fusion signal was identified indicating t(14;18)(q32;q21) or a variant thereof (Figure 10.6).

Classical cytogenetics

A 3-way translocation was identified between chromosomes 8, 14 and 18 (Figure 10.7) in addition to trisomy 7 (not shown) with the karyotype being 45,XY,+7, t(8;14;18)(q24; q32;q21).

Clinical course

The patient commenced R-CHOP therapy with a plan for CNS prophylaxis using high dose systemic methotrexate. An early response was seen in terms of nodal resolution with clearance of circulating disease cells. However, after five cycles of treatment (including one cycle of methotrexate) had been completed, the patient was admitted with swallowing difficulty and new onset right third cranial nerve palsy. The clinical impression was of a bulbar palsy. MRI of the brain showed no clear abnormality, so CSF was taken and submitted for flow cytometry studies.

The CSF cell count was 0.25×10^9/L and a cytospin showed large pleomorphic lymphoid cells with nucleoli and basophilic cytoplasm (Figure 10.8). These resembled the disease cells involving blood and bone marrow at the outset and were surface lambda-restricted, CD10$^+$ and HLA-DR$^+$ B cells now lacking FMC7 expression. The findings were in keeping with meningeal relapse during therapy.

Discussion

The morphology and immunophenotype were those of a high grade B-cell lymphoma, germinal centre subtype, but with an atypical CD19^{dim} and FMC7^{dim} phenotype. The features are

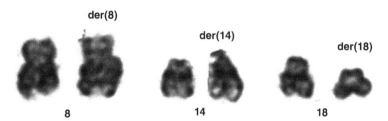

Figure 10.7 Metaphase cytogenetic preparation showing a three-way translocation, t(8;14;18)(q24;q32;q21).

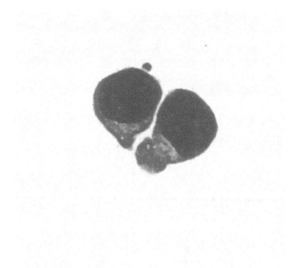

Figure 10.8 MGG, ×1000.

not classical for Burkitt lymphoma in view of the pleomorphic morphology, BCL2 positivity, the complex cytogenetic abnormalities and the proliferation fraction, which though elevated is not as strikingly abnormal as in BL. The atypical morphology, immunohistochemistry showing a BCL2$^+$ germinal centre type mature B-cell neoplasm, together with the FISH and cytogenetic findings, are in keeping with a diagnosis of B-cell lymphoma, unclassifiable (BCLU), with features intermediate between DLBCL and Burkitt lymphoma.

A translocation involving *MYC* (8q24) together with a second translocation involving *BCL2* (18q21) or, less commonly, *BCL6* (3q27) is found in approximately 5–10% of patients with DLBCL, being known as 'dual translocation' or 'double-hit' lymphoma (1). The morphology and immunophenotype of such lymphomas are often those of BCLU. These patients typically present with advanced stage disease often with blood and bone marrow involvement and have an increased incidence of CNS disease. In the reported cases, the outcome was very poor with a median survival of approximately 8 months.

There are also increasing reports of an atypical phenotype by flow cytometry of BCLU, with partial or dim expression of

CD19, CD20, FMC7 and surface Ig being characteristic findings (2, 3).

The three-way translocation in this case is an interesting finding as it has rarely been described before. The same chromosome 14 is involved in both the t(8;14) and t(14;18) translocations resulting in a complex three-way translocation, t(8;14;18)(q24;q32;q21). The small number of such cases in the literature have, like the current case, behaved aggressively and therefore should be classified along with double-hit lymphomas (4). This appears to be just one of the possible mechanisms through which this phenotype can be achieved. Such lymphomas are being increasingly reported but there is little current evidence to indicate how they might be most effectively managed.

Final diagnosis

B-cell lymphoma unclassifiable, intermediate between DLBCL and Burkitt lymphoma with blood and bone marrow involvement followed by CNS relapse during treatment.

References

1 Li, S., Lin, P., Young, K.H., Kanagal-Shamanna, R., Yin, C.C. & Medeiros, L.J. (2013) MYC/BCL2 double-hit high-grade B-cell lymphoma. *Advances in Anatomic Pathology*, **20** (5), 315–326. PubMed PMID: 23939148.

2 Wu, D., Wood, B.L., Dorer, R. & Fromm, J.R. (2010) "Double-Hit" mature B-cell lymphomas show a common immunophenotype by flow cytometry that includes decreased CD20 expression. *American Journal of Clinical Pathology*, **134** (2), 258–265. PubMed PMID: 20660329.

3 Harrington, A.M., Olteanu, H., Kroft, S.H. & Eshoa, C. (2011) The unique immunophenotype of double-hit lymphomas. *American Journal of Clinical Pathology*, **135** (4), 649–650. PubMed PMID: 21411790.

4 Liu, D., Shimonov, J., Primanneni, S., Lai, Y., Ahmed, T. & Seiter, K. (2007) t(8;14;18): a 3-way chromosome translocation in two patients with Burkitt's lymphoma/leukemia. *Molecular cancer*, **6**, 35. PubMed PMID: 17547754. Pubmed Central PMCID: 1904237.

Case 11

11

A 72-year-old man with a history of chronic renal impairment and hypertension presented with anorexia, dyspnoea and ankle swelling. Clinical examination revealed generalised lymphadenopathy and splenomegaly.

Laboratory results

FBC: Hb 131 g/L, WBC 245 × 10^9/L (neutrophils 4.9 × 10^9/L) and platelets 54 × 10^9/L.

U&Es: Creatinine 246 μmol/L, eGFR 23 mL/min.

Bone profile was normal.

LFTs: bilirubin 62 μmol/L, alkaline phosphatase 670 U/L.

Serum LDH: 725 U/L.

Blood film

This showed a marked lymphocytosis with medium to large cells, many with prominent and multiple nucleoli. Some nuclei had prominent clefts and smear cells were common (Figures 11.1–11.4). The chromatin pattern was quite delicate. Thrombocytopenia was confirmed.

Flow cytometry (peripheral blood)

A mature clonal (kappa^{bright} restricted) CD5$^+$ B-cell lymphoproliferative disorder was identified. The cells co-expressed CD20^{bright}, CD38, FMC7, CD79b and HLA-DR. CD10 and CD23 were negative.

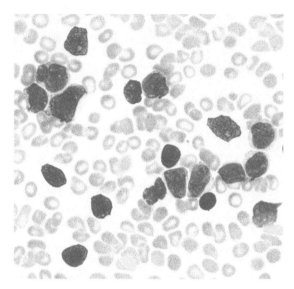

Figure 11.1 MGG, ×500.

FISH

This identified the presence of a t(11;14)(q13;q32) translocation.

Imaging

A CT scan showed widespread small volume (<2 cm) lymphadenopathy in neck, axillae, mediastinum, abdomen and pelvis. The spleen was also enlarged at 21 cm.

Practical Flow Cytometry in Haematology: 100 Worked Examples, First Edition. Mike Leach, Mark Drummond, Allyson Doig, Pam McKay, Bob Jackson and Barbara J. Bain.
© 2015 John Wiley & Sons, Ltd. Published 2015 by John Wiley & Sons, Ltd.

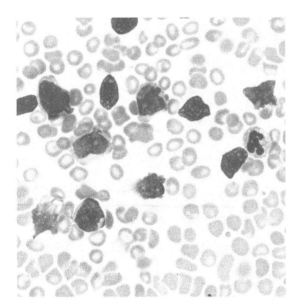

Figure 11.2 MGG, ×500.

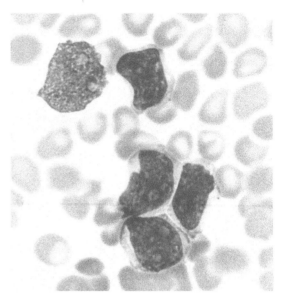

Figure 11.4 MGG, ×1000.

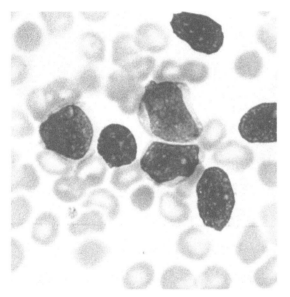

Figure 11.3 MGG, ×1000.

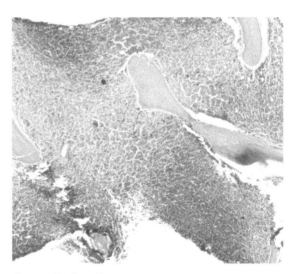

Figure 11.5 H&E, ×40.

Histopathology

Bone marrow trephine biopsy sections showed maximal cellularity due to diffuse infiltration by abnormal lymphoid cells (Figures 11.5 and 11.6). The abnormal cells were medium to large and many showed nucleoli (Figure 11.7).

The proliferation index was high (Ki-67 50%, not shown). The phenotype was identical to that noted above and cyclin D1 was expressed (Figure 11.8).

Discussion

Cell marker studies identified a CD5$^+$ lymphoproliferative disorder in a patient with a high leucocyte count,

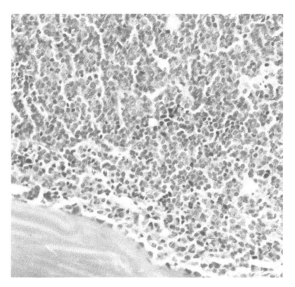

Figure 11.6 H&E, ×200.

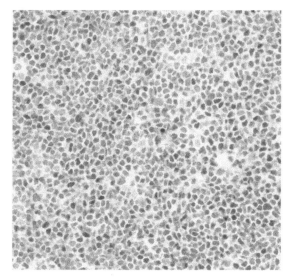

Figure 11.8 Cyclin D1, ×200.

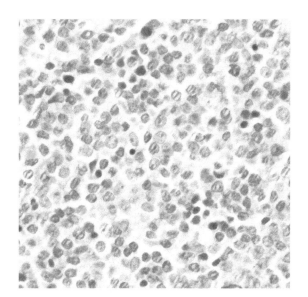

Figure 11.7 H&E, ×400.

lymphadenopathy and splenomegaly. The differential diagnosis included chronic lymphocytic leukaemia (CLL), mantle cell lymphoma (MCL) and marginal zone lymphoma (MZL). The immunophenotype was not indicative of CLL (CLL score 1/5). Marginal zone lymphoma was unlikely in view of the morphology and marked lymphocytosis. The most likely diagnosis was MCL and this was confirmed by the cyclin D1 positivity and the presence of t(11;14)(q13;q32)

which translocates the *CCND1* gene (11q13) so that it is adjacent to the *IGH* gene (14q32).

Mantle cell lymphoma is a rare disease accounting for <10% of all non-Hodgkin lymphomas. It is usually a disease of the elderly, especially males, and presents with advanced stage disease. Bone marrow and gastrointestinal tract involvement are common. Peripheral blood involvement is common but the lymphocytosis is usually mild. Marked lymphocytosis, as in this case, is unusual but well described; the morphology and immunophenotype may mimic B-cell prolymphocytic leukaemia.

The blastoid variant of MCL accounts for <10% of cases and is usually associated with a more aggressive clinical course, marked leucocytosis, transient responses to treatment and shortened overall survival. Marked leucocytosis is associated with often multiple additional cytogenetic and molecular abnormalities, including rearrangement of oncogenes or tumour suppressor genes such as *MYC* at 8q24, *CDKN2A* (p16) at 9p22-24 and *TP53* at 17p13. Mantle cell lymphoma with blastoid morphology often shows high proliferation rates, p53 overexpression and variant mRNA cyclin D1 isoforms (1, 2). The immunophenotype is often typical (expression of pan-B-cell markers with CD5) but loss of CD5 expression and CD10 positivity (3) may be seen in the blastoid variant.

Responses to treatment with first-line chemotherapy are typically short (2) and, as yet, there is no evidence that intensive regimens using high dose cytarabine yield better results. We are now entering an era where new therapies such as Bruton's kinase inhibitors, such as ibrutinib, which act on intracellular signalling, are becoming available for the treatment of MCL and excellent results in relapsed and refractory patients are being reported with overall response rates approaching 70% (4). It remains to be seen how they are integrated into therapy alongside or instead of standard chemotherapy approaches. It also remains to be seen how they might impact on the more highly proliferative blastoid subtype of MCL as described here.

Final diagnosis

Mantle cell lymphoma (MCL), blastoid variant.

References

1 Slotta-Huspenina, J., Koch, I., de Leval, L. *et al.* (2012) The impact of cyclin D1 mRNA isoforms, morphology and p53 in mantle cell lymphoma: p53 alterations and blastoid mor-

phology are strong predictors of a high proliferation index. *Haematologica*, **97** (**9**) 1422–1430. PubMed PMID: 22315488.

2 Parrens, M., Belaud-Rotureau, M.A., Fitoussi, O. *et al.* (2006 Mar) Blastoid and common variants of mantle cell lymphoma exhibit distinct immunophenotypic and interphase FISH features. *Histopathology*, **48** (**4**), 353–362. PubMed PMID: 16487357.

3 Zanetto ,U., Dong, H., Huang, Y. *et al.* (2008) Mantle cell lymphoma with aberrant expression of CD10. *Histopathology*, **53** (**1**), 20–29. PubMed PMID: 18518902.

4 Wang, M.L., Rule, S., Martin, P. *et al.* (2013 Aug 8) Targeting BTK with ibrutinib in relapsed or refractory mantle-cell lymphoma. *The New England Journal of Medicine*, **369** (**6**), 507–516. PubMed PMID: 23782157.

12

Case 12

A frail 77-year-old female presented with fatigue, weight loss, 2-cm palpable splenomegaly and an abnormal full blood count showing Hb 92 g/L, WBC 18.4 × 10⁹/L (neutrophils and precursors 16 × 10⁹/L, basophils 0.6 × 10⁹/L) and platelets 1324 × 10⁹/L. She was diagnosed with chronic phase (CP) CML, with the p210 *BCR-ABL1* transcript (B3A2 splice variant) being demonstrated by RT-PCR. No additional cytogenetic abnormalities were detected beyond the Philadelphia (Ph) chromosome (present in 20/20 cells) and the bone marrow blast cell count was 2%. Her Sokal risk-score was calculated as high. Unfortunately the patient was intolerant of all available tyrosine kinase inhibitors (TKI), and her preference was for palliation with hydroxycarbamide. After 18 months on therapy thrombocytopenia was noted, unresponsive to hydroxycarbamide dose interruption. Examination of a blood film was undertaken.

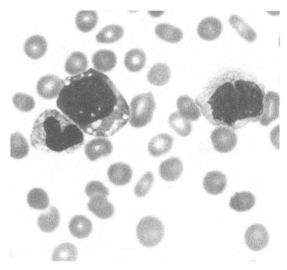

Figure 12.1 MGG, ×1000.

Laboratory data

FBC: Hb 96 g/L, WBC 42.9 × 10⁹/L and platelets 59 × 10⁹/L.

U&Es, LFTs and bone profile: normal. Serum LDH was 550 U/L.

Blood film

A manual differential demonstrated 70% blast cells. These were large cells with basophilic cytoplasm, frequent small cytoplasmic vacuoles and occasional small azurophilic granules (Figures 12.1–12.4). A myeloid left shift was noted (Figure 12.1) along with occasional dysplastic monocytoid and myeloid cells (Figures 12.1 and 12.3). Note the hypogranular basophil in Figure 12.4.

Bone marrow aspirate

This was not performed due to patient frailty and a palliative treatment approach.

Flow cytometry

Blast cells were CD34⁻, CD117⁻, HLA-DR^{dim}, CD38⁺, CD15⁺, CD33⁺, CD13⁺, MPO⁺, CD64⁺⁺ and CD14^{dim}. They were therefore identified as being of monoblastic lineage.

Practical Flow Cytometry in Haematology: 100 Worked Examples, First Edition. Mike Leach, Mark Drummond, Allyson Doig, Pam McKay, Bob Jackson and Barbara J. Bain.
© 2015 John Wiley & Sons, Ltd. Published 2015 by John Wiley & Sons, Ltd.

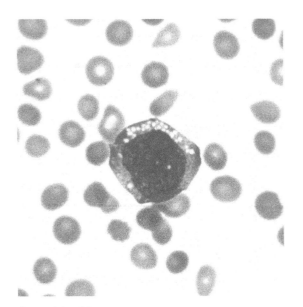

Figure 12.2 MGG, ×1000.

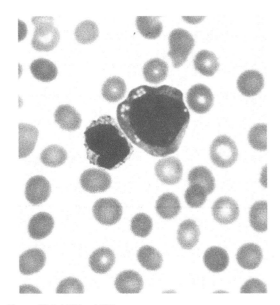

Figure 12.4 MGG, ×1000.

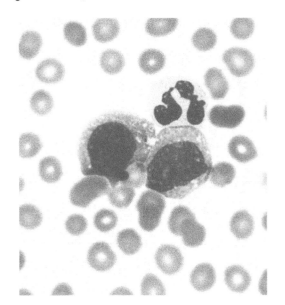

Figure 12.3 MGG, ×1000.

Cytogenetic analysis

47,XX,+19,t(9;22)(q34;q11).

Discussion

This patient presented with symptoms and clinical signs perfectly in keeping with CML. The marked thrombocytosis and relatively modest leucocytosis is not unusual in CML, although to the unwary these parameters may be more suggestive of a Ph⁻ MPN. In this case, however, a careful review of the blood count and film at diagnosis noted the marked basophilia that is highly suggestive of CML and prompted the appropriate cytogenetic and molecular analyses. CML presenting with extreme thrombocytosis ($>1000 \times 10^9$/L) is well described in the literature (perhaps comprising as many as 5% of cases) and the authors have seen several instances, often with platelet counts in the region of $2000-3000 \times 10^9$/L. In fact, the initial description of this entity described it as Ph⁺ essential thrombocythaemia (ET) (1), which we would of course now classify as CML due to the overriding diagnostic importance of the *BCR-ABL1* translocation when present. Overall however, the incidence of thrombosis or haemorrhage is low in CML (estimated at 1% and 3%, respectively) (2). A recent case series of CML with extreme thrombocytosis demonstrated the frequent presence of laboratory features of acquired von Willebrand syndrome (3), but no clinically evident bleeding problems. It is therefore difficult to advocate any particular prophylaxis strategy for these patients and this should be driven by individual patient circumstances, although it would seem appropriate to reduce the platelet count towards normal as rapidly as possible using appropriate CML-directed therapy. It is clearly important not to miss cases of CML in this guise; recent guidance from the BCSH has recommended testing for *BCR-ABL1* in cases of thrombocytosis that are negative for *JAK2* V617F, *MPL* (4) and, given recent publications (5), *CALR* mutations.

As compared to the pre-TKI era, CML-BP is comparatively speaking a relatively rare event. This patient was intolerant of available TKI therapy, and although initial haematological response was obtained with reduced dose dasatinib (resolution of splenomegaly and normalisation of leucocytosis and thrombocytosis) haematological relapse was evident shortly after stopping all TKI therapy (because of toxicity). Thus cessation of disease-modifying therapy in the context of a high-risk Sokal score culminated in relatively rapid evolution of BP disease. The Sokal risk score (incorporating age, spleen size, blast count and platelet count as continuous variables) was developed in the era of conventional chemotherapy treatment (predominantly busulphan) yet continues to offer some degree of prognostic stratification in the TKI era (6). Upfront treatment is rarely altered on the basis of baseline risk score, however, with response to TKI therapy being the single most important determinant of outcome in chronic phase CML. The more recent EUTOS score (which simply incorporates % blood basophils and spleen size as continuous variables) was developed from cohorts of imatinib-treated patients (7). It predicts the likelihood of cytogenetic remission at 18 months (a good surrogate marker for clinical outcome) and has been advocated as more relevant to modern treatment approaches. Prognostic score calculators can be found at http://www.leukemia-net.org.

Flow cytometry is of no routine diagnostic value in the chronic phase of the disease. In blast phase, however, it is applied to determine the precursor cell nature and lineage of the blast cell population. The majority of cases are myeloid (60–80%), with a smaller proportion being lymphoid and mainly of B-cell lineage (20–30%). It may arise and progress extremely rapidly and indeed may be difficult (even impossible) to differentiate from Ph⁺ ALL or AML (see Case 80). Cytogenetic evolution, as evident in our case, is typical. Irrespective of cell lineage, management of blast phase CML remains extremely challenging with outcomes far inferior to those of *de novo* acute leukaemia. Current approaches generally incorporate high-dose TKI therapy with intensive chemotherapy induction regimens (according to cell lineage) and consideration of allogeneic transplantation. Given the dire outlook for our patient, a palliative approach was chosen and the patient succumbed to the disease within a few weeks.

Final diagnosis

Blast phase of chronic myeloid leukaemia (monoblastic transformation).

References

1 LeBrun, D.P., Pinkerton, P.H., Sheridan, B.L., Chen-Lai, J., Dube, I.D., Poldre, P.A. (1991) Essential thrombocythemia with the Philadelphia chromosome and BCR-ABL gene rearrangement. An entity distinct from chronic myeloid leukemia and Philadelphia chromosome-negative essential thrombocythemia. *Cancer Genetics and Cytogenetics*, **54**, 21–25.

2 Schafer, A.I. (1984) Bleeding and thrombosis in the myeloproliferative disorders. *Blood*, **64**, 1–12.

3 Sora, F., Autore, F., Chiusolo, P. *et al.* (2014) Extreme thrombocytosis in chronic myeloid leukemia in the era of tyrosine kinase inhibitors. Leukemia & Lymphoma, epub ahead of print.

4 Harrison, C.N., Butt, N., Campbell, P. *et al.* (2013) Diagnostic pathway for the investigation of thrombocytosis. *British Journal of Haematology,* **161**, 604–606.

5 Nangalia, J., Massie, C.E., Baxter, E.J. *et al.* (2013) Somatic CALR mutations in myeloproliferative neoplasms with nonmutated JAK2. *The New England Journal of Medicine*, **369**, 2391–2405.

6 Sokal, J.E., Cox, E.B., Baccarani, M. *et al.* (1984) Prognostic discrimination in "good-risk" chronic granulocytic leukemia. *Blood*, **63**, 789–799.

7 Hasford, J., Baccarani, M., Hoffmann, V. *et al.* Predicting complete cytogenetic response and subsequent progression-free survival in 2060 patients with CML on imatinib treatment: the EUTOS score. *Blood*, **118**, 686–692.

13

Case 13

A 57-year-old female patient was admitted with fatigue. There were no other specific symptoms and clinical examination was unremarkable. There was no past medical history of note.

Laboratory investigations

FBC: Hb 64 g/L, MCV 94 fl, WBC 7×10^9/L, neutrophils 4×10^9/L and platelets 24×10^9/L.

Coagulation screen: PT 12 s, APTT 30 s, TT 12 s, fibrinogen 9 g/L, D-dimer 1500 ng/mL.

U&Es, LFTs and LDH were normal.

Blood film

The blood film showed nucleated red cells and a myeloid left shift. No red cell fragments or blasts were seen. The thrombocytopenia was confirmed.

Bone marrow aspirate

The bone marrow aspirate was difficult to acquire and appeared aparticulate and hypocellular. There was much cell debris and free nuclei. A number of undifferentiated cells with pleomorphic nuclei with occasional nuclear clefts and without cytoplasmic granules were identified (Figures 13.1–13.4). Clumps of cells displaying nuclear moulding (Figure 13.2) were evident in some parts of the film.

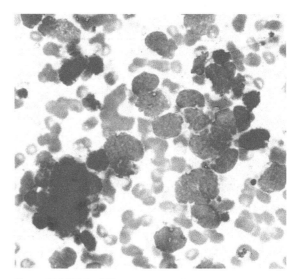

Figure 13.1 MGG, ×500.

Flow cytometry

A non-haemopoietic tumour was suspected so an initial approach to analysis of the marrow aspirate was using a CD45 versus SSC analysis (Figure 13.5).

Note the significant number of events (shown in red) in the CD45⁻ zone. It must be remembered that cell debris and free nuclei will also appear in this area but the number of events appeared too high for this to be the sole explanation and the unidentified cells seen in the film could not be accounted for elsewhere in the plot. Note the small populations of lymphocytes, monocytes and myeloid cells and an absence of cells in the CD45^{dim} gate/region. The CD45⁻ gate

Practical Flow Cytometry in Haematology: 100 Worked Examples, First Edition. Mike Leach, Mark Drummond, Allyson Doig, Pam McKay, Bob Jackson and Barbara J. Bain.
© 2015 John Wiley & Sons, Ltd. Published 2015 by John Wiley & Sons, Ltd.

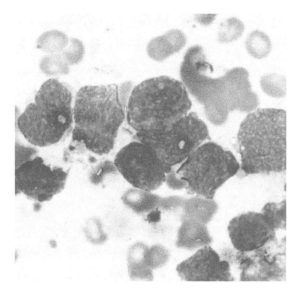

Figure 13.2 MGG, ×1000.

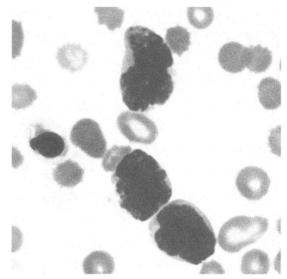

Figure 13.4 MGG, ×1000.

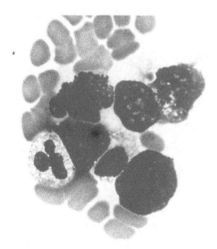

Figure 13.3 MGG, ×1000.

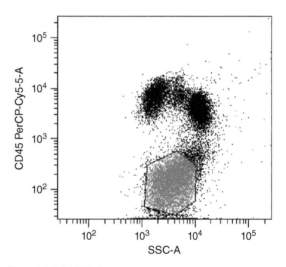

Figure 13.5 CD45/SSC.

was therefore used for subsequent analysis using an acute leukaemia panel covering a spectrum of myeloid and lymphoid antigens. Occasionally, a primitive precursor lymphoid leukaemia can fail to express CD45 so this entity had to be excluded. The gated cells showed limited antigen expression but the following were shown: CD56^{bright}, CD117^{dim} and CD15^{dim}. MPO, cCD3 and cCD79a, lineage-specific antigens for haemopoietic tumours, were not expressed. CD56 is expressed by a number of non-haemopoietic tumours including small cell lung cancer, neuroblastoma and some sarcomas.

The patient had a smoking history and a CXR was organised. This showed a mass at the left hilum (Figure 13.6).

Histopathology

The bone marrow trephine biopsy sections showed virtually complete replacement with tumour and very little residual normal haemopoiesis remained (Figures 13.7 and 13.8).

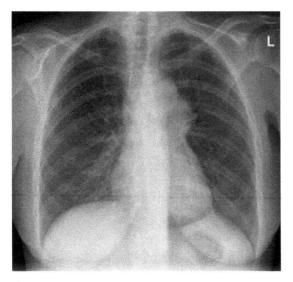

Figure 13.6 CXR.

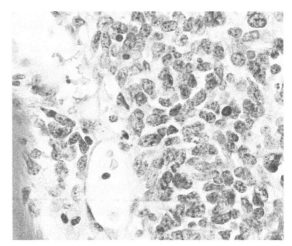

Figure 13.8 H&E, ×500.

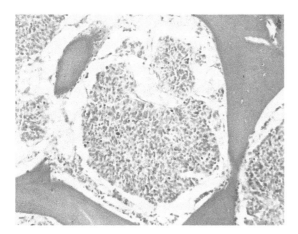

Figure 13.7 H&E, ×100.

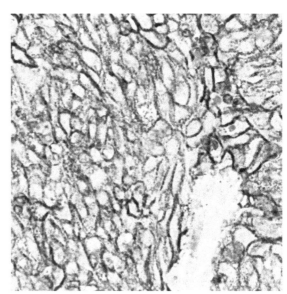

Figure 13.9 CD56, ×400.

Immunohistochemistry showed a phenotype in keeping with a diagnosis of small cell anaplastic carcinoma consistent with an origin from lung: the tumour expressed CD56 (neural cell adhesion molecule [NCAM]) (Figure 13.9) and CAM5.2 (an epithelial marker) (Figure 13.10) and showed positivity for synaptophysin and neuron-specific enolase, further markers of neuroendocrine differentiation.

Discussion

It is not uncommon to see patients presenting with bone marrow failure due to involvement by metastatic carcinoma.

Some, patients have yet to develop direct symptoms from the tumour at the primary site. Small cell carcinoma of lung is an aggressive neoplasm derived from cells of basal bronchial epithelium that have a particular tendency to behave in this way. Many patients have metastatic disease at the time of first presentation. It is important to consider the possibility of marrow involvement by non-haemopoietic tumour in patients in whom the blood film is leucoery-throblastic and marrow is physically difficult to aspirate and, when aspirated, appears aparticulate and hypocellular.

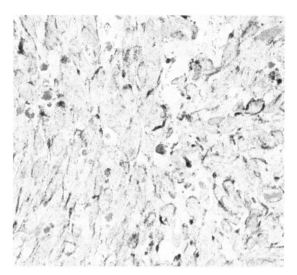

Figure 13.10 CAM5.2, ×400.

In addition, if the aspirate shows atypical cells that are difficult to identify, particularly if they appear in clumps, a metastatic tumour should always be considered. Nuclear moulding is a characteristic feature of small cell carcinoma. Flow cytometry analysis of these aspirates can be rewarding. Non-haemopoietic tumours are always CD45⁻. Certain precursor leukaemias can sometimes be CD45⁻ rather than CD45^{dim} but these should still show lineage-specific antigen expression, namely CCD79a/CD19, CD3 or MPO. CD56, CD117 and CD15 are not lineage specific and can be expressed by a variety of non-haemic tumours. It is important to recognise this when reporting flow cytometry studies. Of course the bone marrow trephine biopsy is essential in these cases and although small cell carcinoma was suspected from the flow cytometric data a definitive diagnosis was only possible using extended immunohistochemistry on the trephine core.

Final diagnosis

Small cell carcinoma of lung with bone marrow metastasis.

14

Case 14

An 82-year-old man was attending his general practitioner for management of his diabetes mellitus and hypertension. A full blood count was taken and an incidental lymphocytosis was noted. He was referred for further assessment.

Laboratory results

FBC: Hb 133 g/L, WBC 15×10^9/L (lymphocytes 11×10^9/L, neutrophils 3×10^9/L) and platelets 189×10^9/L.

U&Es, bone profile, LFTs and serum LDH: normal.

Normal immunoglobulins with no paraprotein.

Blood film

The film showed prominent medium to large lymphoid cells with condensed nuclear chromatin, with occasional nucleoli and nuclear clefts. The pale blue cytoplasm showed irregular margins in some cells (Figures 14.1 and 14.2).

Flow cytometry

The abnormal lymphocytes were shown to be B cells with a mature phenotype expressing CD19, CD20^{dim}, FMC7^{dim}, CD23, HLA-DR, CD79b, CD22 and surface lambda^{bright}. CD5, CD10, CD11c, CD25, CD103, CD123 and CD38 were not expressed. The morphology and immunophenotype did not allow a specific diagnosis at this stage but the findings were not those expected in chronic lymphocytic leukaemia, despite weak expression of FMC7 and positivity for CD23 (CLL score 2/5).

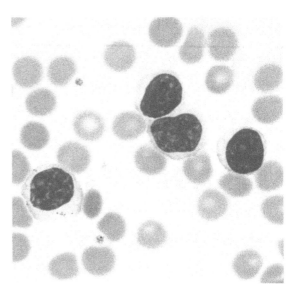

Figure 14.1 MGG, ×1000.

Imaging

A CT scan showed small volume (maximum 1.4 cm) lymphadenopathy in the axillae, iliac regions and groins.

Clinical course

As the patient was well and without disease-related symptoms or cytopenias, he was initially managed by simple observation.

One year later he became less well, having developed anorexia and weight loss. The white blood cell count had

Practical Flow Cytometry in Haematology: 100 Worked Examples, First Edition. Mike Leach, Mark Drummond, Allyson Doig, Pam McKay, Bob Jackson and Barbara J. Bain.
© 2015 John Wiley & Sons, Ltd. Published 2015 by John Wiley & Sons, Ltd.

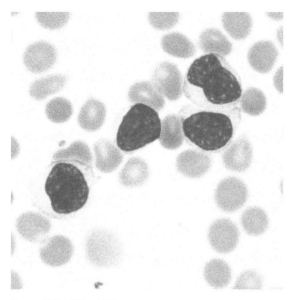

Figure 14.2 MGG, ×1000.

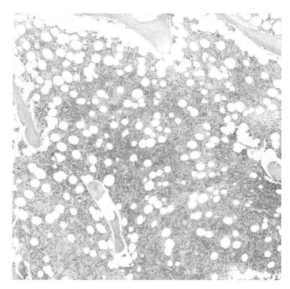

Figure 14.3 H&E, ×40.

risen to 73×10^9/L (lymphocytes 66×10^9/L) with mild anaemia (Hb 113 g/L) and thrombocytopenia (137×10^9/L). A repeat CT scan showed increasing lymphadenopathy and splenomegaly (16 cm). A bone marrow aspirate and trephine biopsy were taken and a cervical lymph node was excised in order to more accurately classify his disease as it now required treatment.

Bone marrow aspirate and trephine biopsy

The bone marrow aspirate was involved by small mature lymphoid cells having the same phenotype as those described in blood. The trephine biopsy sections showed an overall cellularity approaching 80% with much of this due to an interstitial infiltrate of small lymphoid cells (Figures 14.3 and 14.4). These cells expressed CD20 (Figure 14.5) and BCL2. CD23 (Figure 14.6) was expressed weakly in only a minority of cells whilst CD5, CD10 and cyclin D1 were not expressed. The normal haemopoietic elements were consequently reduced.

Cervical lymph node biopsy

The node was effaced by a nodular infiltrate of small/medium-sized lymphoid cells (Figure 14.7) with elongated occasionally cleaved nuclei with relatively abundant cytoplasm. These cells were positive for CD20 (Figure 14.8)

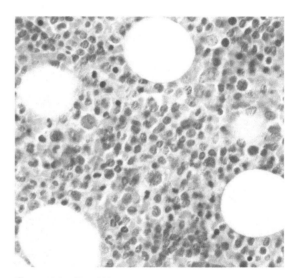

Figure 14.4 H&E, ×400.

and BCL2 and focally for CD23 (5–10%). CD21 mainly highlighted abundant follicular dendritic cells within the nodules (Figure 14.9). The infiltrate was negative for CD5, CD10, BCL6, cyclin D1 and CD30. The proliferation fraction was low at 15% (Figure 14.10).

In view of the nodular architecture, cell morphology and lack of evidence of germinal centre marker expression, the features were considered to be most in keeping with a diagnosis of nodal low-grade marginal zone lymphoma (MZL).

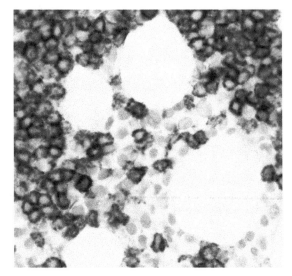

Figure 14.5 CD20, ×400.

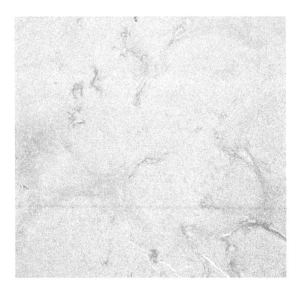

Figure 14.7 H&E, ×20.

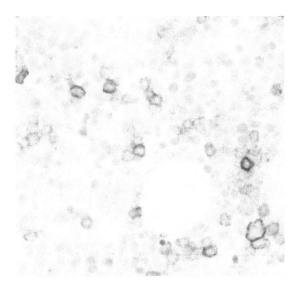

Figure 14.6 CD23, ×400.

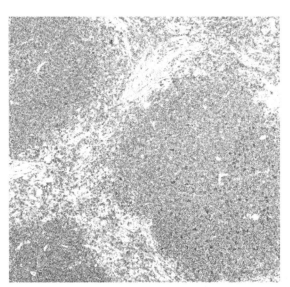

Figure 14.8 CD20, ×40.

Discussion

This case illustrates two important points. Firstly, in patients with an incidental presentation, particularly if they are elderly it may be satisfactory to formulate a working, but not specific, diagnosis. The morphology and immunophenotyping of the mature clonal B cells in the peripheral blood did not show features that could permit a precise diagnosis but they did allow certain conditions to be excluded (CLL,

follicular lymphoma, hairy cell leukaemia and mantle cell lymphoma). Secondly, as the disease progressed causing systemic symptoms and anaemia, it was appropriate to undertake a biopsy of the bone marrow and to excise a lymph node; the latter is still the gold standard in terms of classifying nodal lymphoma. When all the pathological data were interpreted in the light of the clinical presentation and imaging, a precise diagnosis could be formulated.

Figure 14.9 CD21, ×40.

Nodal marginal zone lymphoma is an uncommon disease accounting for only 2% of non-Hodgkin lymphomas. It is less common than the splenic and extranodal MZL variants. Infiltration is initially in the marginal zone of follicles but subsequent follicular colonisation can occur. Peripheral blood involvement, as the terminology suggests, is also unusual. Nodal MZL is often managed using first-line treatments akin to those used in follicular lymphoma (e.g., R-CVP) but the responses seen are often only partial and lack durability.

Final diagnosis

Nodal marginal zone lymphoma with peripheral blood spread.

Figure 14.10 Ki-67, ×40.

Case 15

A 64-year-old man presented to his GP with fatigue and night sweats. A full blood count identified anaemia and marked leucocytosis so he was referred for assessment. On examination, the spleen was just palpable but there were no other notable findings.

Laboratory data

FBC: Hb 79 g/L, WBC 78 × 10^9/L (neutrophils 4.5 × 10^9/L, lymphocytes 5.3 × 10^9/L, monocytes 15 × 10^9/L, eosinophils 53 × 10^9/L) and platelets 30 × 10^9/L.

U&Es: Na 142 mmol/L, K 3.8 mmol/L, urea 6.7 mmol/L, creatinine 79 μmol/L.

LFTs and bone profile: normal except albumin 30 g/L.

Serum LDH 625 U/L and urate 0.59 mmol/L.

ESR 7 mm/h. Autoimmune serology and cANCA/pANCA (cytoplasmic and perinuclear antineutrophil cytoplasmic antibodies) were negative.

Imaging

Assessment using CT was essentially normal apart from showing 16-cm splenomegaly.

Blood film

This showed a number of important abnormalities (Figures 15.1 to 15.4). Firstly, there was a marked eosinophilia, these cells showing large but relatively sparse granules. Second, there was a large monocyte population and some of these had abnormal nuclei. Thirdly, the film showed a

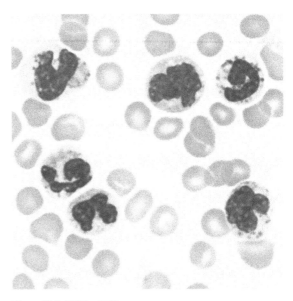

Figure 15.1 MGG, ×1000.

myeloid left shift and nucleated red blood cells with nuclear irregularities and cytoplasmic stippling.

Bone marrow aspirate

The bone marrow aspirate was rather dilute and aparticulate but showed similar features to the peripheral blood in terms of eosinophilia with eosinophil precursors, monocytosis and dysplasia of the erythroid series (Figures 15.5–15.7). Note that some of the eosinophils have dark proeosinophilic granules, a feature of immaturity. Standard myeloid series activity with maturation to neutrophils appeared reduced

Practical Flow Cytometry in Haematology: 100 Worked Examples, First Edition. Mike Leach, Mark Drummond, Allyson Doig, Pam McKay, Bob Jackson and Barbara J. Bain.
© 2015 John Wiley & Sons, Ltd. Published 2015 by John Wiley & Sons, Ltd.

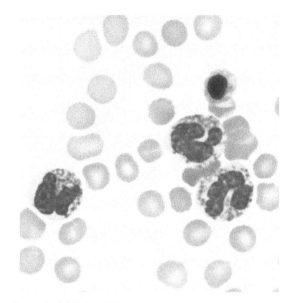

Figure 15.2 MGG, ×1000.

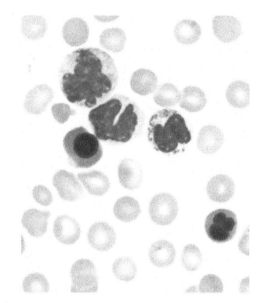

Figure 15.4 MGG, ×1000.

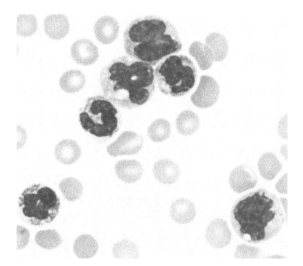

Figure 15.3 MGG, ×1000.

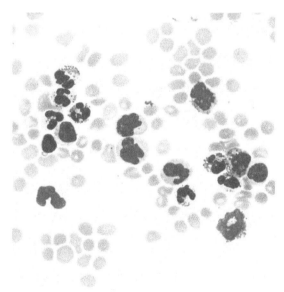

Figure 15.5 MGG, ×500.

and megakaryocytes were scarce. There was no excess of blasts, lymphoid cells, plasma cells or mast cells.

Flow cytometry (peripheral blood and marrow)

No excess of myeloid or lymphoid blasts or aberrant T-cell or B-cell population was identified; CD34$^+$ cells comprised just

1.3%, T cells 0.3% and B cells 3.2% of events. The FSC/SSC analysis showed a gross excess of eosinophils (blue) and their precursors (approximately 70% of events) together with monocytes and promonocytes (red) (25% of events) (Figure 15.8). The CD45/SSC plot shows the position of the monocytes and eosinophils but also the absence of a significant CD45^{dim} population (green) (Figure 15.9). Of all cells

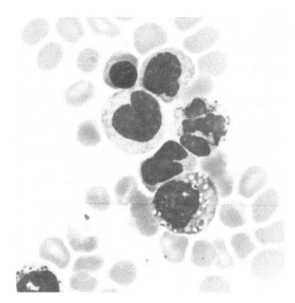

Figure 15.6 MGG, ×1000.

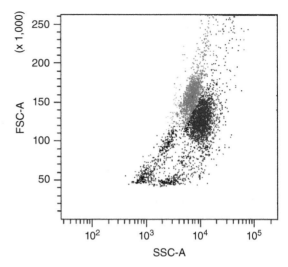

Figure 15.8 FSC/SSC.

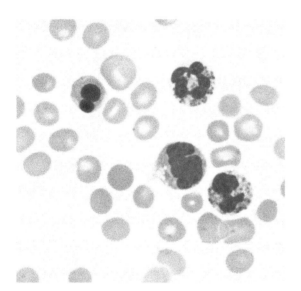

Figure 15.7 MGG, ×1000.

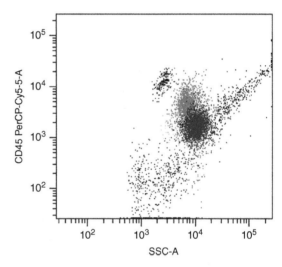

Figure 15.9 CD45/SSC.

of monocytic lineage, 75% were CD15$^+$ CD14^{dim} CD64$^+$ and 25% were CD15$^+$, CD14$^-$ CD64$^+$. CD56 was expressed in a proportion of monocytes in each of these groups.

Histopathology

The trephine biopsy sections were hypercellular with prominent eosinophils and eosinophil precursors and a notable interstitial monocyte population (Figures 15.10 and 15.11). No excess of blasts was identified. Reticulin staining was grade 1.

Cytogenetic analysis

Standard metaphase cytogenetics showed 46,XY. In particular there was no rearrangement of *PDGRFB* at 5q33 or *FGFR1* at 8p11.

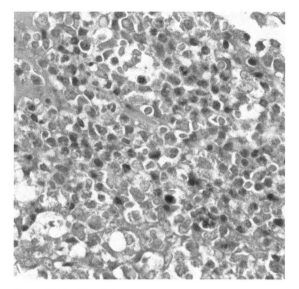

Figure 15.10 H&E, ×400.

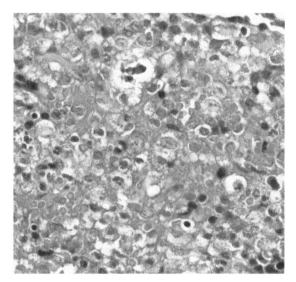

Figure 15.11 H&E, ×400.

Molecular studies

RT-PCR studies did not identify a *JAK2* V617F mutation, *FIP1L1-PDGRFA* or p190 or p210 *BCR-ABL1* transcripts.

Discussion

This is an interesting case of an eosinophilic leukaemia with an abnormal monocyte proliferation and features of dysplasia. This mixed presentation could therefore be described as an MDS/MPN. It was anticipated that a rearrangement of *PDGRFB* at 5q31-33 might be identified (most commonly seen as t(5;12)(q33;p13) generating an *ETV6-PDGRFB* fusion though many additional partners have been described). The haematological consequence is often that of a chronic myelomonocytic leukaemia or occasionally an atypical CML/MPN with an associated eosinophilia. Anaemia and thrombocytopenia are common. In its typical non-transformed state, blasts are not seen in excess. This condition is typically seen in middle-aged males, often generates splenomegaly and can induce eosinophil-related organ damage as it develops chronicity. Although this syndrome is genetically diverse, *PDGFRB* translocations can usually be identified using standard metaphase cytogenetics. *PDGFRB*-related neoplasms are important to identify as they frequently respond to imatinib. Prior to imatinib, the disease inexorably progressed with progressive tissue infiltration, eosinophil-mediated injury and marrow failure but with imatinib therapy the disease comes under control with resolution of eosinophilia, cytopenias and organomegaly. In fact, if the clinical presentation is suggestive of this syndrome, a trial of imatinib is probably justified in cases with normal cytogenetics. If the patient responds to treatment, a cryptic *PDGFRB* fusion is likely.

In the case described, no cytogenetic or molecular signature was identified but there is little doubt that this represents a clonal disorder. The dysplasia, monocytosis and eosinophilia with unusual morphology, marrow fibrosis and organomegaly all suggest a primary haematological disorder. Furthermore, there was no evidence of any other disease process that could have been driving this picture as a reaction. Although not yet included in the WHO classification, a number of other clonal eosinophilias have been reported including translocations of the *PCM1* gene to partners such as *JAK2* (1).

So how should this case be classified? Certainly not as 'idiopathic hypereosinophilic syndrome' since there are many features of a MDS/MPN type of neoplasm. Assignment to the WHO category of chronic eosinophilic leukaemia, not otherwise specified could be considered. However that umbrella seems inadequate in these circumstances. The designation of chronic myelomonocytic leukaemia with eosinophilia seems preferable. In due course further molecular mechanisms will be identified to explain these remaining monocytic and eosinophilic disorders and importantly will inform the pathophysiology and guide development of relevant therapies.

The patient was treated with a trial of imatinib but failed to respond. The disease progressed over the subsequent months with progressive tissue infiltration and respiratory failure.

There were transient responses to steroids, interferon and vincristine but the patient died just 12 months from diagnosis.

Final diagnosis

Chronic myelomonocytic leukaemia with eosinophilia.

Reference

1 Patterer, V., Schnittger, S., Kern, W., Haferlach, T. & Haferlach, C. (2013) Hematologic malignancies with PCM1-JAK2 gene fusion share characteristics with myeloid and lymphoid neoplasms with eosinophilia and abnormalities of PDGFRA, PDGFRB, and FGFR1. *Annals of Hematology*, **92** (**6**), 759–769. PubMed PMID: 23400675.

16

Case 16

A 7-year-old boy presented with a rash, fever and pallor of a few days duration. He had no past medical history of note apart from neonatal jaundice that had resolved with supportive care. He had reached normal developmental milestones and was up to date with all recommended vaccinations. On examination he was pale, unwell and irritable with a fever of 38°C. A fine erythematous rash was noted affecting his face, forearms and trunk. There was neither hepatomegaly nor lymphadenopathy but the spleen tip was just palpable.

Laboratory data

FBC: Hb 30 g/L, MCV 92 fl, WBC 2.98 × 10^9/L, neutrophils 1.34 × 10^9/L, lymphocytes 1.32 × 10^9/L, monocytes 0.32 × 10^9/L and platelets 97 × 10^9/L.

Reticulocyte count 11 × 10^9/L. Direct Coombs test was negative.

U&Es, LFTs normal except bilirubin 23 μmol/L. Serum LDH: normal.

Blood film

The blood film showed prominent spherocytes but polychromasia was absent (Figures 16.1 and 16.2). In addition there was a population of pincered (or mushroom) cells as illustrated in Figure 16.3. Red cell agglutinates and erythrophagocytosis were not seen. The film was not leucoerythroblastic and leukaemic blasts were not seen.

Bone marrow aspirate

In view of the profound anaemia with mild pancytopenia and reticulocytopenia a bone marrow aspirate was taken to

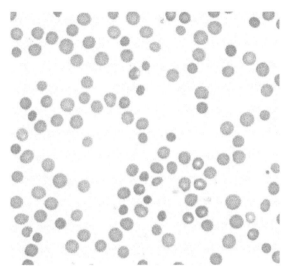

Figure 16.1 MGG, ×500.

exclude an acute leukaemia. This yielded a cellular aspirate with erythroid left shift and maturation arrest (Figure 16.4). Very large proerythroblasts were seen, some with cytoplasmic vacuolation (Figures 16.5 and 16.6). An abnormal infiltrate was not present. It is clearly important that these proerythroblasts are identified as such and not mistaken for cells of a malignant disorder such as acute monoblastic leukaemia.

Flow cytometry

The working diagnosis was now that of an acute erythrovirus (parvovirus B19) infection on a probable background of hereditary spherocytosis. Flow cytometry studies of EMA

Practical Flow Cytometry in Haematology: 100 Worked Examples, First Edition. Mike Leach, Mark Drummond, Allyson Doig, Pam McKay, Bob Jackson and Barbara J. Bain.
© 2015 John Wiley & Sons, Ltd. Published 2015 by John Wiley & Sons, Ltd.

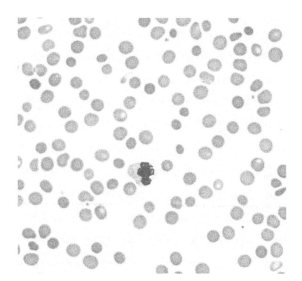

Figure 16.2 MGG, ×500.

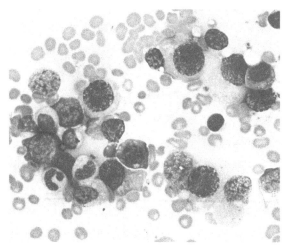

Figure 16.4 MGG, ×500.

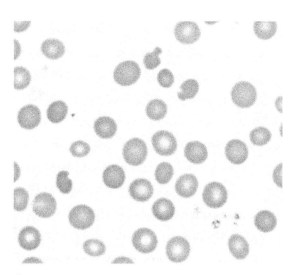

Figure 16.3 MGG, ×1000.

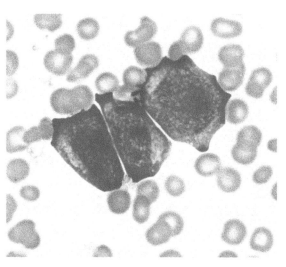

Figure 16.5 MGG, ×1000.

(eosin-5-maleimide) binding on red cells showed an abnormally low ratio of 0.65 (NR > 0.8). This is in keeping with a diagnosis of hereditary spherocytosis.

Discussion

This case illustrates a number of important points. The presentation with a severe anaemia in the presence of a mild pancytopenia generates a fairly restricted differential

diagnosis. An acute leukaemia certainly needed to be excluded, particularly in an unwell febrile child. Iron deficiency anaemia is common in childhood but the red cell indices and blood film morphology did not support this diagnosis, and the leucopenia and thrombocytopenia would not be expected. Paroxysmal cold haemoglobinuria is another important diagnosis to consider in any child presenting with severe anaemia with a history of a febrile illness. This is an acute disorder causing intravascular haemolysis as a result of the biphasic IgG Donath–Landsteiner antibody. The blood film typically shows spherocytosis but also polychromasia, red cell agglutinates and sometimes

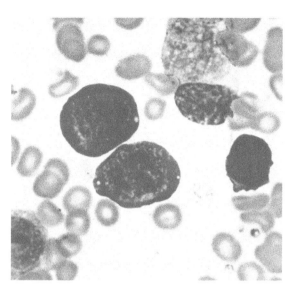

Figure 16.6 MGG, ×1000.

erythrophagocytosis. These additional features were not seen and the reticulocytopenia indicated bone marrow pathology in this case. A possible unifying diagnosis was of transient red cell aplasia due to erythrovirus infection; this may also cause mild leucopenia and thrombocytopenia as it generates a mild haemophagocytic syndrome in the bone marrow milieu. The bone marrow morphology was typical of this though such aspirates are rarely necessary in that most of those affected are known to have a pre-existing red cell disorder. In the knowledge of this, the triad of a worsening anaemia, reticulocytopenia and positive serology is normally conclusive. Erythrovirus infects metabolically active, replicating cells and this drives infected erythroid precursors to premature apoptosis. The abnormal red cell EMA binding in the context of a blood film typical of hereditary spherocytosis with band 3 deficiency (prominent pincered cells) brought this case to a conclusion. The patient's serum was subsequently confirmed to contain IgM antibodies to erythrovirus. He required red cell transfusion but the fever, rash and reticulocytopenia had all resolved 7 days later.

Final diagnosis

Acute erythrovirus infection in the context of previously undiagnosed hereditary spherocytosis.

17

Case 17

A 94-year-old woman was admitted to a surgical unit with abdominal pain and vomiting secondary to transient bowel obstruction in a large inguinal hernia. Her symptoms settled spontaneously with conservative management. She was noted to have a leucocytosis and the initial impression from the consulted haematologist was that this could represent a reactive phenomenon.

Laboratory results

FBC: Hb 110 g/L, WBC 35 × 10^9/L (lymphocytes 19.5 × 10^9/L) and platelets 218 × 10^9/L.

U&Es, LFTs were normal.

Serum LDH was 350 U/L.

Blood film

The film showed an abnormal population of medium to large lymphoid cells with convoluted nuclei and prominent large nucleoli. Some nuclei were hyperchromatic. Cytoplasmic blebs and irregularities were common (Figures 17.1–17.4).

Imaging

CT imaging to assess the small bowel obstruction showed incidental hepatosplenomegaly, widespread small volume lymphadenopathy and bilateral pleural effusions.

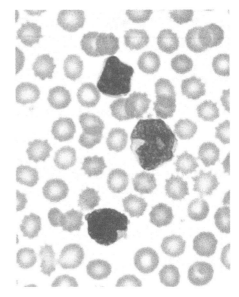

Figure 17.1 MGG, ×500.

Flow cytometry (peripheral blood)

By using a lymphoid gating strategy (Figure 17.5) the abnormal lymphoid cells were shown to be CD4$^+$ T cells co-expressing CD2, CD3, CD5 and CD7^{dim}. CD26 expression was uniformly positive (Figure 17.6). CD7 expression was demonstrated but at low intensity (Figure 17.7).

Practical Flow Cytometry in Haematology: 100 Worked Examples, First Edition. Mike Leach, Mark Drummond, Allyson Doig, Pam McKay, Bob Jackson and Barbara J. Bain.
© 2015 John Wiley & Sons, Ltd. Published 2015 by John Wiley & Sons, Ltd.

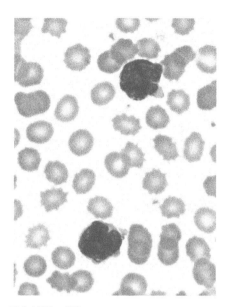

Figure 17.2 MGG, ×500.

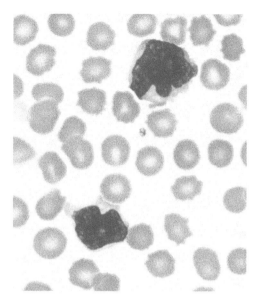

Figure 17.4 MGG, ×1000.

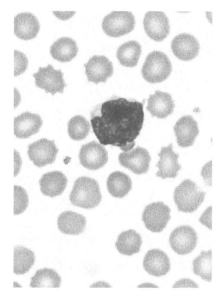

Figure 17.3 MGG, ×1000.

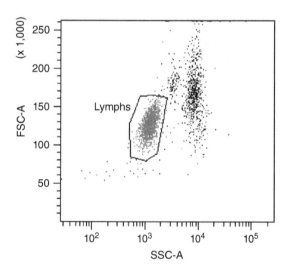

Figure 17.5 FSC/SSC.

Discussion

The blood film morphology was not in keeping with a reactive phenomenon. A stress lymphocytosis can be seen in patients with acute medical and surgical presentations but the features here were suggestive of a lymphoproliferative disorder (LPD). The pleomorphic lymphoid cells with nuclear lobulation and a large single nucleolus together with cytoplasmic blebbing are strongly suggestive of a diagnosis of T-prolymphocytic leukaemia (T-PLL). T-prolymphocytic leukaemia is most commonly a CD4$^+$ disorder but CD8$^+$ and CD4$^+$/CD8$^+$ cases are also seen. It is the only T-cell LPD to frequently retain positivity for the other pan-T antigens (CD2, CD3, CD5 and CD7). In contrast, CD7 expression is often lost in other T-cell leukaemias. The intensity of

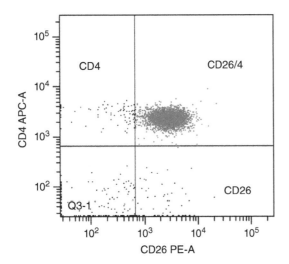

Figure 17.6 CD4/CD26.

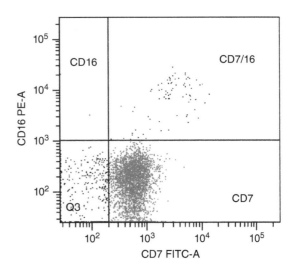

Figure 17.7 CD7/CD16.

expression of CD7 and other pan-T markers, however, is variable between cases and often differs from that seen on normal T cells (1). The CD26 expression is usually uniformly positive in T-PLL, in keeping with the clonal nature of this disorder. Normal T cells show a range of CD26 expression.

Cytogenetic studies were not performed on this case but inv(14)(q11.2q32) or t(14;14)(q11.2;q32) is frequently present and strongly supports this diagnosis if uncertainty exists.

The diagnosis was therefore T-PLL, which in this case was, unusually, an incidental diagnosis at the time of a surgical presentation. A reactive lymphocytosis should not be proposed with peripheral blood morphology as seen in this case. The management of T-PLL presents great difficulties in a patient of any age. Supportive care only was proposed for this patient. The disease progressed rapidly with a leucocytosis up to $253 \times 10^9/L$ and the patient died peacefully 2 months after presentation.

Final diagnosis

T-cell prolymphocytic leukaemia.

Reference

1 Chen, X. & Cherian, S. (2013) Immunophenotypic characterization of T-cell prolymphocytic leukemia. *American Journal of Clinical Pathology*, **140** (**5**), 727–735. PubMed PMID: 24124154.

Case 18

A 37-year-old female attended her GP with a short history of fatigue and breathlessness. The GP noted pallor and some small, scattered bruises and an FBC was taken. A cardiology assessment had noted global left ventricular dysfunction without clear evidence of ischaemic heart disease, valvular disease or recent toxic insult.

Laboratory data

FBC: Hb 64 g/L, WBC 7.0×10^9/L (neutrophils 3.1×10^9/L) and platelets 75×10^9/L.

U&Es, LFTs and bone profile: normal.

Blood film

This was highly informative showing frequent myeloblasts with faintly granular cytoplasm and occasional fine Auer rods (Figures 18.1 and 18.2). Some blast cells showed a prominent Golgi zone within a nuclear indentation (Figure 18.2). Neutrophils were abnormal with abnormal nuclear morphology including hyposegmented, nonsegmented and ring forms (Figures 18.3–18.5). The features were therefore indicative of an acute myeloid leukaemia with dysplastic maturation.

Bone marrow aspirate

Myeloblasts comprised 55% of bone marrow cells; there was abnormal myeloid maturation as in the peripheral blood (not shown). No significant dysplastic changes in other cell lines were noted.

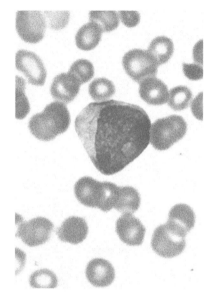

Figure 18.1 MGG, ×1000.

Flow cytometry (bone marrow aspirate)

The CD34+ myeloblasts (red events) were easily separated from the more mature granulocytic elements (blue events) by CD34 and SSC (Figure 18.6). Asynchronous expression of CD15 was present on some of the CD117+ CD34+ population, while asynchronous expression of CD117 was noted on some of the more mature CD15^bright granulocytic component (Figure 18.7). CD19 expression was noted in 20% of the CD34+ cells (not shown), in addition to CD13, CD33 and HLA-DR.

Practical Flow Cytometry in Haematology: 100 Worked Examples, First Edition. Mike Leach, Mark Drummond, Allyson Doig, Pam McKay, Bob Jackson and Barbara J. Bain.
© 2015 John Wiley & Sons, Ltd. Published 2015 by John Wiley & Sons, Ltd.

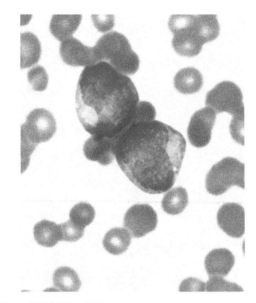

Figure 18.2 MGG, ×1000.

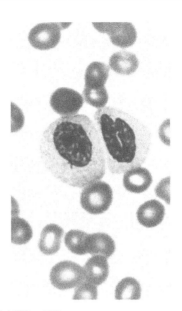

Figure 18.4 MGG, ×1000.

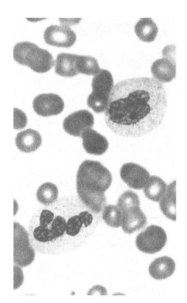

Figure 18.3 MGG, ×1000.

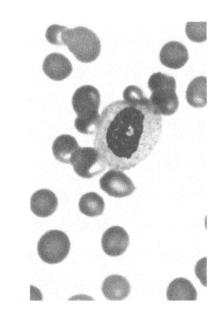

Figure 18.5 MGG, ×1000.

Cytogenetic analysis

Metaphase studies on the bone marrow aspirate showed t(8;21)(q22;q22) in 4/10 cells.

Discussion

AML with t(8;21)(q22;q22) exhibits variable morphology with regards to features of maturation. In this case blast cell features were relatively subtle, with fine granules and

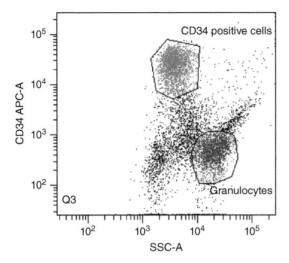

Figure 18.6 CD34/SSC.

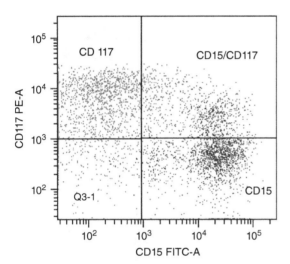

Figure 18.7 CD117/CD15.

occasional slender Auer rods. Large numbers of prominent azurophilic granules, or even the large so-called pseudo-Chédiak-Higashi granules as seen in some cases, were lacking. The prominent Golgi zone is, however, very typical. Note that neutrophil numbers were normal at diagnosis and dysgranulopoietic changes were striking in blood and marrow, a well-recognised feature of this AML subtype.

In keeping with the visual impression of disordered myeloid maturation, asynchronous co-expression of anti-

gens typical of precursor and more mature cell types was noted (CD34, CD117 and CD15). In normal myeloid maturation CD34 is rapidly lost beyond the myeloblast stage, while CD117 continues to be expressed on normal promyelocytes and is then lost. CD15 is first expressed at the late promyelocyte stage. Thus during normal haemopoiesis CD34 and CD15 are not found on the same cell types. The phenotype CD34[+], CD19[+] and CD56[+] is extremely rare in normal marrow (<0.01% of cells) and is typical and highly predictive for AML with t(8;21)(q22;q22) (1, 2).

This subgroup of AML is associated with a good response to treatment and long-term disease-free survival. The presence of an apparent cardiomyopathy at the time of presentation posed serious challenges in terms of optimal therapy. We elected to avoid anthracyclines and used FLA (fludarabine/cytarabine) for induction and consolidation using single agent cytarabine for consolidation cycles 3 and 4. With the knowledge of this recurrent cytogenetic abnormality good prognosis subtype of AML, we were confident that this non-anthracycline-based regimen could yield a successful outcome.

This patient completed chemotherapy without intercurrent cardiac complications and her left ventricular function has subsequently improved. No clear cause for the transient myocardial disorder was identified. She remains well and in continued remission at the time of reporting.

Final diagnosis

Acute myeloid leukaemia with t(8;21)(q22;q22); *RUNX1-RUNX1T1*.

References

1 Kita, K., Nakase, K., Miwa, H. *et al*. (1992) Phenotypical characteristics of acute myelocytic leukemia associated with the t(8;21)(q22;q22) chromosomal abnormality: frequent expression of immature B-cell antigen CD19 together with stem cell antigen CD34. *Blood*, **80** (**2**), 470–477.

2 Coustan-Smith, E., Behm, F.G., Hurwitz, C.A., Rivera, G.K. & Campana, D. (1993) N-CAM (CD56) expression by CD34+ malignant myeloblasts has implications for minimal residual disease detection in acute myeloid leukemia. *Leukemia*, **7** (**6**), 853–858.

19

Case 19

A 65-year-old man presented to his general practitioner with non-specific aches and pains. He had previously worked as a labourer so much of this might have been attributable to simple osteoarthritis. On examination there were no specific findings apart from Heberden's nodes.

Laboratory data

FBC: Hb 133 g/l, WBC 9.3×10^9/L, platelets 363×10^9/L.
    U&Es, bone profile and LFTs: normal.
    Immunoglobulins: IgG 12.5 g/L, IgA 2.1 g/L, IgM 1.55 g/L.
    Serum protein electrophoresis: IgA paraprotein 8 g/L.
    Serum-free light chains: kappa 26 mg/L, lambda 70 mg/L.
    Urine-free light chains were not detected.
    The blood film was normal.

Imaging

A skeletal survey was normal.

Bone marrow aspirate

A bone marrow aspirate was taken to exclude a diagnosis of multiple myeloma. Morphologically this was normal; the plasma cell population was not expanded and normal haemopoiesis was well preserved.

Flow cytometry

Flow cytometry studies may not be necessary where morphological review of a marrow aspirate shows a very

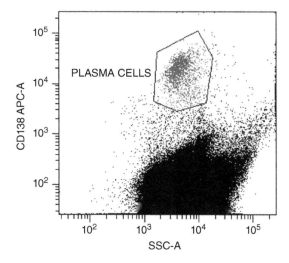

Figure 19.1 CD138/SSC.

low-level plasma cell population. In cases where the diagnosis is not clear and particularly where a lymphoid neoplasm remains a possibility it seems prudent to refer such specimens for review at the regional flow cytometry laboratory. Examination of this aspirate showed a number of important findings. Firstly, using a CD138 versus SSC approach the total plasma cell population was low at only 0.5% of marrow events (Figure 19.1). We do know that flow cytometry often underestimates plasma cell proportions as these cells are fragile and tend to be disrupted on handling. Secondly, however, two distinct plasma cell populations were seen. The first was comprised of normal plasma cells being CD19+, CD45dim, CD56− (53%, blue events) and the second was a neoplastic population with a CD19−, CD45−, CD56+ phenotype (43%, red events) (Figures 19.1–19.3).

Practical Flow Cytometry in Haematology: 100 Worked Examples, First Edition. Mike Leach, Mark Drummond, Allyson Doig, Pam McKay, Bob Jackson and Barbara J. Bain.
© 2015 John Wiley & Sons, Ltd. Published 2015 by John Wiley & Sons, Ltd.

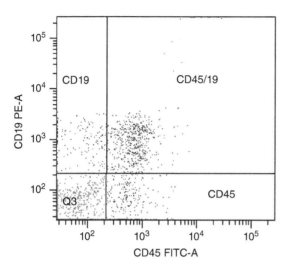

Figure 19.2 CD19/CD45.

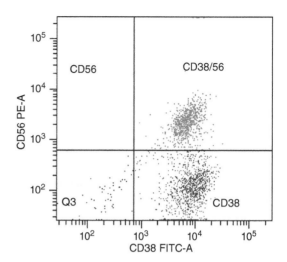

Figure 19.3 CD56/CD38.

Discussion

The diagnosis here is monoclonal gammopathy of undetermined significance (MGUS). A small clonal population of plasma cells, responsible for the paraprotein, was identified but importantly this comprised a small percentage of all bone marrow cells. There was no compromise of bone marrow function, hypercalcaemia, renal failure or bone disease. Typically in good prognosis MGUS, a normal polyclonal plasma cell population is preserved, as in this case (1). Incidental paraproteins are a common finding in modern medicine. Decisions regarding the extent of appropriate investigation in this situation remain a common issue for discussion in the haematology clinic.

Final diagnosis

Monoclonal gammopathy of undetermined significance (MGUS) with preserved polyclonal plasma cells.

Reference

1 Perez-Persona, E., Vidriales, M.B., Mateo, G. *et al.* (2007) New criteria to identify risk of progression in monoclonal gammopathy of uncertain significance and smoldering multiple myeloma based on multiparameter flow cytometry analysis of bone marrow plasma cells. *Blood*, **110** (7), 2586–2592. PubMed PMID: 17576818.

20

Case 20

A 74-year-old man presented with fatigue and cold peripheries during the winter weather. There was no evidence of skin rash, digital ischaemia, lymphadenopathy or splenomegaly on clinical examination.

Laboratory results

FBC: Hb 103 g/L, WBC 6.5 × 10⁹/L (neutrophils 2.4 × 10⁹/L, lymphocytes 3.3 × 10⁹/L) and platelets 175 × 10⁹/L.

U&Es, bone profile and LDH were normal.

Plasma viscosity was borderline at 1.77 centipoise (1.5–1.7).

Immunoglobulin: IgG 2.1 g/L, IgA 0.42 g/L, IgM 16.79 g/L.

No paraprotein was identified in serum separated from a blood specimen that had cooled to room temperature.

Immunofixation carried out on a warm collected specimen analysed at 37°C identified an IgM lambda paraprotein (quantified at 20 g/L) and this was identified as a type I cryoglobulin.

Free lambda light chains were raised at 451.6 mg/L (5.7–26.3) with a low kappa/lambda ratio at 0.06 (0.26–1.65).

Blood film

This showed a number of abnormal lymphoid cells with ovoid nuclei, sometimes eccentric, and variable amounts of medium blue cytoplasm which, in some cells, exhibited a bipolar prominence (Figures 20.1–20.4). Rouleaux formation was obvious and there was an immunoglobulin-related blue tinge to the background plasma staining.

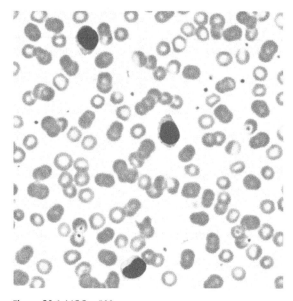

Figure 20.1 MGG, ×500.

Flow cytometry (peripheral blood)

Although the majority of lymphocytes were T cells, gating on the CD19-positive cells revealed a monoclonal kappa-restricted B-cell population. These B cells had the phenotype kappa^mod, CD20⁺, CD5⁺, FMC7⁺, CD23⁺, CD79b⁺, CD10⁻ and CD22⁺. A secondary panel consisting of CD25, CD11c, CD103 and CD123 was negative. This indicated a CD5⁺ mature B-cell disorder that was not chronic lymphocytic (CLL score 2/5) and the possibilities included a splenic marginal zone lymphoma or lymphoplasmacytic lymphoma. Both of the latter can generate IgM paraproteins.

Practical Flow Cytometry in Haematology: 100 Worked Examples, First Edition. Mike Leach, Mark Drummond, Allyson Doig, Pam McKay, Bob Jackson and Barbara J. Bain.
© 2015 John Wiley & Sons, Ltd. Published 2015 by John Wiley & Sons, Ltd.

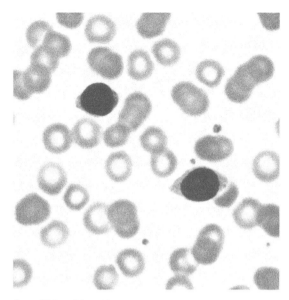

Figure 20.2 MGG, ×1000.

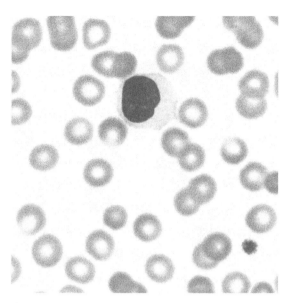

Figure 20.4 MGG, ×1000.

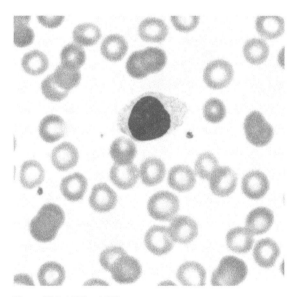

Figure 20.3 MGG, ×1000.

Imaging

A CT scan showed a cuff of tissue around the bifurcation of the aorta and small volume lymphadenopathy in the right groin. There was no organomegaly and the imaging was otherwise unremarkable.

Bone marrow trephine biopsy

An 18-mm specimen was hypercellular with 70% cellularity overall. There was a diffuse interstitial infiltrate of small lymphoid cells accounting for approximately 50% of the cellularity but over 90% in places (Figure 20.5). The cells were positive for CD20 (Figure 20.6), CD79a and BCL2. They were negative for CD5, CD23, CD10, BCL6, CD43 and cyclin D1. Plasma cell differentiation was demonstrated by CD138 positivity; note that this highlights the larger plasma cells amongst the more uniform small lymphoid cells in the background (Figure 20.7). Lambda light chain restriction was demonstrated (Figure 20.8). The proliferation index was low. Appearances were in keeping with marrow infiltration by a low-grade B-cell non-Hodgkin lymphoma with plasmacytic differentiation with the differential lying between splenic marginal zone and lymphoplasmacytic lymphoma. The diffuse marrow infiltration without clear sinusoidal involvement and the absence of splenomegaly were features less in keeping with a splenic marginal zone lymphoma.

Discussion

Cryoglobulins are proteins that precipitate as serum is cooled and that re-dissolve on warming. Patients may be asymptomatic or may have symptoms relating to the *in*

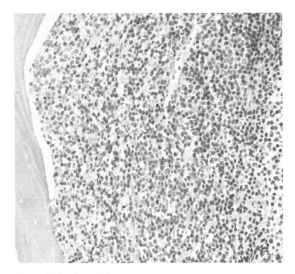

Figure 20.5 H&E, ×200.

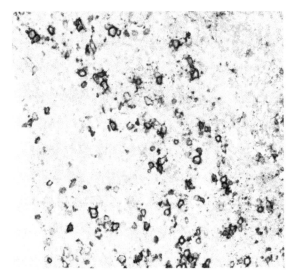

Figure 20.7 CD138, ×200.

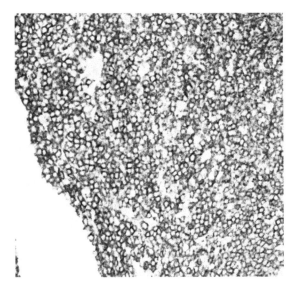

Figure 20.6 CD20, ×200.

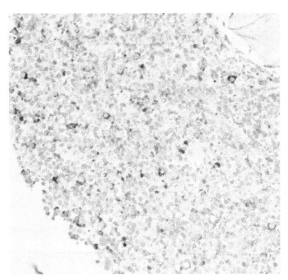

Figure 20.8 Lambda, ×200.

vivo effects of cryoprotein formation affecting the vasculature serving the peripheries inducing purpura, ulcers or Raynaud's phenomenon. There are three sub-types of cryoglobulinaemia. Type I is usually seen in patients with multiple myeloma (MM) or lymphoplasmacytic lymphoma (LPL) and the cryoglobulin is a simple, monoclonal protein (the paraprotein). Type II is usually seen in association with chronic active hepatitis or autoimmune disease. In this sub-type, there are two types of immunoglobulin, usually

polyclonal IgG and monoclonal IgM, which form complexes since the IgM paraprotein has antibody activity against IgG (analogous to a rheumatoid factor). Type III is also associated with chronic infection and autoimmune disease but both the IgG and IgM cryoglobulins are polyclonal.

In the described case, the cryoglobulin was monoclonal IgM lambda consistent with type I cryoglobulinaemia. This occurs incidentally in patients with a paraproteinaemic disorder, where the clonal protein has the capacity to come out of solution on cooling (cryoprecipitate). There was a discrepancy between immunophenotyping by flow cytometry (CD5$^+$ and CD23$^+$) and immunohistochemistry on paraffin-embedded tissue (CD5$^-$ and CD23$^-$), which can be explained by the reduced sensitivity of staining in decalcified formalin-fixed tissue. CD5 positivity may be seen in up to 9% of cases of LPL by flow cytometry [1].

The management of such patients is guided by the behaviour of the underlying lymphoma and the clinical consequences of the cryoglobulin. In this case, the lymphoma was responsible for a mild anaemia though this was well tolerated. The cryoglobulin was responsible for some cold-related symptoms but these were not incapacitating and were easily managed by the use of gloves in cold weather. The patient has therefore been managed by simple observation to the time of reporting.

Final diagnosis

Lymphoplasmacytic lymphoma, with an associated IgM cryoglobulin.

Reference

1 Hunter, Z.R., Branagan, A.R., Manning, R. *et al.* (2005) CD5, CD10, and CD23 expression in Waldenstrom's macroglobulinemia. *Clinical Lymphoma*, **5** (**4**), 246–249.

Case 21

A 43-year-old female sought the help of her general practitioner with regard to discomfort and nocturnal tingling in the right hand. A diagnosis of carpal tunnel syndrome was made but some routine blood tests were scheduled.

Laboratory data

FBC: Hb 122 g/l, WBC 12.2 × 10⁹/L (neutrophils 5.86 × 10⁹/L, lymphocytes 5.78 × 10⁹/L, monocytes 0.46 × 10⁹/L) and platelets 264 × 10⁹/L.

$$FBC: Hb\ 122\,g/l,\ WBC\ 12.2 \times 10^9/L\ (neutrophils\ 5.86 \times 10^9/L,\ lymphocytes\ 5.78 \times 10^9/L,\ monocytes\ 0.46 \times 10^9/L)\ and\ platelets\ 264 \times 10^9/L.$$

U&Es and LFTs: normal.

Flow cytometry studies were requested, on account of the lymphocytosis, by the laboratory processing the sample and reviewing the blood film.

Blood film

This showed a population of atypical, mature, medium sized to large lymphoid cells that frequently demonstrated bi-lobed nuclei often separated by a thin chromatin strand (Figures 21.1–21.4). The film was otherwise normal.

Flow cytometry (peripheral blood)

A lymphocyte-gated CD2 versus CD19 analysis gave equal proportions of T and B cells indicating a low-level B-cell lymphocytosis. These cells showed a pan-B phenotype with no immunophenotypic aberrancy: CD19⁺, CD20⁺, HLA-DR⁺, CD79b⁺, CD22⁺ but without CD5, CD10, CD11c, CD25,

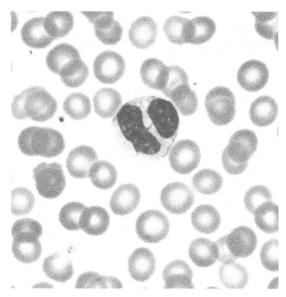

Figure 21.1 MGG, ×1000.

CD103 or CD123. Importantly, the surface immunoglobulin profile showed 58% lambda^mod and 37% kappa^mod. There was therefore a reversed kappa:lamda ratio but no evidence of an abnormal clonal population. This therefore represents a polyclonal B-cell proliferation/reaction.

Discussion

Persistent polyclonal B-cell lymphocytosis is an infrequent cause of lymphocytosis in adults. The lymphocytosis is

Practical Flow Cytometry in Haematology: 100 Worked Examples, First Edition. Mike Leach,
Mark Drummond, Allyson Doig, Pam McKay, Bob Jackson and Barbara J. Bain.
© 2015 John Wiley & Sons, Ltd. Published 2015 by John Wiley & Sons, Ltd.

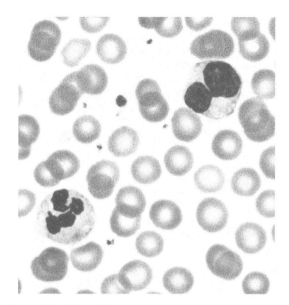

Figure 21.2 MGG, ×1000.

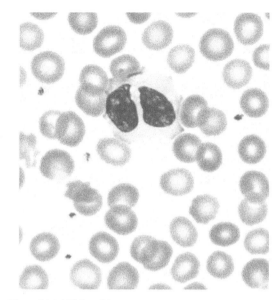

Figure 21.4 MGG, ×1000.

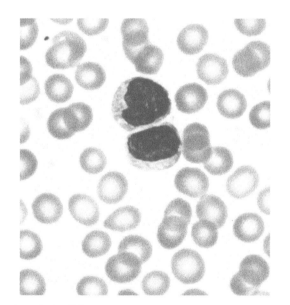

Figure 21.3 MGG, ×1000.

cytosis appears to be due to an expansion of memory B cells, sometimes associated with an increase in polyclonal serum IgM. A reversed kappa:lambda ratio is not uncommon. Most patients are adult females who smoke cigarettes. There may be a genetic predisposition to this reaction, there being an association with HLA-DR7 and familial cases having been reported. In most cases the disease follows a benign clinical course and has been shown to regress with cessation of smoking though mild splenomegaly has been noted in some cases. The exact mechanism remains to be determined but it has been proposed that the lymphocytic reaction is secondary to chronic immune stimulation, presumably to an agent in tobacco. To complicate matters, however, some patients harbour abnormalities of chromosome 3q, typically isochromosome 3q or trisomy 3 (2); in an individual patient these abnormalities may be present in both kappa-expressing and lambda-expressing B cells (3). Despite this there is no definite increase in subsequent lymphoid neoplasms; importantly these patients are more likely to succumb to the pulmonary and cardiovascular sequelae of cigarette smoking. On further questioning this patient was confirmed to be a cigarette smoker; she has agreed to make a determined attempt to give up the habit.

generally in the region of 5 to 15 × 10^9/L and bi-nucleate lymphoid cells and lymphocytes with two widely separated lobes joined by a filament are typically seen (1). The lympho-

Final diagnosis

Persistent polyclonal B-cell lymphocytosis as a reaction to cigarette smoking.

References

1 Deplano, S., Nadel-Melsió, E. & Bain, B.J. (2014) Persistent polyclonal B lymphocytosis. *American Journal of Hematology*, **89**, 224.

2 Callet-Bauchu, E., Gazzo, S., Poncet, C. *et al.* (2000) Distinct chromosome 3 abnormalities in persistent polyclonal B-cell lymphocytosis. *Genes Chromosomes Cancer*, **26**, 221–228.

3 Mossafa, H., Malaure, H., Maynadie, M. *et al.* (1999) Persistent polyclonal B lymphocytosis with binucleated lymphocytes: a study of 25 cases. *Groupe Français d'Hématologie Cellulaire*. *British Journal of Haematology*, **104**, 486–493.

Case 22

A 42-year-old male, previously well, attended his GP because of fatigue. A history of a nosebleed the previous day was reported. Bruising was noted on examination and an FBC was taken.

Laboratory data

FBC: Hb 88 g/L, WBC 5.43 × 10^9/L (neutrophils 0.5 × 10^9/L) and platelets 56 × 10^9/L.

U&Es, LFTs, bone profile and LDH: normal.

Coagulation screen: PT 14 seconds, APTT 29 seconds, TT 20 seconds, fibrinogen 0.9 g/L and D-dimer 15,100 ng/mL.

Blood film/bone marrow aspirate

Blood film examination (Figures 22.1 and 22.2) demonstrated abnormal promyelocytes with many exhibiting bilobed nuclei. Auer rods were frequent, sometimes with multiple rods in one cell, termed a faggot cell (after the old French term, *fagot*, meaning "bundles of sticks") (Figure 22.1).

Bone marrow aspiration was technically difficult, with aspirated material clotting in the needle. Examination of this limited material demonstrated marrow replacement by abnormal promyelocytes; Auer rods were frequent whilst more faggot cells and hypergranular forms were noted (Figures 22.3–22.5). Note that bi-lobed forms are less apparent in the marrow than in the blood in this case and occasional smaller myeloblasts are present.

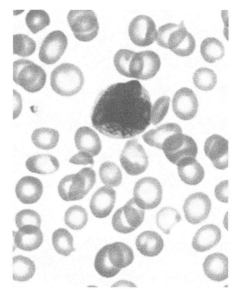

Figure 22.1 MGG, ×1000.

Flow cytometry

Flow cytometry, initially on peripheral blood, confirmed the presence of large numbers of primitive cells with high FSC and SSC (due to size and granularity, respectively). These were CD117$^+$, CD64$^+$, CD33$^+$, CD13$^+$ and MPO$^+$ but HLA-DR and CD34 were negative. The finding of a precursor myeloid proliferation with promyelocyte morphology, cytoplasmic granulation with Auer rods and faggot cells without CD34 and HLA-DR expression is highly suggestive of acute promyelocytic leukaemia.

Practical Flow Cytometry in Haematology: 100 Worked Examples, First Edition. Mike Leach,
Mark Drummond, Allyson Doig, Pam McKay, Bob Jackson and Barbara J. Bain.
© 2015 John Wiley & Sons, Ltd. Published 2015 by John Wiley & Sons, Ltd.

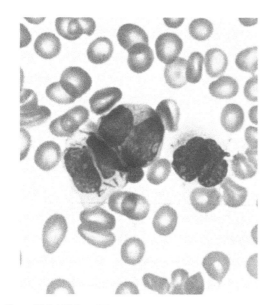

Figure 22.2 MGG, ×1000.

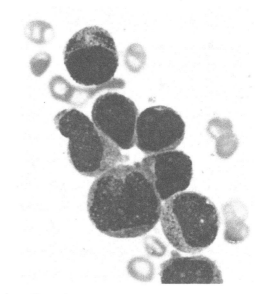

Figure 22.4 MGG, ×1000.

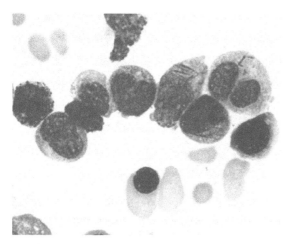

Figure 22.3 MGG, ×1000.

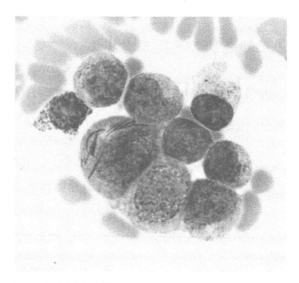

Figure 22.5 MGG, ×1000.

Genetic studies

Urgent FISH studies on marrow cells confirmed a *PML-RARA* rearrangement in 75% of nuclei (fusion signals arrowed, Figure 22.6) and the t(15;17)(q22;q12) translocation was confirmed by metaphase cytogenetics (Figure 22.7).

RT-PCR for the fusion gene was also performed, to establish the *PML* breakpoint and allow subsequent MRD analysis.

Discussion

Even prior to blood film examination, clinical suspicion should have been aroused by the history of nosebleeds despite an acceptable (albeit low) platelet count. The coagulation results are, in the authors' experience, entirely typical and indicate very active fibrinolysis: a normal PT and APTT (which are in fact often shortened and may

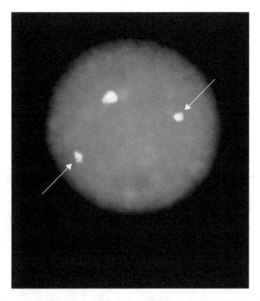

Figure 22.6 FISH, *PML* (15q24.1)/*RARA* (17q21.1-17q21.2) translocation dual fusion probes. This cell shows a single red and a single green signal representing the normal chromosomes 15 and 17, respectively. The arrows indicate the two fusion signals representing the reciprocal translocations.

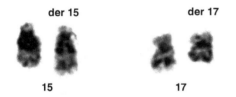

der 15   der 17

15   17

Figure 22.7 Metaphase cytogenetics.

be falsely reassuring), with low fibrinogen and markedly raised D-dimers. Variable prolongation of the PT and APTT may be seen (1) (and may predict for more significant bleeding). It should be borne in mind that leukaemia-related disseminated intravascular coagulation (DIC) is not only associated with APL, but may be seen in other cases of AML (most notably of the monocytic lineage), NK/T lymphoma/leukaemia and even very occasional cases of ALL.

The flow cytometry profile in this case is typical for APL, with a 'pan-myeloid' pattern evident (expression of CD13, CD33, CD117 and MPO) as well as the lack of HLA-DR and CD34. HLA-DR negativity is seen in 15% or so of all AML and it should be remembered that this finding is not specific to APL: in one large study half of HLA-DR negative cases were non-APL, with a majority also lacking CD34 (2). Although morphological and detailed flow cytometric analyses are generally able to differentiate true APL from these cases, molecular characterisation is clearly important.

The importance of early institution of treatment pending diagnostic confirmation, in the form of ATRA, cannot be overestimated. Early haemorrhagic deaths remain a significant problem in this condition; these are measurable by utilising leukaemia registry data (3) (which identify patients at diagnosis) but are often not measurable in clinical trial data (where only patients who survive until trial entry are recorded). Real-world overall survival for this condition therefore remains well below that reported using modern trial protocols (4).

Final diagnosis

Acute promyelocytic leukaemia.

References

1 Chang, H., Kuo, M.C., Shih, L.Y. *et al.* (2012) Clinical bleeding events and laboratory **coagulation** profiles in acute promyelocytic leukemia. *European Journal of Haematology*, **88**, 321–328.

2 Oelschlaegel, U., Mohr, B., Schaich, M. *et al.* (2009) HLA-DRneg patients without acute promyelocytic leukemia show distinct immunophenotypic, genetic, molecular, and cytomorphologic characteristics compared to acute promyelocytic leukemia. *Cytometry Part B: Clinical Cytometry*, **76**, 321–327.

3 Lehmann, S., Ravn, A., Carlsson, L. *et al.* (2011) Continuing high early death rate in acute promyelocytic leukemia: a population-based report from the Swedish Adult Acute Leukemia Registry. *Leukemia*, **25**, 1128–1134.

4 McClellan, J.S., Kohrt, H.E., Coutre, S. *et al.* (2012) Treatment advances have not improved the early death rate in acute promyelocytic leukemia. *Haematologica*, **97**, 133–136.

Case 23

A 58-year-old woman with a history of stage 4B activated B-cell subtype diffuse large B-cell lymphoma (DLBCL) treated with six cycles of R-CHOP chemotherapy re-presented with sweats and recurrence of a left pleural effusion within a few weeks of chemotherapy completion.

Laboratory results

FBC: Hb 125 g/L, WBC 2.9×10^9/L (neutrophils 1.2×10^9/L, lymphocytes 0.9×10^9/L) and platelets 322×10^9/L.

Renal and hepatic function were normal apart from a low albumin at 31 g/L.

Blood glucose was 20 mmol/L (patient diabetic) and LDH was raised at 419 U/L.

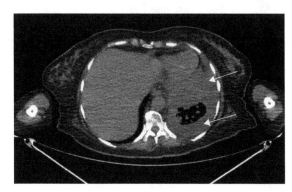

Figure 23.1 Contrast CT.

Imaging

PET/CT scan showed extensive lymphomatous involvement above and below the diaphragm with both nodal and extranodal (pleural and bone) disease. Figures 23.1 and 23.2 show sections through the chest using CT and PET/CT, respectively, where glucose avid tissue is seen along the left thoracic periphery/pleura around the effusion (arrows).

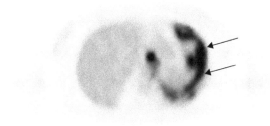

Figure 23.2 PET/CT.

Flow cytometry (pleural fluid)

The protein content of the fluid was 45 g/L, glucose 12.6 mmol/L, triglyceride 0.63 mmol/L and LDH 206 U/L. The total white cell count of the pleural fluid was 0.11×10^9/L. On the FSC/SSC plot, two distinct populations were noted (Figure 23.3).

The first population, in the small lymphoid gate with low FSC/SSC, consisted of normal-sized lymphocytes with the immunophenotype of reactive T cells with a mixture of CD4- and CD8-positive cells and no antigen loss. Gating on the large cells (P1) using the same lymphoid panel was done to exclude the presence of large clonal B cells. This approach showed cells with a CD4+, HLA -DR+, CD14+

Practical Flow Cytometry in Haematology: 100 Worked Examples, First Edition. Mike Leach,
Mark Drummond, Allyson Doig, Pam McKay, Bob Jackson and Barbara J. Bain.
© 2015 John Wiley & Sons, Ltd. Published 2015 by John Wiley & Sons, Ltd.

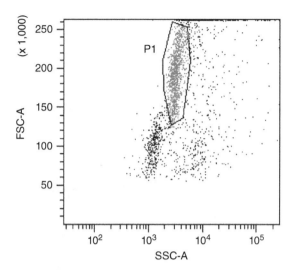

Figure 23.3

phenotype: other T- and B-cell antigens were not expressed. These cells are macrophages that are often present in reactive effusions. It is important not to misinterpret them as aberrant T cells.

The fluid therefore contained a mixture of reactive, activated T lymphocytes and a significant monocyte/macrophage population. No abnormal B cells were identified.

Discussion

There are two main mechanisms for pleural effusions in lymphoid malignancy. Firstly, direct disease involvement of pleural surfaces causes serosal irritation typically producing a cellular proteinaceous exudate, sometimes blood stained, with a high LDH level and low glucose. Malignant cells can usually be identified in this situation by either flow cytometry or cytology. The second mechanism is through direct obstruction to lymphatic drainage due to disease involvement of mediastinal nodes and/or obstruction of the thoracic duct. The latter may cause a chylous effusion (milky appearing pleural fluid due to the high lipid content) or a serous effusion; the LDH level may not be elevated and

glucose levels are similar to blood levels. Malignant cells are often not seen.

It might be anticipated that in this case a clonal B-cell population would be identified using flow studies on the pleural fluid. The protein level was high and the specimen was cellular but the LDH level was lower than blood whilst the glucose level was elevated due to diabetes. PET-avid disease was evident along the pleura and it might be expected that exfoliating disease cells would be demonstrated at least as a low percentage of the total cell count. Flow cytometry is far more sensitive than fluid cytology in this respect and can identify clonal B cells present at very low levels. There are good examples of this principle applied to other worked examples discussed in this book (see Cases 1, 2 and 99).

The reasons for the possible failure of detection in this case might be due to increased adhesion characteristics of lymphoma cells to the pleura or more likely that shed neoplastic cells underwent early apoptosis and disintegration losing cytoplasm and surface antigens and generating nuclear debris. This is one reason why macrophages are attracted to such fluids. Flow cytometry needs fresh effusion specimens delivered promptly to the laboratory in order to offer the best chance of characterising intact lymphoma cells. Delays in delivery, for whatever reason, can impair the quality and reliability of the analysis.

These studies did however identify a reactive pleural fluid and the characteristics of this reaction with polyclonal, activated T cells together with macrophages was identical to that seen at presentation when the diffuse large B-cell lymphoma was first identified. The recurrence of the effusion with the same fluid characteristics was therefore highly suggestive of relapse. Further imaging with CT and PET/CT showed mediastinal and pleural abnormalities in keeping with this interpretation and clinical disease progression was subsequently seen. Of course, if relapse is in doubt it is essential to confirm this with tissue biopsy before fully informed management decisions are possible.

Final diagnosis

Reactive pleural effusion due to relapsed diffuse large B-cell lymphoma.

Case 24

A 60-year-old man presented with severe back pain, nausea, anorexia and constipation. He had also noted recent bilateral leg weakness. There was no past medical history of note. On examination he was pale and tired and was in obvious pain when undertaking any simple activity.

Laboratory data

FBC: Hb 66 g/L, WBC 10 × 10⁹/L (neutrophils 6.7 × 10⁹/L, lymphocytes 2 × 10⁹/L, monocytes 1.1 × 10⁹/L) and platelets 95 × 10⁹/L.

U&Es: Na 137 mmol/L, K 5 mmol/L, urea 18.4 mmol/L, creatinine 145 µmol/L.

Bone profile: calcium 4.0 mmol/L, phosphate 1.6 mmol/L, ALP 70 U/L.

LFTs: normal except albumin 30 g/L, total protein 80 g/L.

Immunoglobulins: IgG 3.7 g/L, IgA not assessable, IgM 0.43 g/L.

Serum electrophoresis: IgA lambda paraprotein quantified at 50.9 g/L.

Blood film

The film was unremarkable showing a normocytic anaemia, prominent rouleaux and background protein staining.

Imaging

Urgent imaging of the spine was clearly indicated in view of the clinical presentation and the hypercalcaemia. The CT images showed an abnormal mottled appearance of the

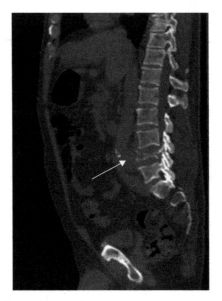

Figure 24.1 CT bone windows.

vertebral bodies with collapse of the fourth lumbar vertebra with an associated soft tissue mass (arrow, Figure 24.1). This was more clearly shown using MRI where the normal bone marrow fat signal was clearly attenuated by disease and the collapsed vertebra had retro-pulsed causing compression of the cauda equina (arrow, Figure 24.2). A diagnosis of multiple myeloma seemed very likely.

Morphology (bone marrow aspirate)

A cellular aspirate was easily obtained and the patient's bone texture was noted to be very soft at the time of the cortical

Practical Flow Cytometry in Haematology: 100 Worked Examples, First Edition. Mike Leach,
Mark Drummond, Allyson Doig, Pam McKay, Bob Jackson and Barbara J. Bain.
© 2015 John Wiley & Sons, Ltd. Published 2015 by John Wiley & Sons, Ltd.

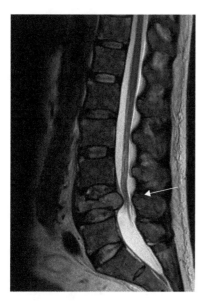

Figure 24.2 MRI.

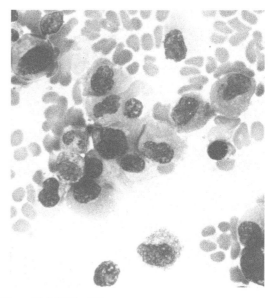

Figure 24.4 MGG, ×500.

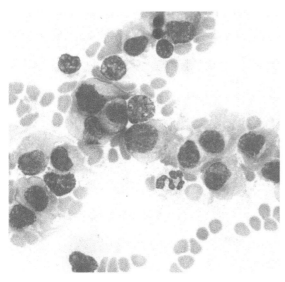

Figure 24.3 MGG, ×500.

puncture. The aspirate was clearly involved by a pleomorphic population of large plasma cells with little remaining haemopoietic reserve (Figures 24.3–24.6).

Flow cytometry (bone marrow aspirate)

The malignant plasma cell population comprised over 50% of all bone marrow events using a CD138 versus SSC analysis

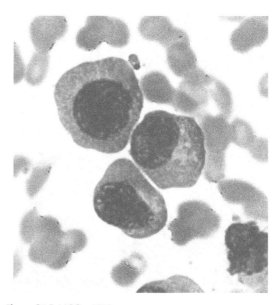

Figure 24.5 MGG, ×1000.

(Figure 24.7). The very large size of the plasma cells is shown by their position in the high blast gate in Figure 24.8. These cells had a typical malignant plasma cell phenotype with loss of CD19 and CD45 (Figure 24.9) and expression of CD56 (Figure 24.10).

Trephine biopsy
Sections showed almost maximal cellularity as a consequence of a diffuse plasma cell infiltrate (Figure 24.11). These cells

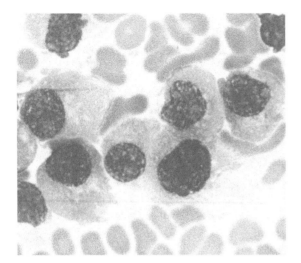

Figure 24.6 MGG, x1000.

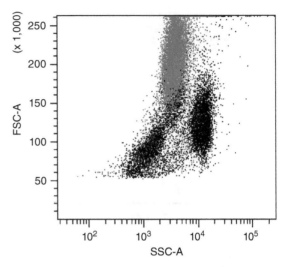

Figure 24.8 FSC/SSC.

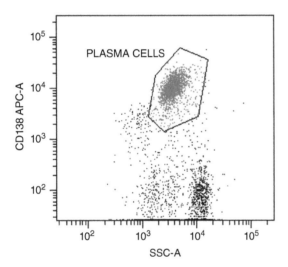

Figure 24.7 CD138/SSC.

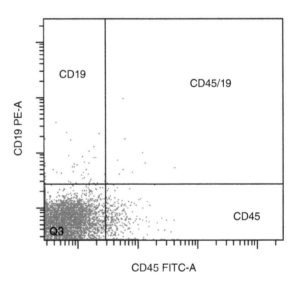

Figure 24.9 CD45/CD19.

were large with prominent nucleoli (Figure 24.12). There was little remaining normal haemopoietic activity.

The malignant plasma cells had a typical phenotype expressing CD138 (Figure 24.13) and CD56 (Figure 24.14) with cytoplasmic lambda restriction (Figure 24.15). The proliferation fraction was high at 60% (Figure 24.16); multiple myeloma and plasmacytomas are normally low proliferation neoplasms with Ki-67 nuclear protein expression in less than 20% of cells.

Cytogenetic analysis

Standard metaphase preparations and FISH studies using a panel of selected hybridisation probes identified a hypodiploid karyotype with a t(4;14)(p16;q32), del(17p) and del(1p) with amplified 1q. *FGFR3* and *IGH* were involved in the translocation.

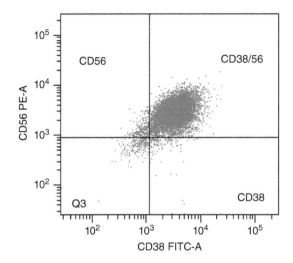

Figure 24.10 CD38/CD56.

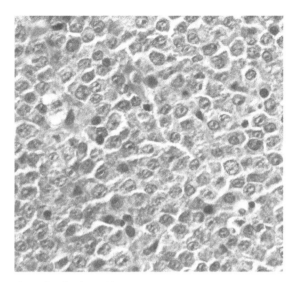

Figure 24.12 H&E, ×400.

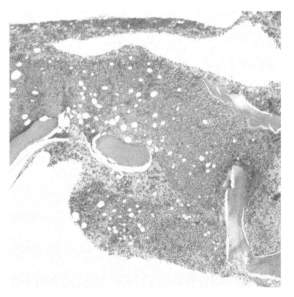

Figure 24.11 H&E, ×40.

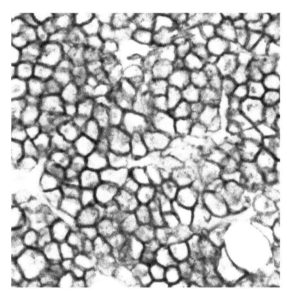

Figure 24.13 CD138, ×400.

Discussion

This case should present no diagnostic difficulty for the experienced haematology trainee. The presentation with hypercalcaemia, renal failure, anaemia and bone related symptoms (CRAB) is very familiar. In addition, this patient also had neurological compromise at the outset due to ver-

tebral collapse/displacement and cauda equina compression. The fitness of such patients and their suitability for treatment is often compromised at the outset.

This case is unusual, however, in showing blastoid morphology; almost complete effacement of haemopoietic tissue in the biopsy specimen and a high proliferation fraction of

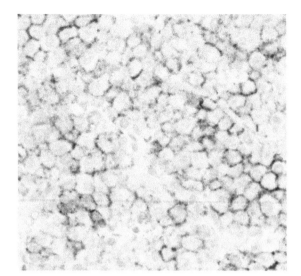

Figure 24.14 CD56, ×400.

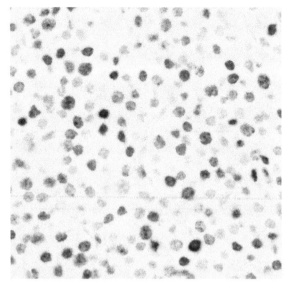

Figure 24.16 Ki-67, ×400.

abnormalities may occur during evolution of the disease, including *MYC* rearrangement, del(13q), del(17p), del(1p) and amplification of 1q. This patient had poor risk disease with evidence of primary and secondary aberrations at the time of diagnosis. His disease was refractory to initial treatment using bortezomib and subsequent lenalidomide.

Final diagnosis

Multiple myeloma with blastoid morphology and poor risk cytogenetics.

Reference

1 Sawyer, J.R. (2011) The prognostic significance of cytogenetics and molecular profiling in multiple myeloma. *Cancer Genetics*, **204** (**1**), 3–12. PubMed PMID: 21356186.

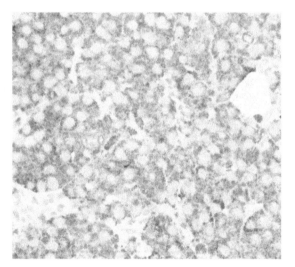

Figure 24.15 Lambda, ×400.

the tumour. Such cases often show an adverse cytogenetic profile as demonstrated here. The chromosome ploidy profile and the presence of *IGH* gene translocations, particularly t(4;14)(p16;q32) and t(14;16)(q32;q23), are the two main criteria used to stratify patients at the outset. Secondary

Case 25

A 76-year-old man was referred by gastroenterology for investigation of marrow failure and 10 kg weight loss. He gave a 4-month history of anorexia, daily diarrhoea and disabling fatigue but denied any other symptoms. His past medical history included stable ischaemic heart disease. Examination demonstrated cachexia but no skin changes, lymphadenopathy or organomegaly. Routine investigations were performed as below, including a bone marrow aspirate and trephine biopsy.

Laboratory data

FBC: Hb 114 g/L, WBC 19.2 × 10^9/L (neutrophils 14.2 × 10^9/L) and platelets 35 × 10^9/L.

U&Es: Na$^+$ 140 mmol/L, K$^+$ 3.0 mmol/L, urea 10.7 mmol/L, creatinine 98 μmol/L.

LFTs: ALP 264 U/L, ALT 65 U/L, AST 9 U/L, GGT 364 U/L, albumin 28 g/L, bilirubin 22 μmol/L. Serum LDH was 213 U/L.

Imaging

CT imaging, undertaken by the referring team, had shown widespread low-volume intra-abdominal lymphadenopathy (1–2 cm diameter lymph nodes), a bulky spleen (14 cm in long axis) and sclerotic bone lesions with an abnormal bone marrow signal (Figure 25.1).

Blood film

Leucoerythroblastic changes were noted but no abnormal population was seen (not shown).

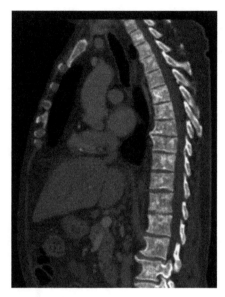

Figure 25.1 CT (bone windows).

Marrow aspirate

Marrow aspiration was dry and no material was obtained.

Bone marrow trephine biopsy

The marrow sample was completely replaced by a diffuse spindled cell infiltrate, with a suggestion of accompanying fibrosis, generating 100% cellularity (Figure 25.2). The bony trabeculae appeared irregular and thickened. There were some residual neutrophils, histiocytes and eosinophils interspersed between the spindled cells (Figure 25.3). The nuclei of the latter appeared long and thin and in some

Practical Flow Cytometry in Haematology: 100 Worked Examples, First Edition. Mike Leach, Mark Drummond, Allyson Doig, Pam McKay, Bob Jackson and Barbara J. Bain.
© 2015 John Wiley & Sons, Ltd. Published 2015 by John Wiley & Sons, Ltd.

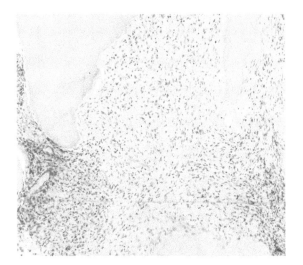

Figure 25.2 MGG, ×100.

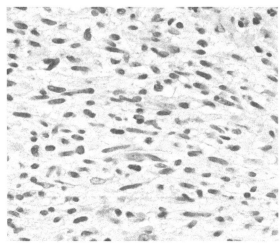

Figure 25.4 H&E, ×500.

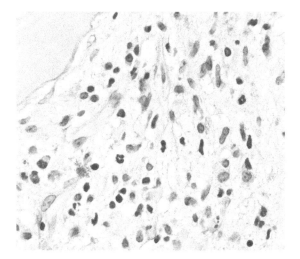

Figure 25.3 H&E, ×500.

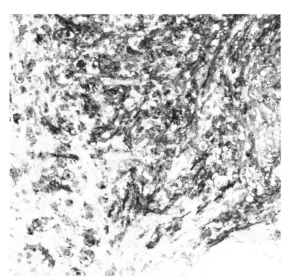

Figure 25.5 CD117, ×200.

areas apparently drawn in the direction of the cutting microtome (Figure 25.4). This can occur as an artefact in fibrotic marrows but the spindle morphology was real in this case as adjacent polymorphs and eosinophils were unaffected (Figure 25.3). For the inexperienced, the trephine biopsy histology on H&E staining can be puzzling and could be misinterpreted as marrow infiltration by carcinoma or sarcoma. In this situation, and in the light of the clinical history, mast cell disease should always be considered. Immunohistochemistry for CD117 and mast cell tryptase showed strong positive staining (Figures 25.5 and 25.6).

Given the marrow findings a serum tryptase was requested and found to be grossly elevated at 452 ng/mL. Unfortunately material for molecular studies was unobtainable (marrow dry tap).

Discussion

This patient presented with nonspecific symptoms highly suggestive of underlying malignancy. A diagnostic marrow

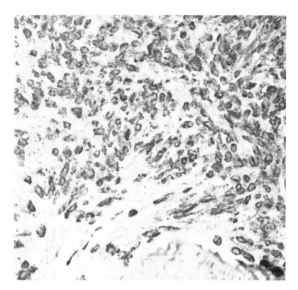

Figure 25.6 Mast cell tryptase, ×200.

biopsy was considered as the investigation of choice because of the constellation of thrombocytopenia, splenomegaly and lymphadenopathy. The full work-up of such a case includes molecular analysis for the typical mutation of *KIT* (D816V) present in almost all cases; material for this analysis was not available. This is not a prerequisite for the diagnosis of systemic mastocytosis (SM) (and is classed only as a minor criterion in the WHO classification, which relies primarily upon the histological demonstration of dense multifocal mast-cell tissue infiltrates). This, in addition to raised serum tryptase (>20 ng/mL, an additional minor criterion), is diagnostic of SM. Note that elevated serum tryptase is not specific to SM and may be seen with other myeloid disorders and following anaphylactoid reactions (1). Systemic mastocytosis usually presents as an indolent disorder (ISM) with skin lesions (urticaria pigmentosa) and mediator-type symptoms (flushing, abdominal pain, syncope, anaphylactoid reactions, etc.). The full blood count in these cases is usually normal and patients lack evidence of end-organ-damaging mast-cell infiltrates. In this case, however, the patient was progressively unwell with severe weight loss, marked thrombocytopenia, splenomegaly and bone lesions but no skin rash. These features are more typical of aggressive disease (ASM), and qualify as so-called 'C' findings. Indolent systemic mastocytosis is associated with an excellent prognosis and normal life expectancy, whereas ASM exhibits a progressive clinical course (median survival 3.5 years) (2).

Normal mast cells comprise <1% of marrow cells and on aspirates are usually seen in and around the particles as round mononuclear cells with heavily granulated cytoplasm.

They are only occasionally spindle shaped. Increased mast cell numbers may occasionally be hard to appreciate on marrow aspirates. Flow cytometry is a useful adjunct to diagnosis, with demonstration of an abnormal mast cell phenotype (CD2⁺ CD25⁺). Trephine (or other tissue) biopsy with IHC remains the gold standard for diagnosis, however. Normal mast cells appear in small numbers, scattered throughout the marrow with mainly a round mononuclear appearance, with clumped chromatin. Abnormal mast cells are found in aggregates, with spindled morphology and on occasion hypogranularity and/or immature chromatin. They are often paratrabecular or periarteriolar in distribution. IHC for tryptase, CD117, CD2 and CD25 are important for their identification.

Bone imaging using CT and MRI frequently identifies abnormalities such as osteoclerosis or altered bone marrow signal in patients with systemic mastocytosis (3). Osteolytic lesions can coexist with sclerotic lesions. In patients presenting with systemic upset, weight loss and anaemia imaging is often requested as part of the search for an underlying neoplasm. The authors have identified a number of patients, ultimately diagnosed with mast cell disorders, referred to our department from medical specialties on account of abnormal bone radiology. This is an important phenomenon and its recognition can expedite the diagnostic process.

Treatment of ASM remains challenging. This patient was treated with midostaurin (PKC412), a multi-tyrosine kinase inhibitor, but was intolerant of treatment and he died of disease 10 months from presentation.

Diagnosis

Aggressive systemic mastocytosis.
See also Case 64.

References

1 Sperr, W.R., El-Samahi, A., Kundi, M. *et al.* (2009) Elevated tryptase levels selectively cluster in myeloid neoplasms: a novel diagnostic approach and screen marker in clinical haematology. *European Journal of Clinical Investigation,* **39** (**10**), 914–923. PubMed PMID: 19522836.

2 Lim, K.H., Tefferi, A., Lasho, T.L. *et al.* (2009) Systemic mastocytosis in 342 consecutive adults: survival studies and prognostic factors. *Blood,* **113** (**23**), 5727–5736. PubMed PMID: 19363219.

3 Fritz, J., Fishman, E.K., Carrino, J.A. & Horger, M.S. (2012) Advanced imaging of skeletal manifestations of systemic mastocytosis. *Skeletal Radiology,* **41** (**8**), 887–897. PubMed PMID: 22366736.

Case 26

A 24-year-old man developed left upper quadrant pain following a fall down stairs at home. He was found to have a tender left upper quadrant mass and was referred for ultrasound examination. This showed a haematoma in an enlarged spleen.

Laboratory investigations

FBC: Hb 161 g/L, WBC 20.2×10^9/L (lymphocytes 17.2×10^9/L) and platelets 137×10^9/L.

U&Es and LFTs normal. LDH normal.

Serum immunoglobulins were normal with no paraprotein evident on serum electrophoresis.

The blood film showed an abnormal lymphoid population of small to medium-sized lymphocytes with irregular nuclei and variable amounts of cytoplasm (Figures 26.1 and 26.2).

Imaging

CT scan showed splenomegaly (18 cm) but no significant lymphadenopathy. There was a notable low-density lesion in the lower pole of the spleen (arrow, Figure 26.3) in keeping with a splenic tear from trauma and a subsequent haematoma.

Flow cytometry

A CD2 versus CD19 analysis showed an excess of B cells with surface lambda[strong] and a CD20+, CD5+, FMC7+, CD23+, HLA-DR+, CD79b+ and CD22+ phenotype. The differential diagnosis of a CD5+ B-cell lymphoproliferative disorder includes chronic lymphocytic leukaemia (CLL),

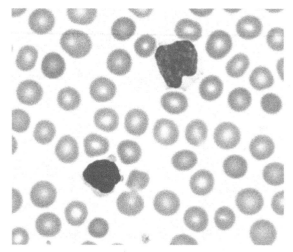

Figure 26.1 MGG, ×1000.

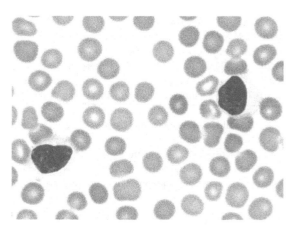

Figure 26.2 MGG, ×1000.

Practical Flow Cytometry in Haematology: 100 Worked Examples, First Edition. Mike Leach, Mark Drummond, Allyson Doig, Pam McKay, Bob Jackson and Barbara J. Bain.
© 2015 John Wiley & Sons, Ltd. Published 2015 by John Wiley & Sons, Ltd.

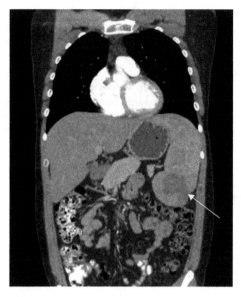

Figure 26.3 CT.

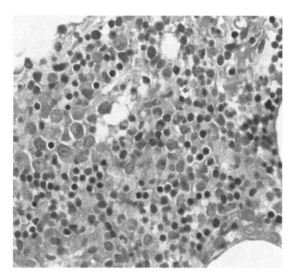

Figure 26.4 H&E, ×400.

mantle cell lymphoma (MCL) and less commonly marginal zone lymphoma (MZL). The presence of strong surface Ig, FMC7, CD22 and CD79b positivity is against a diagnosis of CLL, making MZL and MCL the favoured diagnoses. CD23 positivity is more frequently seen in MZL.

Bone marrow trephine biopsy

The trephine core was of normal cellularity with no obvious lymphoid infiltration on H&E-stained sections (Figure 26.4). However, immunohistochemistry demonstrated an interstitial infiltrate of small CD20$^+$ lymphoid cells accounting for approximately 20% of all cells (Figure 26.5). These cells co-expressed CD5 (Figure 26.6) and cyclin D1 (Figure 26.7) suggesting a diagnosis of mantle cell lymphoma (MCL).

FISH studies

A t(11;14)(q13;q32) translocation was confirmed by FISH studies on peripheral blood.

Discussion

Cell marker studies on peripheral blood demonstrated a CD5$^+$ B-cell lymphoproliferative disorder, which was clearly

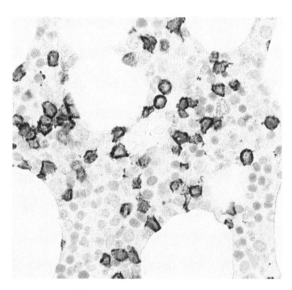

Figure 26.5 CD20, ×400.

not CLL on account of the moderately strong CD20, FMC7 and CD79b and strong SIg expression. The most likely differential diagnosis was MCL or a CD5$^+$ variant of MZL. Although both of these conditions are rare in a 24-year-old man, MZL was thought more likely. The expression of cyclin D1 and the demonstration of t(11;14)(q13;q32), however, showed the diagnosis to be MCL.

The presentation in this case with splenomegaly and peripheral blood lymphocytosis without significant

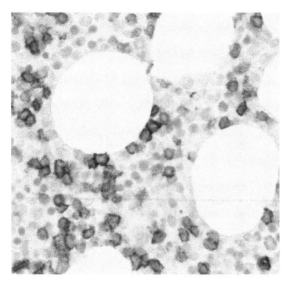

Figure 26.6 CD5, ×400.

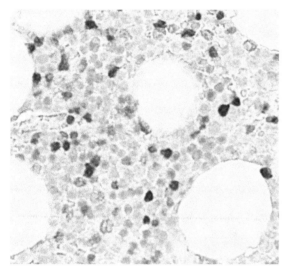

Figure 26.7 Cyclin D1, ×400.

lymphadenopathy conforms to the recently described entity of indolent mantle cell leukaemia, a condition characterised by only slow progression (1, 2). The only atypical features were the presence of lambda rather than kappa restriction and the young age of the patient. The diagnosis of MCL in a 24-year-old man, however, poses significant difficulties in terms of optimal management. He made an uneventful recovery from the fall and splenic trauma. He currently remains well and is being managed by close observation at the time of reporting.

Final diagnosis

Indolent mantle cell leukaemia

References

1 Ondrejka, S.L., Lai, R., Smith, S.D. & His, E.D. (2011) Indolent mantle cell leukaemia: a clinicopathological variant characterised by isolated lymphocytosis, interstitial bone marrow involvement, kappa light chain restriction and good prognosis. *Haematologica*, **96** (8), 1121–1127.
2 Royo, C., Navarro, A., Clot, G. *et al.* (2012) Non-nodal type of mantle cell lymphoma is a specific biological and clinical subgroup of the disease. *Leukemia.* **26** (8), 1895–1898.

Case 27

A 29-year-old man, previously lost to follow up, was re-referred to the Haematology clinic. He had a long history of thrombocytopenia from childhood that had been partially responsive to steroid therapy. He described simple bruising and cutaneous petechiae in relation to trauma. He reported no excess of infection, no other significant past history and no family history of a platelet disorder. Physical examination confirmed minor bruising, fine petechiae over the forearms and a generally dry skin but without signs of inflammation or excoriation.

Laboratory data

FBC: Hb 155 g/L, WBC 6.2×10^9/L, neutrophils 4.0×10^9/L, lymphocytes 1.5×10^9/L, platelets 31×10^9/L.
    U&Es, LFTs, LDH and CRP were normal.
    Serum immunoglobulins were normal.

Blood film

The blood film showed a true thrombocytopenia. The platelets were generally small (Figures 27.1 and 27.2). The film was otherwise normal.

Flow cytometry

Analysis of T-cell, B-cell and NK-cell subsets was normal.

Differential diagnosis

The working diagnosis of autoimmune thrombocytopenic purpura (ITP) was certainly possible but there are a few

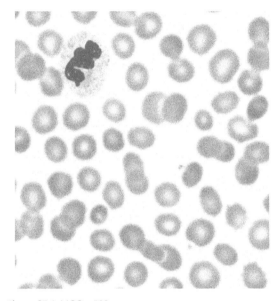

Figure 27.1 MGG, ×500.

atypical features in this case. Firstly, the history dated back to childhood and although chronic ITP can first present at an early age this is unusual. Secondly, the patient did appear to have a mild bleeding tendency despite a platelet count of between 30 and 40×10^9/L; this again would not be expected in ITP where significant bruising and petechiae are infrequent unless the platelet count falls below 20×10^9/L. Finally, mean platelet volume in ITP is generally increased and this is thought to be due to shortened platelet half life and increased platelet turnover. Here the platelets were notable for their very small size at 7 fl (normal 12–18 fl). Despite this the patient did report an improvement in platelet count in response to oral steroid therapy, with maximal responses to between 80 and 100×10^9/L. He had never been treated

Practical Flow Cytometry in Haematology: 100 Worked Examples, First Edition. Mike Leach, Mark Drummond, Allyson Doig, Pam McKay, Bob Jackson and Barbara J. Bain.
© 2015 John Wiley & Sons, Ltd. Published 2015 by John Wiley & Sons, Ltd.

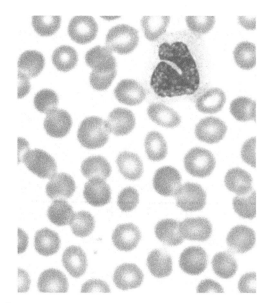

Figure 27.2 MGG, ×500.

with intravenous immunoglobulin but had been treated with platelet transfusion following a facial injury at the age of 13 years. This scenario should give rise to consideration of the possibility of the X-linked thrombocytopenia subset of Wiskott–Aldrich syndrome (WAS).

Molecular studies

Blood was submitted from the patient and his mother to Great Ormond Street Hospital where leucocyte DNA was analysed at the *WAS* gene locus on the X chromosome at Xp11.22-23. This indicated a missense mutation in exon 2 c.G223A; pVal75Met in the patient whilst his mother was a carrier for the same mutation.

Discussion

Wiskott–Aldrich syndrome is the clinical entity of thrombocytopenia, eczema and recurrent infection. This is an X-linked disorder and affected individuals suffer serious and recurrent bacterial infections from an early age. Mutations completely preventing the production of WAS protein (WASp) typically lead to the classical phenotype, and these patients present early with pyogenic infections consequent of immune deficiency resulting from combined T-cell and B-cell dysfunction with hypogammaglobulinaemia. WASp is solely expressed in haemopoietic cells and is involved in

the organisation of the cellular cytoskeleton, signal transduction and apoptosis. Affected patients are often treated with prophylactic intravenous immunoglobulin therapy and improvements in the platelet count have been noted suggesting that, at least in part, the thrombocytopenia has an immune component. In fact, this is where the notion that such therapy might be useful in true ITP first arose. Classical Wiskott–Aldrich syndrome often results in early death due to infection or bleeding and allogeneic stem cell transplant should be considered early in the disease course.

It is now clear that mutations in the *WAS* gene resulting in the production of reduced quantity of WASp are capable of producing this subsyndrome known as X-linked thrombocytopenia. In this condition, a minor degree of eczema may be apparent but serious infections are infrequent. This entity might be easily confused with ITP and should be considered in all males presenting with a long history and small platelets despite an improvement in platelet counts following steroid or immunoglobulin therapy. It is an important entity to recognise as the treatment options for the thrombocytopenia need to be carefully considered. Although steroids, intravenous immunoglobulins and splenectomy have all been used with good effect in X-linked thrombocytopenia the risks and benefits should be considered carefully in the light of this diagnosis. In addition to the bleeding risks associated with thrombocytopenia and a low platelet mass it is recognised that platelet function is also abnormal in this condition. This should be taken into account when formulating management plans for any surgical intervention in these patients. A comprehensive review of X-linked thrombocytopenia including a review of *WAS* genotype–phenotype clinical correlation is presented by Albert and colleagues (1).

This patient illustrates that even in the presence of normal T-cell subsets, on immunophenotyping the possibility of a *WAS* mutation should not be excluded. When thrombocytopenic patients have features that are not typical of ITP, the possibility of a congenital thrombocytopenia must be considered.

Final diagnosis

X-linked thrombocytopenia due to a mutation in *WAS* gene.

Reference

1 Albert, M.H., Bittner, T.C., Nonoyama, S. *et al.* (2010) X-linked thrombocytopenia (XLT) due to WAS mutations: clinical characteristics, long-term outcome, and treatment options. *Blood*, **115** (**16**), 3231–3238. PubMed PMID: 20173115.

Case 28

A 76-year-old man presented with fatigue, back pain, weight loss and sweats. Physical examination showed a pale, tired looking man but there were no specific findings. In particular there was no palpable lymphadenopathy.

Laboratory results

FBC: Hb 95 g/L, WBC 4.36×10^9/L and platelets 153×10^9/L.

U&Es: normal. LFTs: albumin 24 g/L, alkaline phosphatase 450 U/L, AST 49 U/L, ALT 40 U/L, bilirubin 18 μmol/L. LDH was 1514 U/L.

The blood film was unremarkable.

Imaging

A CT scan showed subcentimetre axillary lymph nodes. The retroperitoneal area showed a diffuse soft tissue abnormality surrounding the aorta and inferior vena cava. It was not clear whether this represented a diffuse nodal mass or retroperitoneal fibrosis. A CT-guided biopsy was planned.

Bone marrow aspirate

In view of the anaemia (and borderline pancytopenia), a bone marrow aspiration and trephine biopsy were performed. The aspirate was cellular and comprised of a population of large lymphoid cells with basophilic cytoplasm admixed with normal haemopoietic precursors (Figures 28.1–28.3). Note the erythrophagocytosis by the large lymphoid cell in Figure 28.2 (arrow).

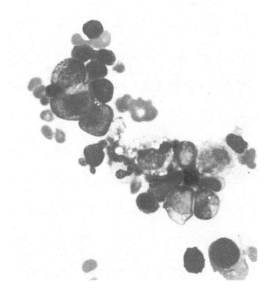

Figure 28.1 MGG, ×500.

Flow cytometry (bone marrow)

The abnormal population fell within the blast gate on the FSC versus SSC analysis. These cells were shown to express CD19, CD20, CD10 (Figure 28.4), HLA-DR, FMC7, CD22 and CD79b with surface lambda^{dim} restriction (Figure 28.5). The cells therefore had a mature CD10+ phenotype with blastoid morphology. A germinal centre-type diffuse large B-cell lymphoma (DLBCL) was a likely diagnosis.

Practical Flow Cytometry in Haematology: 100 Worked Examples, First Edition. Mike Leach, Mark Drummond, Allyson Doig, Pam McKay, Bob Jackson and Barbara J. Bain.
© 2015 John Wiley & Sons, Ltd. Published 2015 by John Wiley & Sons, Ltd.

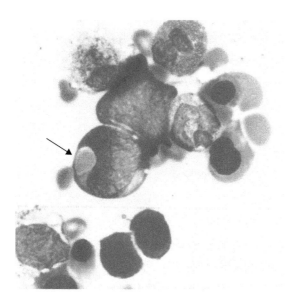

Figure 28.2 MGG, ×1000.

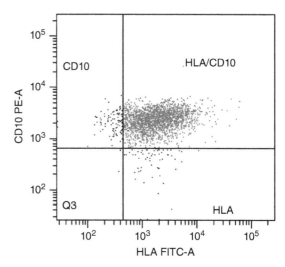

Figure 28.4 CD10/HLA-DR.

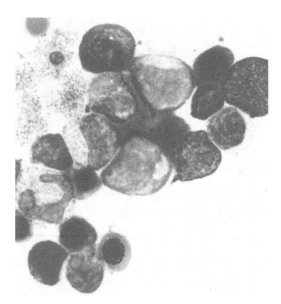

Figure 28.3 MGG, ×1000.

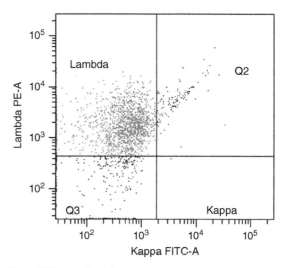

Figure 28.5 Kappa/lambda.

Bone marrow trephine biopsy

This showed a hypercellular core due to a combination of diffuse interstitial and some paratrabecular infiltration (Figures 28.6 and 28.7). There was also an extensive area of coagulative necrosis, shown in Figure 28.6 (arrow).

The majority of cells had centroblastic morphology and were expressing CD20, CD10, BCL2 (Figure 28.8) and BCL6 (Figure 28.9).

All lymphoid cells were positive for CD10. The proliferation fraction was 40–50% in the interstitial areas (Figure 28.10) but only 10% in the paratrabecular regions. These features are therefore suggestive of paratrabecular marrow involvement by a follicular lymphoma (FL) with interstitial involvement by DLBCL.

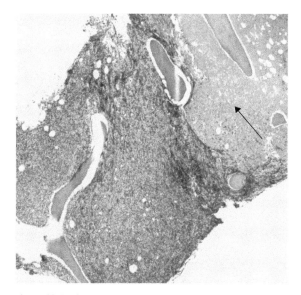

Figure 28.6 H&E, ×40.

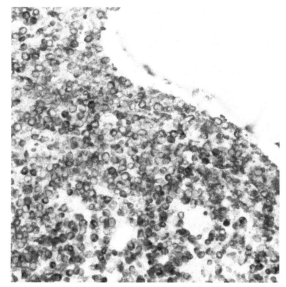

Figure 28.8 BCL2, ×200.

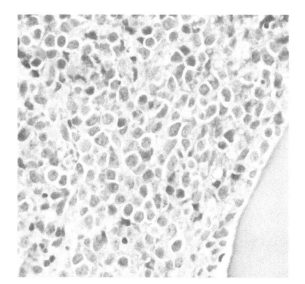

Figure 28.7 H&E, ×400.

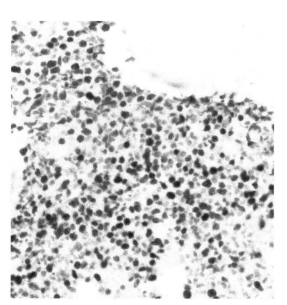

Figure 28.9 BCL6, ×200.

Core biopsy of retroperitoneal tissue

Multiple percutaneous cores were taken from the retroperitoneal mass using CT guidance. These showed a dense lymphoid infiltrate composed of small follicular structures (arrows, Figures 28.11 and 28.12) containing medium-sized centrocytes with occasional centroblasts (Figure 28.13).

These cells were positive for CD20, CD10, BCL6 and BCL2. CD21 highlights follicular dendritic cells within the follicles (Figure 28.14). The proliferation fraction was less than 10% (Figure 28.15). The appearances were consistent with follicular lymphoma, grade 1.

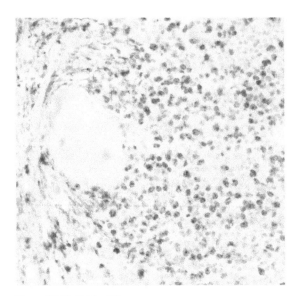

Figure 28.10 Ki-67, ×100.

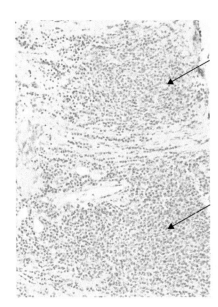

Figure 28.12 H&E, ×100.

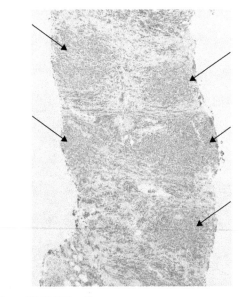

Figure 28.11 H&E, ×40.

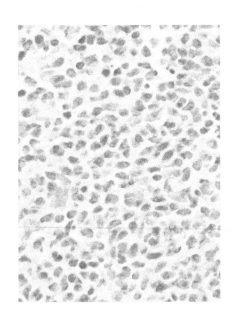

Figure 28.13 H&E, ×400.

Discussion

This case represents a relatively common clinical scenario. The presentation was of an unwell patient with marked B symptoms, mild pancytopenia and raised serum LDH. These features are suggestive of a high-grade neoplasm.

The bone marrow aspirate findings were in keeping with DLBCL whilst the retroperitoneal core biopsy showed FL. The trephine biopsy identified the two pathologies, DLBCL and the FL from which it had evolved, in the same specimen. The DLBCL superimposed on a background of

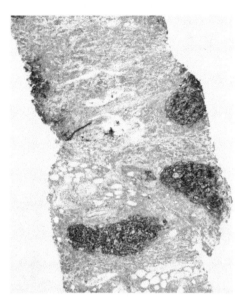

Figure 28.14 CD21, ×40.

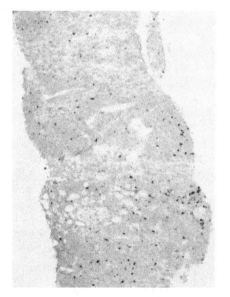

Figure 28.15 Ki-67, ×40.

undiagnosed follicular lymphoma was clearly responsible for the clinical decline. The analysis of different tissues can yield information to fully inform the diagnosis and this guides important decisions on subsequent therapy.

Final diagnosis

High-grade transformation (diffuse large B-cell lymphoma with a germinal centre phenotype) of a follicular lymphoma.

Case 29

A previously well 46-year-old female presented to her GP with a short (2–3 week) history of fatigue and a sore throat. There had been no weight loss, night sweats, bleeding or bruising. There was no palpable organomegaly or lymphadenopathy. Routine blood testing was performed.

Basic laboratory data

FBC: Hb 123 g/L, WBC 41.6 × 10^9/L (monocytes 30.9 × 10^9/L, neutrophils 8.5 × 10^9/L) and platelets 136 ×10^9/L.

Coagulation screen including fibrinogen: normal.

U&Es, LFTs, bone profile: normal.

Blood film

Numerous abnormal cells of monocyte lineage were seen, some with more mature morphology (Figure 29.1), but most being promonocytes (exhibiting more delicately folded and convoluted nuclear margins, with less mature chromatin and some fine granules, Figures 29.2 and 29.3) with an occasional monoblast (Figure 29.4). Dysplastic neutrophils were easily found and an occasional myeloblast was noted including one or two with Auer rods (not shown).

Bone marrow aspirate

The marrow was hypercellular. Eighty percent of cells were monoblasts or promonocytes (monoblasts being the most frequent), with a corresponding marked reduction in other marrow elements (Figures 29.5–29.8). Occasional more mature monocytic forms were noted. Dysplastic myeloid maturation was evident.

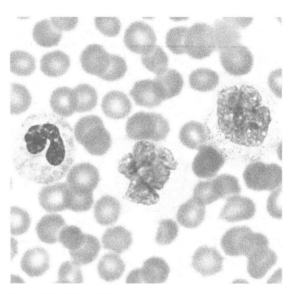

Figure 29.1 MGG, ×1000.

Flow cytometry (blood)

Flow cytometry on peripheral blood revealed an abnormal population of monocytes and promonocytes, with the immunophenotype being CD38$^+$, CD64^{++}, CD14$^+$ and CD56$^+$ (Figures 29.9 and 29.10). No significant myeloblast population was demonstrable by flow cytometry.

Flow cytometry (bone marrow aspirate)

As seen morphologically, cells of monocytic lineage comprised 75% of cells, although with an immunophenotype considerably less mature than that in peripheral blood.

Practical Flow Cytometry in Haematology: 100 Worked Examples, First Edition. Mike Leach, Mark Drummond, Allyson Doig, Pam McKay, Bob Jackson and Barbara J. Bain.
© 2015 John Wiley & Sons, Ltd. Published 2015 by John Wiley & Sons, Ltd.

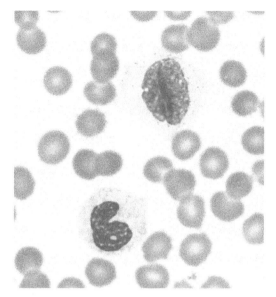

Figure 29.2 MGG, ×1000.

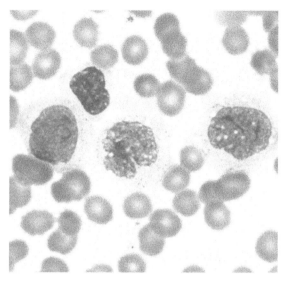

Figure 29.4 MGG, ×1000.

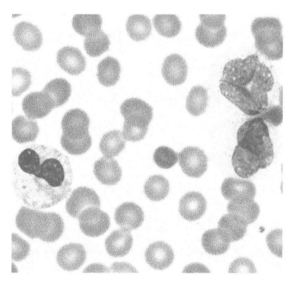

Figure 29.3 MGG, ×1000.

CD14$^-$ CD64^{++} monoblasts comprised >50% of the abnormal population, with the remaining cells showing varying degrees of CD14 positivity (Figure 29.11). Note the 'smear' of CD14 as more mature monoblasts/promonocytes express it, in a parody of normal monocytic maturation.

Cytogenetics

Normal female karyotype, 46,XX.

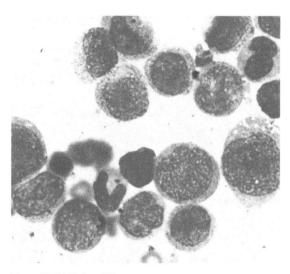

Figure 29.5 MGG, ×1000.

FISH studies

No *MLL* rearrangement was detectable by FISH.

Discussion

At first sight, this case presents some diagnostic difficulty between an acute monoblastic/monocytic leukaemia and CMML. Although neutrophilia is unusual, there are a

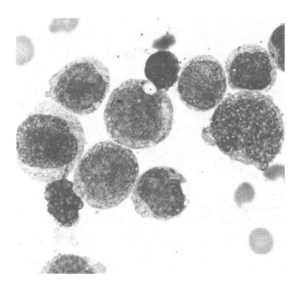

Figure 29.6 MGG, ×1000.

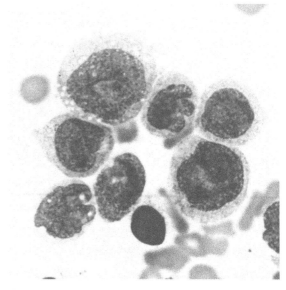

Figure 29.8 MGG, ×1000.

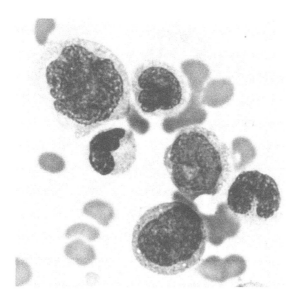

Figure 29.7 MGG, ×1000.

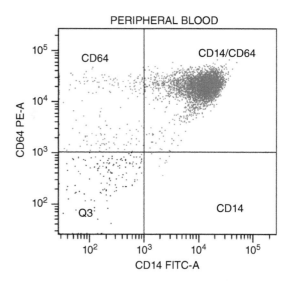

Figure 29.9 CD14/CD64.

number of features that favour the former, not least the young age and female sex of the patient (CMML has a median age of presentation of 75–80 years, and is most often seen in males), short history and lack of organomegaly. Acute leukaemia was indicated by the observation that promonocytes were the dominant cells in peripheral blood. The marrow findings were unequivocal in demonstrating that this was acute monoblastic leukaemia. *MLL* gene rearrangements are not infrequent in this entity (they are

found in 10–25% of AML with a monocytic component (1), but are rare in CMML). Most are identified by standard cytogenetic analysis, although FISH is very useful for confirmatory screening. When present they may be regarded as indicative of AML rather than CMML, although no *MLL* rearrangements were identified in our case.

This case emphasises the importance of an accurate marrow diagnosis for AML, the appearances of which may often

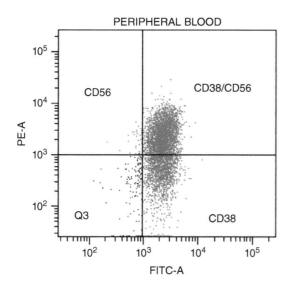

Figure 29.10 CD38/CD56.

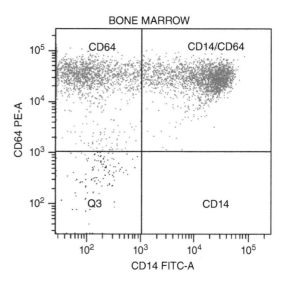

Figure 29.11 CD14/CD64.

be considerably different from that of peripheral blood. It is not rare in acute monocytic/monoblastic leukaemia for the monocyte lineage cells to be considerably more mature in the blood than the marrow as in this patient and the diagnosis of CMML may have to be considered.

The distinction between promonocytes and immature monocytes is very important in distinguishing acute leukaemia from CMML. CD56 is an important antigen to recognise in haematological malignancy. In normal cell populations it is expressed on NK cells and small subsets of T cells. It is promiscuously (and usually aberrantly) expressed on a range of blood cancers as well as solid tumours (the latter comprising small cell/neuroendocrine tumours). It is most frequently seen in CMML (80% or so of cases) and acute monoblastic/monocytic leukaemias (up to 50% of cases). It is also found in other AML subtypes as well as in cases of MDS, T ALL, mature T- and NK-cell neoplasms, myeloma and blastic plasmacytoid dendritic cell neoplasm.

Final diagnosis

Acute monoblastic leukaemia.

Reference

1 De Braekeleer, M., Morel, F., Le Bris, M.J., Herry, A., Douet-Guilbert, N. (2005) The MLL gene and translocations involving chromosomal band 11q23 in acute leukemia. *Anticancer research*, **25** (**3B**), 1931–1944. PubMed PMID: 16158928.

Case 30

A 37-year-old Iranian man presented to the Accident and Emergency department with a short history of fever, myalgia, night sweats and abdominal pain. On examination he was icteric and he had soft low volume nodes palpable in the neck bilaterally. His abdomen was tender maximally in the right upper quadrant but there was no rebound or guarding. An old midline surgical laparotomy scar was evident.

Laboratory data

FBC: Hb 130 g/L, WBC 20 × 10⁹/L, neutrophils 3.6 × 10⁹/L, lymphocytes 13.7 × 10⁹/L, monocytes 2.75 × 10⁹/L and platelets 288 × 10⁹/L. Reticulocytes 200 × 10⁹/L.

Direct Coombs test was negative.

U&Es normal. CRP 28 mg/L.

LFTs: bilirubin 102 μmol/L, AST 379 U/L, ALT 682 U/L, ALP 349 U/L and albumin 32 g/L. Haptoglobin was absent.

Blood film

The blood film showed a number of features (Figures 30.1– 30.4). Firstly, spherocytes were prominent in the film together with Howell–Jolly bodies indicating previous splenectomy or another hyposplenic state. Secondly, large pleomorphic lymphocytes, some with cytoplasmic granulation were noted and were accounting for the noted lymphocytosis.

Differential diagnosis

The presenting features were of an acute illness causing sweats, fever, hepatitis and lymphadenopathy. The blood film

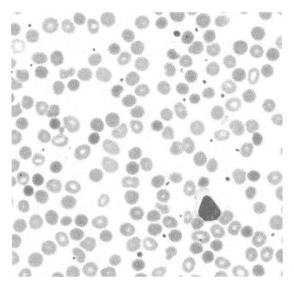

Figure 30.1 MGG, ×500.

morphology suggested a nonimmune spherocytic red cell disorder previously treated by splenectomy and a diagnosis of hereditary spherocytosis seemed likely.

Flow cytometry

Red cell flow cytometry assessment of EMA (eosin-5-maleimide) binding to the red cell membrane showed a reduced ratio of 0.74 (NR > 0.80). Flow analysis of the leucocytes showed an activated CD8⁺ T-cell population with prominent HLA-DR expression and partial loss of CD7. This is typical of the lymphocyte response seen as a result of acute viral infection.

Practical Flow Cytometry in Haematology: 100 Worked Examples, First Edition. Mike Leach, Mark Drummond, Allyson Doig, Pam McKay, Bob Jackson and Barbara J. Bain.

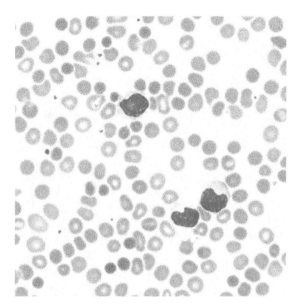

Figure 30.2 MGG, ×500.

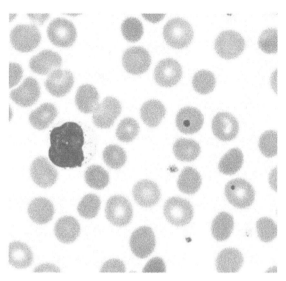

Figure 30.4 MGG, ×1000.

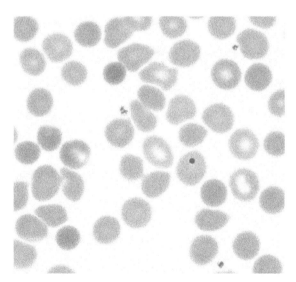

Figure 30.3 MGG, ×1000.

Virology

A glandular fever screening test was positive for heterophile antibodies. Serology showed IgM antibodies to Epstein–Barr virus (EBV) in keeping with recent infection. Serology for HIV, hepatitis B, hepatitis C, toxoplasma and CMV was negative.

Discussion

On further direct questioning, the patient described a surgical procedure in childhood in Iran for a persistent blood condition causing anaemia and tiredness; the condition had also been a problem in other family members. The clinicopathological scenario is therefore in keeping with an acute EBV infection causing an acute hepatitis, fever, lymphadenopathy and sweats in a patient who had undergone a previous splenectomy for hereditary spherocytosis. The hyperbilirubinaemia attributable to viral hepatitis could have been aggravated by an exacerbation of haemolysis typically seen as a result of viral infection in this condition. The patient was treated symptomatically and he made an uneventful recovery.

Final diagnosis

Acute EBV infection in a patient with previous splenectomy for hereditary spherocytosis.

Case 31

A 72-year-old woman presented with general malaise and shortness of breath. There was a non-productive cough. Clinical examination revealed a right-sided pleural effusion but no organomegaly or lymphadenopathy.

Laboratory results

FBC: Hb 118 g/L, WBC 7.8 × 10⁹/L and platelets 209 × 10⁹/L. U&Es, LFTs, bone profile and LDH: normal.

Imaging

A CXR and subsequent CT scan showed a right-sided pleural effusion. There was no clear pleural, mediastinal or pulmonary mass visible on careful scrutiny. Pleural fluid aspiration was performed. This yielded a cellular specimen with a cell count of 10.9 × 10⁹/L and protein level of 40 g/L.

Pleural fluid morphology

There was a population of large pleomorphic cells with irregular nuclei, large nucleoli and abundant basophilic and often vacuolated cytoplasm (Figures 31.1 and 31.2) with a few admixed neutrophils and macrophages.

Pleural fluid flow cytometry

The immunophenotype of these cells was of mature B cells with expression of CD20, CD38, FMC7, HLA-DR and

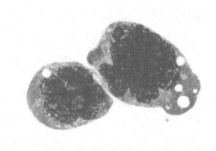

Figure 31.1 MGG, ×1000.

CD79b. No surface immunoglobulin was demonstrated (the inability to demonstrate monoclonality in pleural fluid is not uncommon, possibly due to loss of surface Ig in the fluid environment).

Immunocytochemistry and immunohistochemistry (pleural fluid)

Our histopathology colleagues independently reported the pleural fluid cytology and identified the same large cells using Papanicolaou (Figure 31.3) and Giemsa stains (Figure 31.4).

Practical Flow Cytometry in Haematology: 100 Worked Examples, First Edition. Mike Leach, Mark Drummond, Allyson Doig, Pam McKay, Bob Jackson and Barbara J. Bain.
© 2015 John Wiley & Sons, Ltd. Published 2015 by John Wiley & Sons, Ltd.

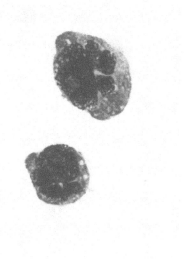

Figure 31.2 MGG, ×1000.

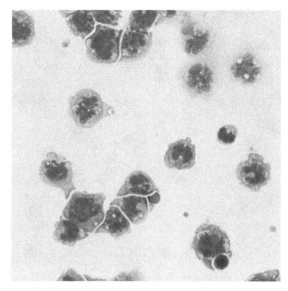

Figure 31.4 Giemsa, ×500.

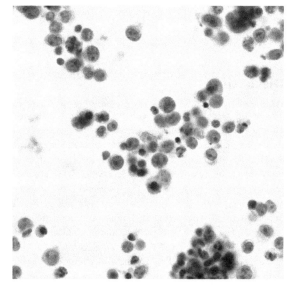

Figure 31.3 Papanicolaou, ×400.

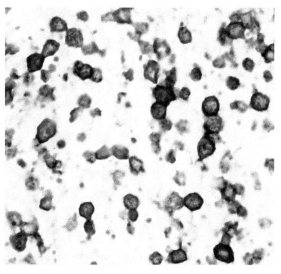

Figure 31.5 CD20, ×400.

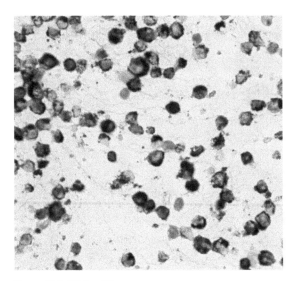

Figure 31.6 BCL2, ×400.

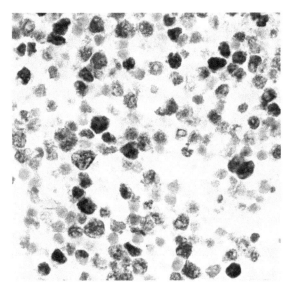

Figure 31.7 BCL6, ×400.

A paraffin-embedded cell block was made from the pleural fluid after centrifugation and immunocytochemistry was performed. The malignant cells expressed CD20 (Figure 31.5), BCL2 (Figure 31.6), BCL6 (Figure 31.7) and MUM-1. The Ki-67-positive proliferation fraction was high at over 90% (Figure 31.8). CD10 was not expressed.

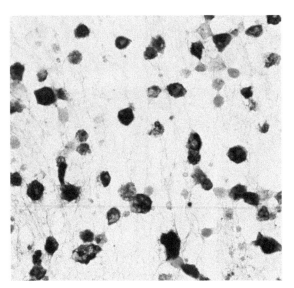

Figure 31.8 Ki-67, ×400.

Cytogenetic analysis (pleural fluid)

This showed a complex karyotype with no evidence of a *MYC* (8q24) translocation.

Discussion

The results were in keeping with diffuse large B-cell lymphoma (DLBCL), activated B-cell (ABC) subtype, confined to the pleura. Immunocytochemistry for human herpesvirus 8 (HHV8) was negative. The isolated involvement of a body cavity, in this case the pleural cavity, in the absence of any tumour mass raises the possibility of primary effusion lymphoma (PEL). This is a rare type of large B-cell neoplasm usually occurring in human immunodeficiency virus-infected patients with severe immunodeficiency. It is associated with HHV8 and there is often co-infection with Epstein – Barr virus (EBV). It can also occur in nonimmunosuppressed patients, usually elderly men and women. The malignant cells in PEL are CD45$^+$ but usually lack B-cell markers; they may express CD30, CD138 and HLA-DR (1). This case is not a PEL given the presence of B-cell antigens and the absence of HHV8.

Whilst biopsy of solid tissue is normally required to make a definitive diagnosis of lymphoma, a diagnosis in this case can be achieved on pleural fluid alone based on the morphology and immunophenotype of the cells together with the chromosomal abnormalities identified.

Final diagnosis

Diffuse large B-cell lymphoma, activated B-cell subtype, of pleura.

Reference

1 Ammari, Z.A., Mollberg, N.M., Abdelhady, K., Mansueto, M.D., Massad, M.G. (2013) Diagnosis and management of primary effusion lymphoma in the immunocompetent and immunocompromised hosts. *The Thoracic and Cardiovascular Surgeon*, **61** (**4**), 343–349. PubMed PMID: 23424065.

Case 32

A 61-year-old female with no prior medical history and on no regular medications complained of fatigue and easy bruising whilst on holiday abroad. Routine blood testing 18 months before had been normal. She was admitted to hospital and after examination of her blood counts/film and bone marrow aspirate, she was flown by air ambulance back to the UK.

Laboratory data

FBC: Hb 94 g/L, WBC 3.9×10^9/L (neutrophils 2.6×10^9/L), platelets 138×10^9/L.

Haematinics (serum ferritin, vitamin B12 and serum folate): normal

U&Es, LFTs, bone profile and LDH: normal

Blood film

Neutrophils exhibited gross dysplastic changes, with abnormal nuclear segmentation (Figure 32.1) including hypolobated forms (Figures 32.2 and 32.3). Hypogranular forms were frequent (Figure 32.3). Blast cells were seen (10% of circulating cells); these had largely agranular cytoplasm and showed little evidence of maturation (Figures 32.4–32.6).

Bone marrow aspirate

The marrow contained hypercellular particles. Myeloblasts were easily seen (comprising 30% of cells) and, as in the blood, exhibited little evidence of maturation (Figure 32.7). Dysplastic myelomonocytic precursor cells with immature chromatin patterns and scanty granules were prominent

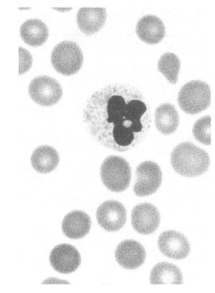

Figure 32.1 MGG, ×1000.

(Figures 32.7–32.9). The lack of nuclear segmentation of maturing cells was apparent. Erythroid precursors demonstrated granular, open chromatin (Figure 32.9) and a left shift. Megakaryocyte nuclei were hypolobated (Figure 32.10).

Flow cytometry (bone marrow aspirate)

CD34$^+$ CD117$^+$ CD33$^+$ CD13$^+$ HLA-DR$^+$ MPO$^+$ myeloblasts accounted for 34% of all events. Aberrant CD34$^+$ CD15$^+$ co-expression was seen on a proportion of these cells (20%).

Practical Flow Cytometry in Haematology: 100 Worked Examples, First Edition. Mike Leach, Mark Drummond, Allyson Doig, Pam McKay, Bob Jackson and Barbara J. Bain.
© 2015 John Wiley & Sons, Ltd. Published 2015 by John Wiley & Sons, Ltd.

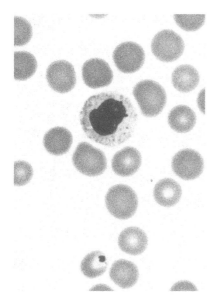

Figure 32.2 MGG, ×1000.

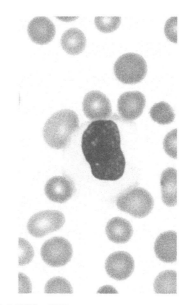

Figure 32.4 MGG, ×1000.

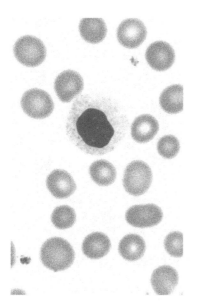

Figure 32.3 MGG, ×1000.

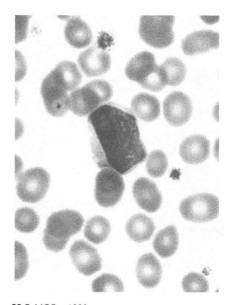

Figure 32.5 MGG, ×1000.

Histopathology

A trephine biopsy was not performed, as the aspirate was particulate.

Cytogenetic analysis

Multiple complex changes were demonstrated including del(5q), monosomy 7 and an undefined abnormality at 3q26 (*EVI1 – ecotropic virus integration-1*).

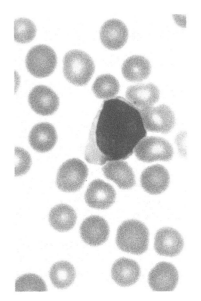

Figure 32.6 MGG, ×1000.

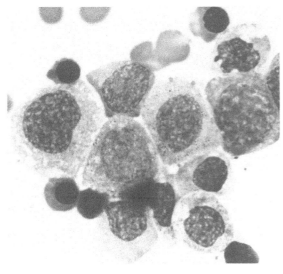

Figure 32.8 MGG, ×1000.

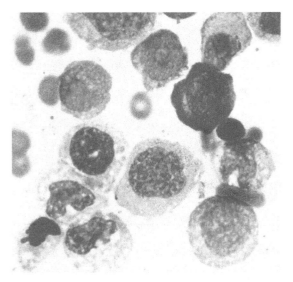

Figure 32.7 MGG, ×1000.

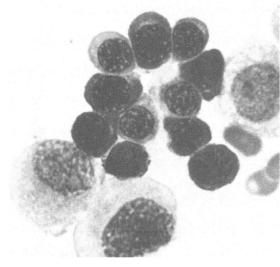

Figure 32.9 MGG, ×1000.

Discussion

The diagnosis in this case was clearly AML, given the percentage of blast cells in the marrow (30%). While some dysplastic change is frequently observed in most cases of AML (and indeed abnormal myeloid morphology in the peripheral blood is a very useful initial clue that a blast population is likely to be of myeloid lineage), the changes noted in this case were striking with few normal cells seen. Gross trilineage dysplasia was evident (i.e., involving myeloid, erythroid and megakaryocytic lineages). There was no history of an antecedent haematological disorder in this case and a normal historical FBC result was available.

Complex cytogenetic changes indicated a poor prognosis. Several authors have reported on the particularly poor outcome of patients with a monosomal karyotype (defined, e.g.,

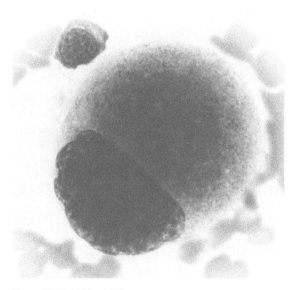

Figure 32.10 MGG, ×1000.

as a karyotype with two or more autosomal monosomies or a single autosomal monosomy plus a structural abnormality) (1, 2). In addition there was an abnormality at 3q26 (*EVI1*), this being another independent adverse cytogenetic finding (significance discussed in Case 80).

The WHO Classification recognises the entity of AML with myelodysplasia-related changes (AML-MRC), be it from a historical, morphological or cytogenetic perspective. Thus, it includes patients who have a prior history of MDS or MDS/MPN, have MDS-type cytogenetic abnormalities or have significant multi-lineage dysplasia. This case qualified as AML-MRC on both the latter parameters. Outcome in such cases is determined largely by the cytogenetic findings; a recent large study demonstrated no independent risk to outcome for the morphological changes alone and noted the poor prognosis associated with prior MDS or poor-risk cytogenetics (1). The predominance of genetic factors in prognosis of AML has also been demonstrated in *NPM1*-mutated AML, where the presence or absence of multilineage dysplasia had no additional prognostic impact (2). Thus, although morphological assessment of such cases might generate concern as to outcome, the message is clear; risk stratification should be based on genetic features and any prior history of MDS rather than morphology in isolation.

Final diagnosis

Acute myeloid leukaemia with myelodysplasia-related changes.

References

1 Grimwade, D. & Mrozek, K. (2011) Diagnostic and prognostic value of cytogenetics in acute myeloid leukemia. *Hematology/Oncology Clinics of North America.*, **25** (**6**), 1135–1161 vii. PubMed PMID: 22093581.

2 Grimwade, D., Hills, R.K., Moorman, A.V. *et al.* (2010) Refinement of cytogenetic classification in acute myeloid leukemia: determination of prognostic significance of rare recurring chromosomal abnormalities among 5876 younger adult patients treated in the United Kingdom Medical Research Council trials. *Blood.*, **116** (**3**), 354–365. PubMed PMID: 20385793.

Case 33

A 68-year-old woman presented with a short history of fatigue and sweats. On admission she appeared pale and unwell but there were no specific findings.

Laboratory data

FBC: Hb 101 g/L, WBC 92 × 10^9/L (automated differential not available) and platelets 68 × 10^9/L.

U&Es: Na 130 mmol/l, K 4.6 mmol/L, urea 14 mmol/L, creatinine 180 μmol/L.

Bone profile: calcium 2.1 mmol/L, phosphate 2.2 mmol/L, ALP 110 U/L.

LFTs: normal except albumin 26 g/L. Serum LDH 1350 U/L and urate 0.8 mmol/L.

Immunoglobulins: normal with no paraprotein.

Blood film

This showed numerous medium to large lymphoid cells with pleomorphic and folded nuclei, nucleoli and basophilic cytoplasm focally containing multiple round vacuoles that are likely to indicate lipid (Figures 33.1 and 33.2). Some circulating cells were undergoing spontaneous apoptosis (arrow, Figure 33.1).

Bone marrow aspirate

The bone marrow aspirate was heavily infiltrated by the same neoplastic cells. The cytoplasmic vacuolation was more prominent (Figure 33.3) and mitotic figures were easily identified (arrow, Figure 33.4). This morphology is typical of that seen in Burkitt lymphoma/leukaemia.

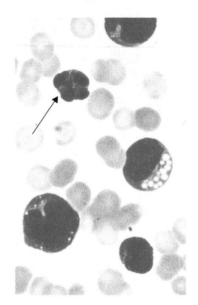

Figure 33.1 MGG, ×500.

Flow cytometry (peripheral blood and bone marrow)

The neoplastic cells had a mature B-cell phenotype expressing CD19, CD20^{mod}, CD10, FMC7, CD22, CD79b, HLA-DR and surface lambda^{bright}. This phenotype is typical of Burkitt lymphoma. Note the mature CD10$^+$ phenotype with moderate to strong expression of CD20 and surface Ig.

Imaging

Imaging using CT did not demonstrate lymphadenopathy or extranodal masses whilst the spleen was borderline enlarged.

Practical Flow Cytometry in Haematology: 100 Worked Examples, First Edition. Mike Leach, Mark Drummond, Allyson Doig, Pam McKay, Bob Jackson and Barbara J. Bain.
© 2015 John Wiley & Sons, Ltd. Published 2015 by John Wiley & Sons, Ltd.

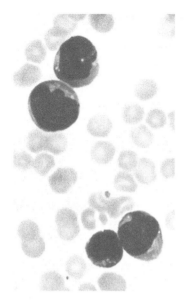

Figure 33.2 MGG, ×500.

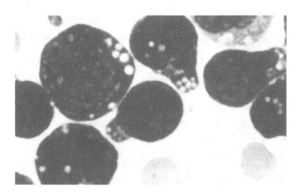

Figure 33.3 MGG, ×1000.

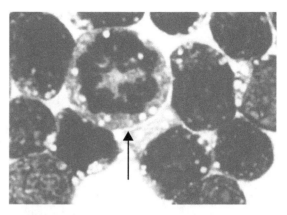

Figure 33.4 MGG, ×1000.

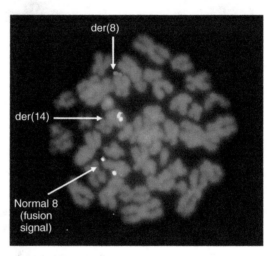

Figure 33.5 Abbott Vysis *MYC* break-apart probe.

Histopathology

Bone marrow trephine biopsy sections showed maximal cellularity due to involvement by the cells described above. These had a CD20$^+$, CD10$^+$, BCL6$^+$, BCL2$^-$ phenotype, typical of Burkitt lymphoma.

FISH studies

FISH profiling using a *MYC* break-apart probe on the bone marrow trephine biopsy section showed a split signal in virtually all cells examined in keeping with a *MYC* rearrangement (Figure 33.5). The translocation partner was *IGH* at 14q32 and this was demonstrated using an *IGH/MYC* dual-fusion FISH probe (Figure 33.6).

Cytogenetics

Standard metaphase karyotyping identified a t(8;14)(q24;q32) (Figure 33.7). No additional abnormalities were identified.

Discussion

The clinical presentation was in keeping with a high-grade neoplasm with a marked leucocytosis, high LDH, hyperuricaemia, bone marrow failure and early renal failure. The peripheral blood and bone marrow morphology were

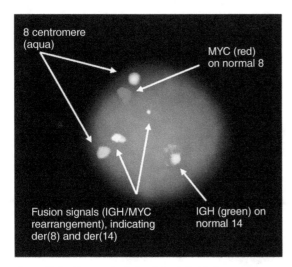

Figure 33.6 Abbott Vysis *IGH/MYC* CEP 8 dual-fusion probe.

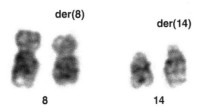

Figure 33.7 Metaphase cytogenetic preparation showing t(8;14) (q24;q32).

typical of Burkitt lymphoma/leukaemia. In this case the presentation was as leukaemia as the disease was primarily affecting bone marrow and blood whilst other 'tissue disease' was not readily apparent. Immunophenotyping and immunohistochemistry studies showed a mature CD10+ BCL2− B-cell phenotype and FISH/cytogenetics identified the classic *MYC/IGH* rearrangement, t(8;14)(q24;q32) without additional abnormalities. *MYC* rearrangement to the kappa gene at 2p12 or lambda gene at 22q11 is seen in a minority of cases but translocations to other sites and additional cytogenetic abnormalities are not in keeping with this diagnosis. Gene expression profiling in BL shows a distinct signature unlike the heterogeneous signatures seen within the entity we call diffuse large B-cell lymphoma.

Burkitt lymphoma (BL) is a highly proliferative neoplasm often presenting with a short history, massive tumour bulk and spontaneous tumour lysis. It occurs in three clinical circumstances. Endemic BL is seen in equatorial Africa, Indonesia and Papua New Guinea mainly in children who typically present with large extranodal tumours affecting the maxillae and mandible. It is Epstein-Barr virus (EBV) driven and occurs in the context of immunodeficiency and immune

stimulation resulting from recurrent malaria infection. Immunodeficiency-associated BL is most frequently seen in association with human immunodeficiency virus (HIV) infection. It can develop early in the disease course and is not necessarily seen in patients with very low CD4 counts unlike many other HIV-related tumours. Sporadic BL, as seen in this patient, occurs worldwide and mainly affects children and young adults without immunodeficiency. It may have a leukaemic or lymphomatous presentation. The latter is more common and multiple extranodal sites are commonly affected. This entity is less often linked to EBV than endemic cases though the virus can be identified in tumour cells in about one third of patients.

All three BL variants have a propensity for central nervous system involvement, either affecting the brain parenchyma, meninges or both. This can occur at presentation or during treatment if CNS-directed therapies are not included in the treatment schedule. All modern BL protocols incorporate cytotoxic drugs capable of crossing the blood brain barrier (methotrexate, ifosfamide, cytarabine) with additional intrathecal injections. Rituximab should also be routinely used in view of the regular moderate to strong expression of CD20.

Sporadic BL is often a rewarding condition to treat as this highly proliferative neoplasm is particularly chemotherapy sensitive. Short intense chemotherapy protocols are capable of inducing high cure rates in BL in children and young adults (including HIV-infected patients) but the co-morbidities and reduced cardiovascular reserve seen in some older patients make treatment more challenging in this group. This tumour is so sensitive to chemotherapy and the response is so rapid, that tumour-lysis syndrome becomes a major consideration. Before urate oxidases were available for clinical use many patients died of acute renal failure and hyperkalaemia after exposure to the first doses of chemotherapy and/or corticosteroids. Recombinant urate oxidase is now routinely used with hyperhydration in the early management of BL alongside chemotherapy and many deaths due to the inevitable tumour-lysis syndrome have been prevented.

Because of the rapid tumour growth and the possibility of tumour-lysis, BL should be regarded as a medical emergency. Suspicion of the diagnosis requires urgent immunophenotyping and FISH analysis.

Final diagnosis

Burkitt lymphoma presenting as leukaemia (previously known as acute lymphoblastic leukaemia, L3 in FAB classification).

Case 34

A 70-year-old woman presented with a recent history of profound fatigue, night sweats and weight loss. She had particularly been troubled by painful bulky cervical lymphadenopathy of recent rapid onset. She was referred for haematology assessment by a medical team who had arranged a core biopsy of a left inguinal lymph node. This node showed typical morphological and immunophenotypic features of mantle cell lymphoma (MCL) with evidence of a t(11;14) in the majority of cells on analysis by FISH.

On examination the patient appeared pale, gaunt and irritable. She had marked bilateral cervical lymphadenopathy. The nodal masses were conglomerate and were firm, warm and tender to touch. She also had large palpable nodes in the axillae and less bulky nodes in the groins.

Laboratory results

FBC: Hb 91 g/L, MCV 90 fl, WBC 13.4 × 10^9/L (neutrophils 9.25 × 10^9/L, lymphocytes 2.39 × 10^9/L) and platelets 36 × 10^9/L. ESR was 105 mm/h.

Immunoglobulins showed a polyclonal increase without a paraprotein.

U&Es and bone profile: normal. LFTs normal except albumin 24 g/L.

Imaging

A CT scan performed by the referring team had shown widespread bulky lymphadenopathy with individual nodes up to 3 cm diameter. The spleen was moderately enlarged at 18 cm but no extra-nodal masses were apparent.

Blood film

The film showed normochromic red cells, rouleaux, a mild neutrophilia and true thrombocytopenia (Figure 34.1). No primitive cells or abnormal lymphoid cells were seen but plasma cells were noted (Figures 34.2–34.4) and these appeared somewhat atypical.

Flow cytometry (peripheral blood)

It was important to screen peripheral blood not only for abnormal lymphoid cells but also to characterise the plasma

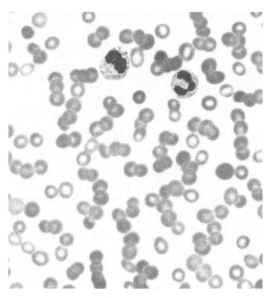

Figure 34.1 MGG, ×500.

Practical Flow Cytometry in Haematology: 100 Worked Examples, First Edition. Mike Leach, Mark Drummond, Allyson Doig, Pam McKay, Bob Jackson and Barbara J. Bain.
© 2015 John Wiley & Sons, Ltd. Published 2015 by John Wiley & Sons, Ltd.

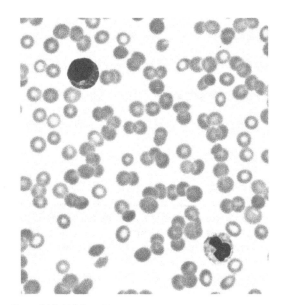

Figure 34.2 MGG, ×500.

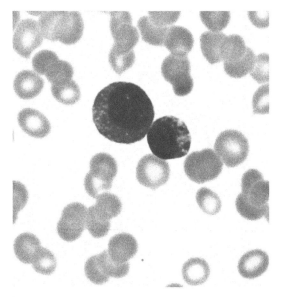

Figure 34.3 MGG, ×1000.

cells that were obvious morphologically. There was no evidence of a monoclonal B-cell population and notably there was no aberrant CD5$^+$/CD19$^+$ clone such as might have been expected in mantle cell lymphoma. No abnormal T cells were apparent. There was a significant plasmacytosis but the cells had a normal phenotype (CD38$^+$, CD138$^+$, CD19$^+$, CD45^{dim} and CD56$^-$).

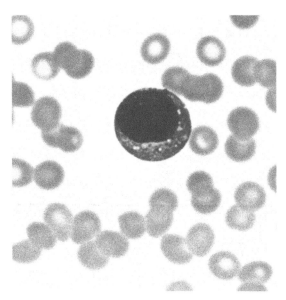

Figure 34.4 MGG, ×1000.

Flow cytometry (bone marrow aspirate)

As in the peripheral blood, an excess of phenotypically normal plasma cells was identified, comprising 10–15% of cells. There was no evidence of a T-cell or B-cell proliferation.

Bone marrow trephine biopsy

Trephine biopsy sections appeared hypercellular and reactive with a prominent myeloid cells (neutrophil and eosinophil series), lymphocytes and plasma cells. Erythroid activity was reduced but megakaryocytes were easily identified. No malignant infiltrate was apparent.

Clinical course

The clinical symptoms seemed disproportionate to the identified pathology. Mantle cell lymphoma is very variable in its presentation and behaviour but a number of features remained unexplained. The anaemia and thrombocytopenia were not due to bone marrow disease. Secondly, there appeared to be a marked inflammatory phenomenon in evolution and finally the extent of clinical deterioration and tenderness of neck nodes was not explained. Despite the documented history of confirmed mantle cell lymphoma, verified on second review, a further biopsy targeting a tender neck node was undertaken. In the interim, due to a progressive clinical decline, the patient was treated with high dose cytarabine and rituximab but with no meaningful improvement.

Histopathology

The second biopsy, taken from a tender neck node, showed complete effacement by a polymorphous lymphoid cell population comprised of small, intermediate and large lymphocytes (Figures 34.5 and 34.6) some with prominent nucleoli (Figure 34.7) admixed with histiocytes and plasma cells. Many cells had a prominent cytoplasmic halo and blood vessels were prominent. The neoplastic population expressed CD2, CD3 (Figure 34.8) and CD5 but CD7 was largely lost (Figure 34.9). Cyclin D1 (normally expressed in endothelial cell nuclei) was not expressed by the lymphoid cells (Figure 34.10) but PD-1 showed strong membrane positivity (Figure 34.11). Programmed death 1 (PD-1, CD279) is normally expressed in germinal centre-associated T helper cells; it is frequently positive in angioimmunoblastic T-cell lymphoma. The features in the second core biopsy indicated a T-cell lymphoma most likely of angioimmunoblastic T-cell lymphoma (AITCL) subtype.

With the knowledge of a second diagnosis of T-cell lymphoma and with the benefit of hindsight the original core biopsy was reviewed. This did show two different zones within the biopsy core, defined clearly by CD20 expression (Figure 34.12).

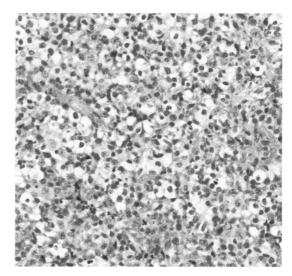

Figure 34.6 H&E, ×200.

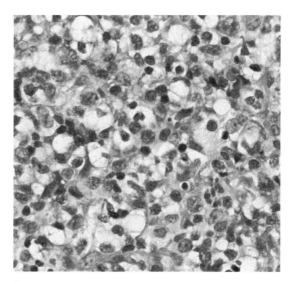

Figure 34.7 H&E, ×400.

The first population was CD20+ with co-expression of CD5 and cyclin D1 (Figures 34.13 and 34.14) in keeping with mantle cell lymphoma.

The second, however, was CD20−, cyclin D1− and expressed T-cell markers and PD-1 in keeping with the diagnosis of AITCL, as described above. This review therefore confirmed the coexistence of unrelated B-cell and T-cell lymphomas in the same lymph node cores.

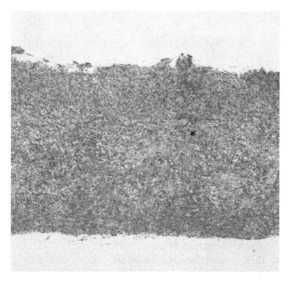

Figure 34.5 H&E, ×40.

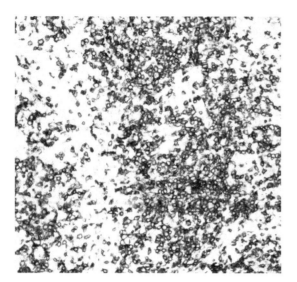

Figure 34.8 CD3, ×100.

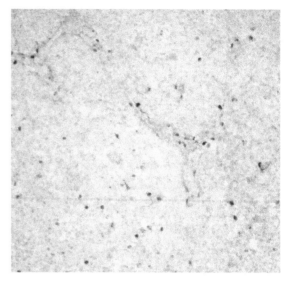

Figure 34.10 Cyclin D1, ×100.

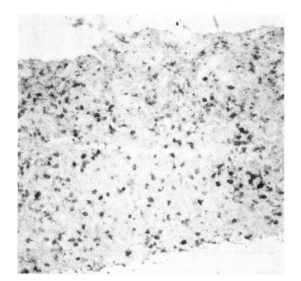

Figure 34.9 CD7, ×100.

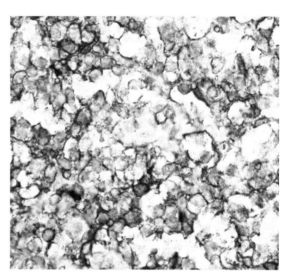

Figure 34.11 PD-1 (CD279), ×400.

Discussion

It is always important to correlate the patient's presenting symptoms and laboratory findings with the working diagnosis based on blood, bone marrow, lymph node, spleen or extra-nodal tissue biopsy. In cases where there is apparent discrepancy one of the following scenarios should be considered:

1. The initial biopsy has been misinterpreted.

2. There is a transformation or complication of the identified disease entity.

3. A second EBV-related lymphoma has developed as a result of immunosuppression caused by the first lymphoma/leukaemia or its treatment (e.g. in some examples of Richter syndrome in CLL).

4. There are two unrelated diagnoses.

This case falls into the fourth group and importantly it appears that the T-cell lymphoma was largely responsible for

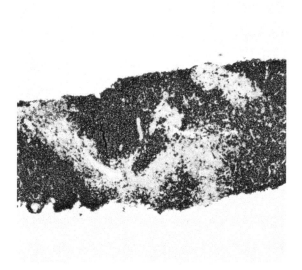

Figure 34.12 CD20, ×40.

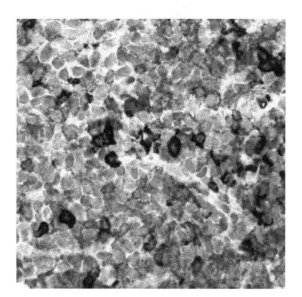

Figure 34.13 CD5, ×400.

her symptoms. Angioimmunoblastic T-cell lymphoma is a great mimic. It is associated with marked systemic upset with fever, rashes, normocytic anaemia, consumptive cytopenias, polyclonal hypergammaglobulinaemia and occasionally circulating reactive plasma cells. Flow cytometry can also identify low levels of circulating neoplastic cells in some cases, these having a CD3+, CD10+ phenotype (1). This case

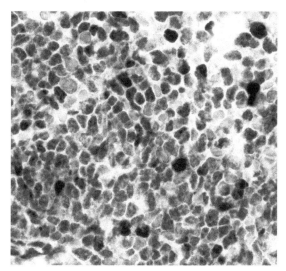

Figure 34.14 Cyclin D1, ×400.

also calls into question the role of core biopsy in assessing patients with lymphadenopathy. Although core biopsy is now commonly employed in the diagnosis of lymphoma with a diagnostic success rate of between 65% and 85%, it is likely that some complex cases are misinterpreted. An initial excision biopsy might have clearly revealed the dual pathology in the patient described. Corticosteroids are an important component of therapy as the T-cell clone appears to generate a systemic inflammatory reaction and monotherapy with corticosteroids can improve performance status in some patients prior to definitive therapy. This patient was subsequently treated with CHOP and showed prompt resolution of all her symptoms, lymphadenopathy and laboratory abnormalities. CT imaging showed a complete response indicating that the chosen treatment has been effective for both disease entities.

Final diagnoses

1. Peripheral T-cell lymphoma, angioimmunoblastic subtype
2. Mantle cell lymphoma

Reference

1 Baseggio, L., Berger, F., Morel, D. *et al.* (2006) Identification of circulating CD10 positive T cells in angioimmunoblastic T-cell lymphoma. *Leukemia, UK*, **20** (**2**), 296–303. PubMed PMID: 16341050.

35

Case 35

An 18-month-old boy had recently become unwell with pallor, irritability and anorexia. On examination he appeared ill, was uninterested in his surroundings and cried easily. Of note he had firm periorbital swellings bilaterally. There was no organomegaly or lymphadenopathy.

Laboratory data

FBC: Hb 68 g/L, WBC 11.8 × 10^9/L (neutrophils 2.4 × 10^9/L, lymphocytes 7.2 × 10^9/L, monocytes 1.6 × 10^9/L) and platelets 109 × 10^9/L.

U&Es: Na 135 mmol/l, K 4.1 mmol/L, urea 5.3 mmol/L, creatinine 18 μmol/L.

Bone profile: calcium 2.45 mmol/L, phosphate 1.72 mmol/L, ALP 233 U/L.

LFTs: normal except albumin 37 g/L and AST 70 U/L.

LDH: 1255 U/L.

Blood film

The film did not show any informative features but blast cells were not seen.

Bone marrow aspirate

The aspirate was aparticulate but hypercellular and showed an infiltrate of medium to large undifferentiated cells forming clumps in some areas of the film (Figure 35.1). The cells had prominent nucleoli and mitotic figures were frequent (Figure 35.2). There was some moulding of nuclei by adjacent cells. There was some fibrillar extracellular

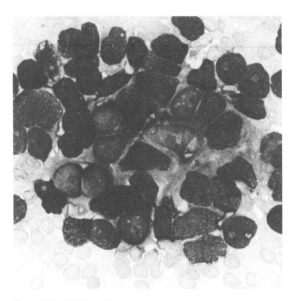

Figure 35.1 MGG, ×500.

material (Figure 35.1). The overall morphology was suggestive of a non-haemopoietic neoplasm rather than acute lymphoblastic leukaemia.

Flow cytometry

A CD45 versus SSC analysis revealed a large population of CD45⁻ cells shown in red (Figure 35.3) in contrast to the residual small populations of lymphocytes (green), monocytes (magenta) and myeloid precursors (blue). These cells did not show lineage-specific haemopoietic markers (cytoplasmic CD3, CD19/79a or MPO) but did express CD15

Practical Flow Cytometry in Haematology: 100 Worked Examples, First Edition. Mike Leach, Mark Drummond, Allyson Doig, Pam McKay, Bob Jackson and Barbara J. Bain.
© 2015 John Wiley & Sons, Ltd. Published 2015 by John Wiley & Sons, Ltd.

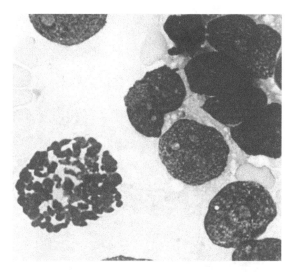

Figure 35.2 MGG, ×1000.

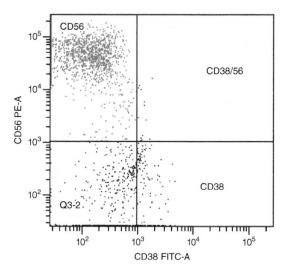

Figure 35.4 CD56/CD38.

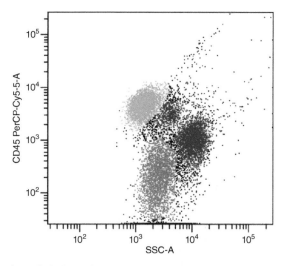

Figure 35.3 CD45/SSC.

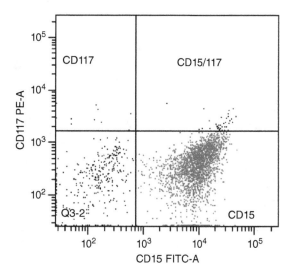

Figure 35.5 CD117/CD15.

and CD56^{strong} (Figures 35.4 and 35.5); these two antigens are not lineage specific and can be expressed by a variety of non-haemopoietic neoplasms. The most likely tumour involving bone marrow and causing periorbital swelling in a child of this age is neuroblastoma. Neuroblastomas frequently show CD56 positivity, often together with CD15.

Imaging

Extensive imaging was undertaken using CT and MRI. Together they identified an irregular lobulated partly calcified mass lesion in the left paravertebral region. It extended from the level of the upper pole of left kidney up toward the arch of the aorta (Figure 35.6, MRI (arrow) and Figure 35.7, CT (arrow)). In addition there appeared to be tumour deposits in a number of ribs, in the skull and within the dura over the frontal cortex of the brain (Figure 35.8, MRI (arrow)).

Bone marrow trephine biopsies (bilateral)

The marrow was extensively infiltrated by a poorly differentiated small spindled 'blue cell' tumour forming

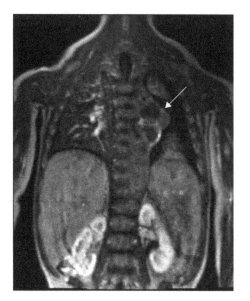

Figure 35.6 MRI.

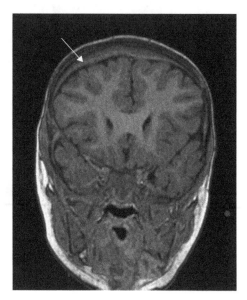

Figure 35.8 MRI.

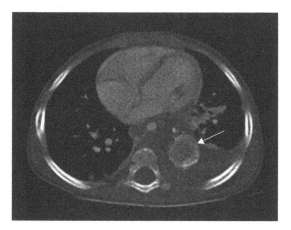

Figure 35.7 CT.

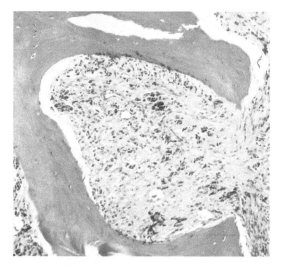

Figure 35.9 H&E, ×100.

neuropil (a fine fibrillary matrix between cells) (Figures 35.9 and 35.10). Rosettes and palisades were not prominent. Immunoreactivity for neural-specific markers (synaptophysin and NB84 (Figure 35.11)) was identified together with CD56 positivity (Figure 35.12). The findings were diagnostic of a metastatic poorly differentiated neuroblastoma with both trephine biopsy specimens being involved.

Discussion

Neuroblastoma is a tumour derived from neural crest cells of the adrenal glands or from the paravertebral sympathetic chain. The median age at diagnosis is 21 months. It has a tendency to develop early widespread metastases to bone marrow and bones of the skull. Anaemia or pancytopenia is common at presentation. The tumour cells are frequently present in bone marrow aspirates and clearly need to be differentiated from lymphoblasts of acute lymphoblastic leukaemia which is the commonest tumour affecting this age group. The morphology can appear similar but the tendency of neuroblastoma to form clumps and the associated

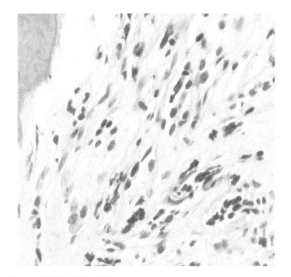

Figure 35.10 H&E, ×500.

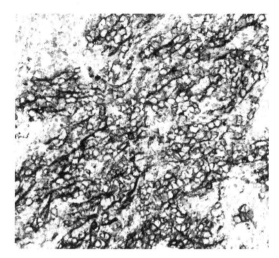

Figure 35.12 CD56, ×200.

neuropil should alert the morphologist to this diagnosis. Furthermore, this tumour is always CD45$^-$ and the presence of non-lineage-specific antigen expression by flow cytometry (CD56 and CD15) should alert the clinician to the diagnosis. In fact the presence of such antigens, in the absence of CD45, cytoplasmic CD3, CD19/cytoplasmic CD79a and MPO, can strengthen the working diagnosis until it is fully confirmed using a full panel of immunohistochemical markers on the trephine biopsy sections.

Final diagnosis

Metastatic neuroblastoma with bone marrow involvement.

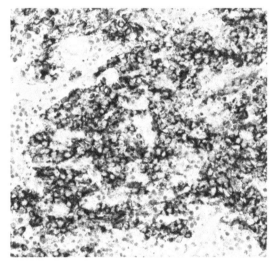

Figure 35.11 NB84, ×200.

36

Case 36

A 24-year-old male was transferred to our unit from another city after presenting with a short history of bruising, epistaxis and visual disturbance. He was found to have bilateral extensive retinal haemorrhages with involvement of the macula of the left eye. There was no palpable lymphadenopathy or organomegaly.

Laboratory data

FBC: Hb 81 g/L, WBC 255 × 10^9/L (neutrophils 0.5 × 10^9/L) and platelets 51 × 10^9/L.

Coagulation screen: PT 15 s, APTT 25 s, TT 25 s, fibrinogen 0.7 g/L and D-dimers 7725 ng/mL.

U&Es, LFTs, bone profile: normal. Serum LDH was 715 U/L.

Blood film

This showed a large population of small compact blasts with nuclear indentations, convolutions and nucleoli (Figures 36.1–36.4). The nucleoli appeared 'cup-like' in some cells (Figure 36.3). There were a small number of residual neutrophils without dysplastic features.

Bone marrow aspirate

This was heavily infiltrated by blasts similar to those described in the blood; erythroid and myeloid activity was significantly reduced (Figures 36.5 and 36.6).

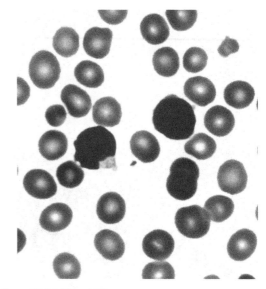

Figure 36.1 MGG, ×1000.

Flow cytometry

The blast cells were easily identified in the CD45^{dim} gate and expressed weak CD34, cCD79a, CD19, HLA-DR and CD15. TdT, CD10, CD20, cCD3, were not expressed. MPO and other myeloid markers were absent.

Histopathology

A bone marrow trephine biopsy was not performed.

Practical Flow Cytometry in Haematology: 100 Worked Examples, First Edition. Mike Leach, Mark Drummond, Allyson Doig, Pam McKay, Bob Jackson and Barbara J. Bain.
© 2015 John Wiley & Sons, Ltd. Published 2015 by John Wiley & Sons, Ltd.

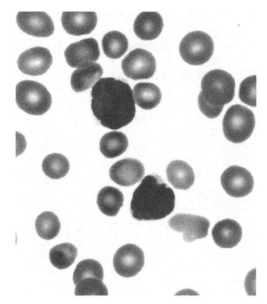

Figure 36.2 MGG, ×1000.

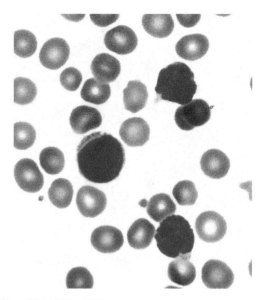

Figure 36.4 MGG, ×1000.

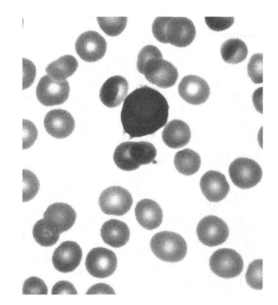

Figure 36.3 MGG, ×1000.

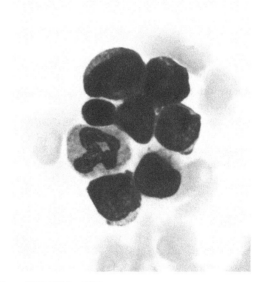

Figure 36.5 MGG, ×1000.

Cytogenetics

46,XY,t(4;11)(q21;q23) was identified in 15/18 cells examined. The remaining cells had a normal karyotype.

FISH studies

A *MLL* break apart probe showed an abnormal pattern in 97/106 cells examined in keeping with the above result.

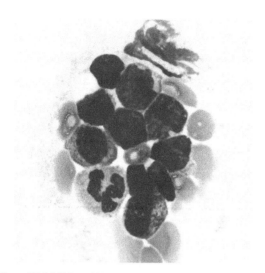

Figure 36.6 MGG, ×1000.

Molecular studies

RT-PCR for *BCR-ABL1* was negative.

Discussion

The presentation here was of a high white cell count acute leukaemia with disseminated intravascular coagulation and associated retinal haemorrhages.

The morphology and immunophenotyping are in keeping with a lymphoblastic leukaemia, more specifically a pro-B cell leukaemia with aberrant expression of CD15. The cells showed B-lineage specificity and the pro-B cell stage of maturation of the cell of origin is indicated by the lack of CD10. Aberrant myeloid markers (CD15, CD13 and CD33) are frequently expressed in pro-B ALL and may be associated with the presence of t(4;11). The only unusual feature here was the absence of the TdT expression that would have been expected in such a primitive lymphoid neoplasm.

Disseminated intravascular coagulation is frequently observed at presentation in patients with AML (particularly APL where it is almost universal) triggered by the procoagulant activity of the myeloid granules and cytoplasmic enzymes. It is seen much less frequently in ALL but has long been recognised in a subset of cases. It has been implicated in haemorrhagic complications (1) (as in this patient) so should be managed accordingly and not be discounted as an incidental laboratory anomaly. It appears to be more common in adults than children but does not appear to be associated with any specific cytogenetic subgroup or phenotype. The coagulopathy can be induced or aggravated by chemotherapy as tissue factor-like procoagulant agents are released at induction of cell death.

Pro-B ALL with aberrant myeloid antigen expression (in particular CD15) is associated with *MLL* gene rearrangement, typically t(4;11)(q21;q23) (2). It has long been recognised as an adverse cytogenetic subgroup in terms of progression-free and overall survival, and historically this finding has been a clear indication for consideration of allogeneic transplantation in first remission (3). However, with the introduction of intensive risk-stratified contemporary ALL regimens, with management decisions modified on the basis of MRD levels following induction and consolidation, transplantation may not be necessary in all patients (4).

Final diagnosis

Pro-B cell acute lymphoblastic leukaemia with t(4;11) and disseminated intravascular coagulation at presentation.

References

1 Higuchi, T., Toyama, D., Hirota, Y. *et al.* (2005) Disseminated intravascular coagulation complicating acute lymphoblastic leukemia: a study of childhood and adult cases. *Leukemia & Lymphoma*, **46** (8), 1169–1176. PubMed PMID: 16085558.

2 Seegmiller, A.C., Kroft, S.H., Karandikar, N.J. & McKenna, R.W. (2009) Characterization of immunophenotypic aberrancies in 200 cases of B acute lymphoblastic leukemia. *American Journal of Clinical Pathology*, **132** (6), 940–949. PubMed PMID: 19926587.

3 Marks, D.I., Moorman, A.V., Chilton, L. *et al.* (2013) The clinical characteristics, therapy and outcome of 85 adults with acute lymphoblastic leukemia and t(4;11)(q21;q23)/MLL-AFF1 prospectively treated in the UKALLXII/ECOG2993 trial. *Haematologica*, **98** (6), 945–952. PubMed PMID: 23349309.

4 Ribera, J.M., Oriol, A., Morgades, M. *et al.* (2014) Treatment of high-risk Philadelphia chromosome-negative acute lymphoblastic leukemia in adolescents and adults according to early cytologic response and minimal residual disease after consolidation assessed by flow cytometry: final results of the PETHEMA ALL-AR-03 trial. *Journal of Clinical Oncology: Official Journal of the American Society of Clinical Oncology*, **32** (15), 1595–1604. PubMed PMID: 24752047.

37

Case 37

A 38-year-old man, previously well, presented to his local Accident & Emergency department with a 4 to 5 week history of thirst, polyuria, fatigue and spontaneous bruising. Routine blood tests were done.

Laboratory data

FBC: Hb 71 g/L, WBC 6.1×10^9/L (neutrophils 1.0×10^9/L, blast cells 1.8×10^9/L) and platelets 422×10^9/L.

Biochemistry: Na$^+$ 149 mmol/L, K$^+$ 5.2 mmol/L, serum osmolality 305 mOsm/L and urine osmolality 201 mOsm/L.

LFTs, bone profile and LDH: normal.

Blood film

This demonstrated neutrophil dysplasia (Figures 37.1 and 37.2), blast cells (Figure 37.3), hypogranular platelets (Figure 37.4) and frequent nucleated red blood cells with some dysplastic forms (Figure 37.5). Some neutrophils showed a single round non-segmented nucleus (Figure 37.6).

Bone marrow aspirate

This was of consistently poor quality and paucicellular. Flow cytometry was performed.

Flow cytometry

This demonstrated a myeloblast population comprising 42% of marrow cells, with the immunophenotype CD34$^+$,

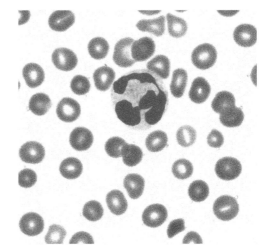

Figure 37.1 MGG, ×1000.

CD117$^+$, CD33$^+$, CD13$^+$, HLA-DR$^+$, CD38$^+$ and MPO$^+$ along with aberrant expression of CD2 and CD7.

This confirmed a hypercellular marrow (80%) with a diffuse infiltrate of myeloblasts on a dysplastic marrow background.

Cytogenetics

45,XY,-7,t(3;3)(q21;q26.2).

Practical Flow Cytometry in Haematology: 100 Worked Examples, First Edition. Mike Leach, Mark Drummond, Allyson Doig, Pam McKay, Bob Jackson and Barbara J. Bain.
© 2015 John Wiley & Sons, Ltd. Published 2015 by John Wiley & Sons, Ltd.

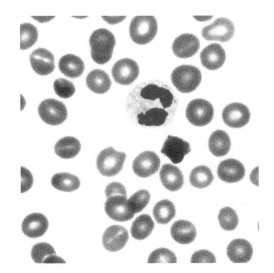

Figure 37.2 MGG, ×1000.

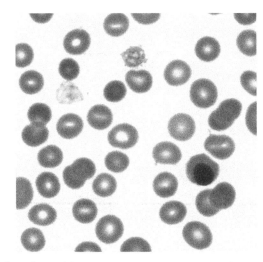

Figure 37.4 MGG, ×1000.

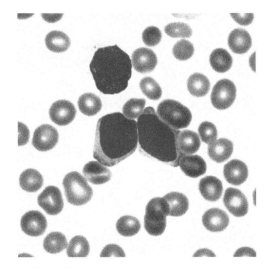

Figure 37.3 MGG, ×1000.

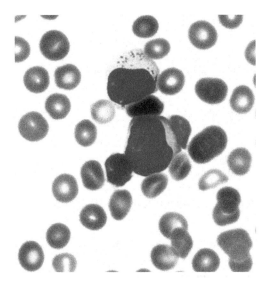

Figure 37.5 MGG, ×1000.

Additional investigations

MRI of pituitary: possibility of early hypophysitis, with an incidental 7 mm pituitary cyst.

Pituitary axis testing: panhypopituitarism.

Discussion

This case illustrates the rare but well-recognised association between diabetes insipidus and AML with specific cytogenetic/molecular genetic abnormalities (−7, 3q rearrangements involving the *EVI1* gene and *RUNX1* mutation) (reviewed in (1)). Panhypopituitarism has also been described in this setting, as in our case. The association of structural chromosomal abnormalities at 3q21 and 3q26 with preservation of a normal platelet count or even thrombocytosis, abnormal megakaryocyte morphology and poor outcome is also well documented. Thrombocytosis is of course unusual in AML, with thrombocytopenia being more usual and its recognition should prompt consideration of these associated cytogenetic abnormalities. The mechanism

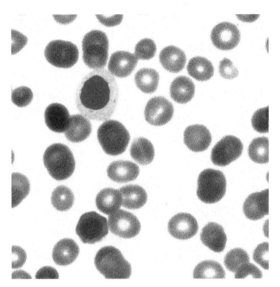

Figure 37.6 MGG, ×1000.

of the diabetes insipidus remains obscure, with MRI imaging of the pituitary gland often being unhelpful in such cases. The prognostic significance of *EVI1* overexpression would seem to extend beyond those patients with cytogenetically detected 3q rearrangements: a recent study has documented increased expression of *EVI1 per se* as a poor risk feature, even in patients lacking typical rearrangements (2).

The prognosis of AML with *EVI1* gene rearrangements is dismal (36% CR rate with intensive induction chemotherapy,

6% 5-year survival (Professor A. Burnett, Personal Communication, 2011)). Accordingly this patient was treated with two courses of FLAG-IDA chemotherapy, with achievement of morphological CR after the first cycle (1.7% blast cells detectable by flow cytometry). A matched unrelated donor transplant was performed in first CR, but unfortunately the patient relapsed after 6 months and died of disease.

Final diagnosis

AML with t(3;3)(q21;q26.2), monosomy 7 and associated diabetes insipidus.

References

1 Cull, E.H., Watts, J.M., Tallman, M.S. *et al.* (2014) Acute myeloid leukemia presenting with panhypopituitarism or diabetes insipidus: a case series with molecular genetic analysis and review of the literature. *Leukemia & Lymphoma*, **55**, (**9**), 2125–2129. PMID: 24286261

2 Groschel, S., Lugthart, S., Schlenk, R.F. *et al.* (2010) High EVI1 expression predicts outcome in younger adult patients with acute myeloid leukemia and is associated with distinct cytogenetic abnormalities. *Journal of Clinical Oncology*, **28**, 2101–2107.

38

Case 38

A 56-year-old female was referred for investigation of chronic neutropenia. She was clinically well and there was no history of significant infection. Her only regular medication was hormone replacement therapy.

Laboratory results

FBC: Hb 125 g/L, WBC 3.19×10^9/L (neutrophils 0.38×10^9/L, lymphocytes 2.5×10^9/L) and platelets 189×10^9/L.

U&Es, LFTs and bone profile were normal.

Rheumatoid factor and anti-nuclear antibody screens were negative.

Blood film

The film confirmed neutropenia. No primitive cells or features of dysplasia were identified. There was a prominent population of large granular lymphocytes (LGLs), medium to large cells with a moderate amount of cytoplasm and numerous distinct azurophilic granules (Figures 38.1 – 38.3).

Flow cytometry

T and NK cells represented 98% of cells in the lymphoid gate with B cells just 2% of events. The T-lymphocyte population was abnormal showing an excess of CD8$^+$ cells (CD4:CD8 ratio 1:3) (Figure 38.4). The CD8-positive cells expressed CD2, CD3 and CD5. About half of them were aberrant with loss or partial expression of CD7, loss of CD26 and combined positivity for CD56 and CD57. Note the two populations of T cells in Figure 38.5. The abnormal

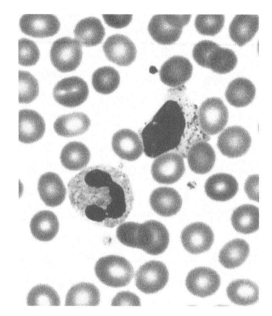

Figure 38.1 MGG, ×1000.

population (P1) shows reduced intensity of CD2 expression with the majority being CD26$^-$. The normal T cells (P2) show brighter CD2 expression and the majority are CD26$^+$. The cells in population P1 expressed CD56 and CD57.

Molecular studies

Polymerase chain reaction (PCR) for T-cell receptor gamma (TCRγ) gene rearrangement was performed on the same peripheral blood sample and detected a peak consistent with the presence of a monoclonal T-cell proliferation.

Practical Flow Cytometry in Haematology: 100 Worked Examples, First Edition. Mike Leach, Mark Drummond, Allyson Doig, Pam McKay, Bob Jackson and Barbara J. Bain.
© 2015 John Wiley & Sons, Ltd. Published 2015 by John Wiley & Sons, Ltd.

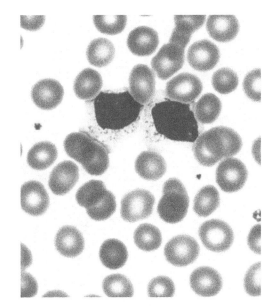

Figure 38.2 MGG, ×1000.

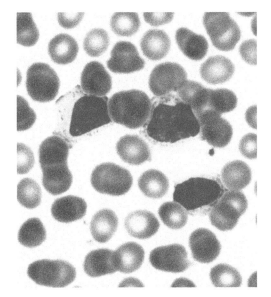

Figure 38.3 MGG, ×1000.

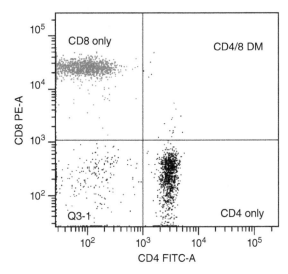

Figure 38.4 CD4/CD8.

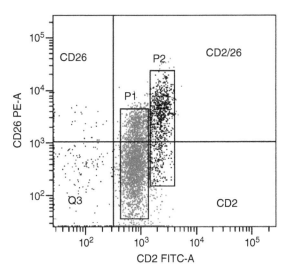

Figure 38.5 CD2/CD26.

Discussion

Large granular lymphocytes are either NK cells or CD8$^+$ cytotoxic T cells, which are important components of the innate immune system. They are capable of responding, without priming by other cells, to a variety of immunological challenges. They are often prominent in peripheral blood as a reaction to infective, inflammatory and neoplastic disorders.

Clonal LGL proliferations, known as LGL leukaemia, may be found incidentally but they can be implicated in the pathogenesis of neutropenia, autoimmune haemolytic anaemia and acquired red cell aplasia (1). This condition rarely causes lymphadenopathy but can cause splenomegaly. Most patients present with an absolute LGL count of greater than 2×10^9/L, with the LGL showing immunophenotypic aberrancy. A monoclonal T-cell population is detectable in

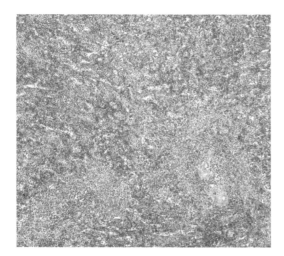

Figure 38.6 H&E, ×40.

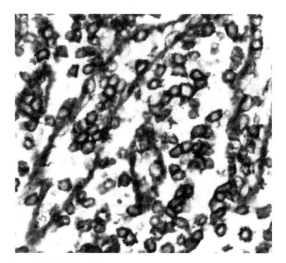

Figure 38.8 CD3, ×400.

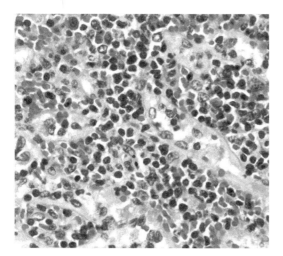

Figure 38.7 H&E, ×400.

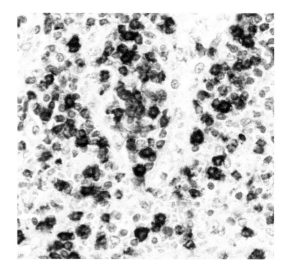

Figure 38.9 CD57, ×400.

the peripheral blood by PCR. Some patients, as in this case, do not show a clear lymphocytosis so the proliferation may be missed unless a blood film is examined carefully. There is an association with autoimmune disorders, particularly rheumatoid arthritis, where the LGL proliferations may be implicated in neutropenia. It can occur in the form of a post-transplant lymphoproliferative disorder and rarely also in association with myeloid disorders and B-cell leukaemias and lymphomas (chronic lymphocytic leukaemia, hairy cell leukaemia and splenic marginal zone lymphoma).

The supplementary images show T-LGL involvement of a spleen removed from another patient with a history of treated marginal zone lymphoma (Figures 38.6 and 38.7).

This shows diffuse infiltration of the red pulp with a striking peri- and intrasinusoidal distribution of the CD3$^+$, CD8$^+$, CD57$^+$ cells (Figures 38.8 and 38.9).

Interestingly, the spleen showed no evidence of involvement by marginal zone lymphoma.

The immunophenotype of the LGL leukaemia in this neutropenic patient was typical: CD8$^+$ with co-expression of CD2, CD3 and CD57, some loss of CD7 and loss of CD26. CD56 is expressed in a proportion of cases of T-cell LGL leukaemia but is more often associated with NK-cell proliferations. In contrast, the latter are usually CD2$^+$, CD16$^+$, CD56$^+$, CD7$^{+/-}$ but importantly CD3$^-$, CD4$^-$

and CD8⁻, whilst *TCR* gene rearrangements are not seen. The differentiation of reactive LGL lymphocytosis from LGL leukaemia can be difficult. The presence of *TCR* gene rearrangements is supportive of clonal proliferation. Flow cytometric evaluation of two TCR targets, TCRbeta and TCRgamma can provide strong evidence of clonality (2). Furthermore, the recent identification of *STAT3* mutations provides the strongest basis yet for defining LGL clonality and importantly appears to predict the cases likely to complicated by red cell aplasia and neutropenia (3, 4).

The management of T-cell LGL leukaemia has to be tailored to the clinical circumstances. The patient described here has not required any intervention so far since, although the neutropenia is a likely consequence of the LGL proliferation, infective complications have not been encountered.

Final diagnosis

T-cell large granular lymphocytic leukaemia.

References

1 Watters, R.J., Liu, X., Loughran, T.P. Jr., (2011) T-cell and natural killer-cell large granular lymphocyte leukemia neoplasias. *Leukemia & Lymphoma*, **52** (**12**), 2217–2225. PubMed PMID: 21749307.

2 Qiu, Z.Y., Wen-Yi, S., Fan, L. *et al.* (2014) Assessment of clonality in T-cell large granular lymphocytic leukemia: flow cytometric T cell receptor Vbeta repertoire and T cell receptor gene rearrangement. *Leukemia & Lymphoma*, **14**, 1–21. PubMed PMID: 24828862.

3 Jerez, A., Clemente, M.J., Makishima, H. *et al.* (2012) STAT3 mutations unify the pathogenesis of chronic lymphoproliferative disorders of NK cells and T-cell large granular lymphocyte leukemia. *Blood*, **120** (**15**), 3048–3057. PubMed PMID: 22859607.

4 Koskela, H.L., Eldfors, S., Ellonen, P. *et al.* (2012) Somatic STAT3 mutations in large granular lymphocytic leukemia. *The New England Journal of Medicine*, **366** (**20**), 1905–1913. PubMed PMID: 22591296. Pubmed Central PMCID: 3693860.

39

Case 39

A 59-year-old man presented with early satiety, abdominal fullness and nausea. In addition, he had developed a sharp left hypochondrial pain a few days earlier which had led him to seek medical advice. On examination, he had marked splenomegaly with tenderness to palpation but no superficial lymphadenopathy.

Laboratory results

FBC: Hb 124 g/L; WBC 8.6 × 10^9/L (neutrophils 2.5 × 10^9/L, lymphocytes 2.5 × 10^9/L, 'monocytes' 2.5 × 10^9/L), platelets 100 × 10^9/L.

U&Es, LFTs normal. LDH was raised at 415 U/L.

Blood film

The film showed a population of very large lymphoid cells with a single large nucleolus and plentiful cytoplasm (Figures 39.1 and 39.2).

Imaging

A CT scan showed marked splenomegaly (23 cm) and small volume abdominal lymphadenopathy. Note the splenic infarct close to the lower pole of the spleen in Figure 39.3.

Flow cytometry (peripheral blood)

The FSC/SSC profile showed these large cells (red events, Figure 39.4). They were clearly B cells accounting for 23% of total leucocytes and expressing CD20^{bright} (Figure 39.5)

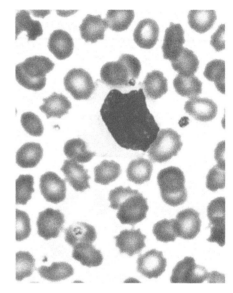

Figure 39.1 MGG, ×1000.

with FMC7, HLA-DR, CD79b and kappa^{bright}. In addition, CD11c and CD103 were expressed whilst CD5, CD38, CD23, CD10, CD25 and CD123 were not. This was therefore a mature B-cell neoplasm with a hairy cell leukaemia score of 2/4. There was no associated neutropenia and a manual monocyte count was normal; the neoplastic cells were counted as monocytes by the automated analyser.

Bone marrow trephine biopsy

Bone marrow involvement was not immediately apparent on examining the trephine sections stained with haematoxylin

Practical Flow Cytometry in Haematology: 100 Worked Examples, First Edition. Mike Leach, Mark Drummond, Allyson Doig, Pam McKay, Bob Jackson and Barbara J. Bain.
© 2015 John Wiley & Sons, Ltd. Published 2015 by John Wiley & Sons, Ltd.

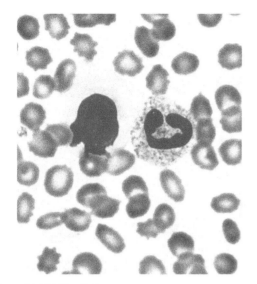

Figure 39.2 MGG, ×1000.

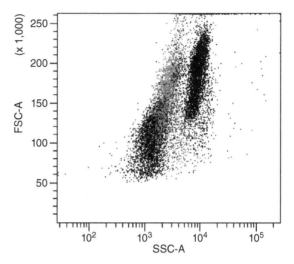

Figure 39.4 FSC/SSC.

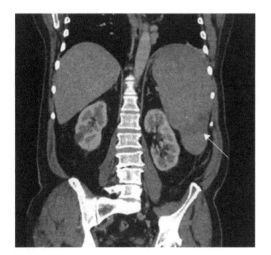

Figure 39.3 CT.

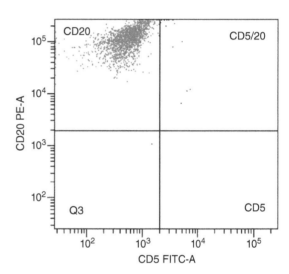

Figure 39.5 CD5/CD20.

and eosin (Figure 39.6) but foci of infiltration were apparent on the CD20 stained sections (Figure 39.7); sinusoidal infiltration was not identified.

The working diagnosis at this point was hairy cell leukaemia variant on account of the clinical presentation, blood film morphology and immunophenotype. The findings were not in keeping with classical hairy cell leukaemia; the absence of neutropenia and monocytopenia, the morphology with prominent nucleoli and the immunophenotype with a hairy cell score of only 2/4 are not typical. Hairy cell leukaemia variant is more usually associated with a marked

leucocytosis at the time of presentation and there is often intrasinusoidal infiltration in the bone marrow, but these were the only atypical features. It should be noted that, despite its name, hairy cell leukaemia variant is not closely related to hairy cell leukaemia.

In view of the profound symptomatic splenomegaly with established infarction and the paucity of effective treatment options in hairy cell leukaemia variant, it was decided, after multi-disciplinary team discussion, to perform a therapeutic splenectomy. The procedure was uneventful and the patient reported resolution of all previous symptoms.

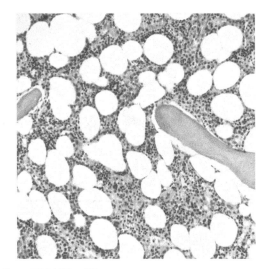

Figure 39.6 H&E, ×100.

Figure 39.8 H&E, ×25.

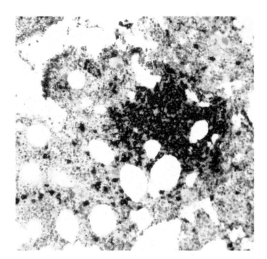

Figure 39.7 CD20, ×100.

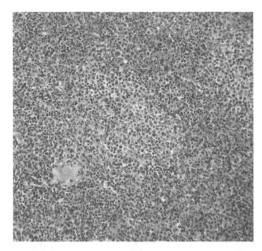

Figure 39.9 H&E, ×100.

Histopathology

Spleen: the excised spleen measured 32 cm × 22 cm × 9 cm and weighed 3 kg. Macroscopically, irregular geographic areas of pale discolouration were noted.

Microscopically, there was a diffuse and focally nodular infiltrate replacing red and white pulp (Figures 39.8 and 39.9). The nodules were composed of intermediate sized lymphoid cells, some with prominent nucleoli and abundant clear cytoplasm (Figures 39.9 and 39.10); these were strongly

positive for CD20 (Figure 39.11). There were also areas of infarction. Blood lakes, typically seen in classical hairy cell leukaemia, were not identified.

The neoplastic cells were also positive for BCL6, BCL2 and tartrate-resistant alkaline phosphatase (TRAP). Staining with the antibody DBA-44 (CD72) was positive in 15–20% of cells. Notably annexin-1, CD25 and CD123 were not expressed; neither were CD3, CD5, CD10, CD23 nor cyclin D1. The proliferation fraction was 10–15%.

Lymph nodes: splenic hilar lymph nodes were also available for examination. The nodes were diffusely involved by cells identical to those described above.

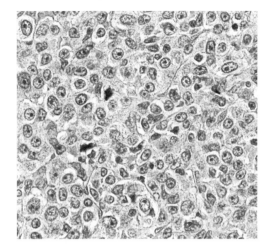

Figure 39.10 H&E, ×400.

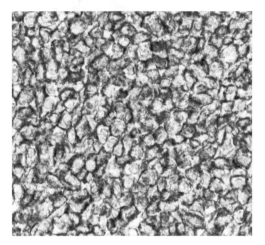

Figure 39.11 CD20, ×400.

Discussion

Hairy cell leukaemia variant is a rare B-cell lymphoproliferative disorder being approximately 100 times less prevalent than CLL and 10 times less common than classic hairy cell leukaemia (HCL). The diagnosis of HCL-V can cause some difficulty as there is no specific immunophenotypic or immunohistochemical marker. HCL has a more consistent immunophenotype showing positivity for CD11c, CD25, CD103 and CD123 (score 4) whereas HCL-V normally scores 1 or 2 (typically showing negativity for CD25 and CD123). On splenic histology, HCL shows diffuse involvement of the red pulp with white pulp atrophy and the cells are positive for TRAP, CD72 and annexin-1. In HCL-V the infiltrate is usually diffuse within the red pulp, obliterating the white pulp and can thus resemble the pattern of infiltration of classic hairy cell leukaemia; whilst the cells can show partial positivity with TRAP and CD72, annexin-1 staining is negative. The pattern of bone marrow involvement, splenic morphology and lack of annexin-1 positivity in the described case excludes a diagnosis of HCL.

The differential diagnosis also includes splenic marginal zone lymphoma (SMZL). There is considerable clinical, morphological and immunophenotypic overlap between HCL-V and SMZL. The morphological features noted in the peripheral blood and the flow cytometric features, although not specific would be in keeping with a diagnosis of HCL-V, but the relatively low peripheral lymphocyte count would be unusual. The changes in the trephine biopsy specimen are somewhat unusual for HCL-V as there are non-paratrabecular nodules of small B cells, a feature found in only 1 of 10 cases of HCL-V in one series described (1). Bone marrow nodules are more typical of SMZL. The lack of sinusoidal spread in the marrow and the nodular pattern of splenic involvement are also features more in keeping with a diagnosis of SMZL although the cytology of the cells in the spleen was more suggestive of HCL-V. Immunophenotyping of paraffin-embedded material in this case showed positivity for some hairy cell markers, a feature that can be seen in both conditions. Accurate classification is therefore difficult and the lymphoma is probably best regarded as splenic B-cell lymphoma/leukaemia unclassifiable.

The therapeutic splenectomy provided symptomatic improvement for the patient but also yielded valuable splenic tissue for extended histopathological examination. Despite this a specific diagnosis could not be attributed in this case.

Final diagnosis

Splenic B-cell lymphoma/leukaemia unclassifiable, probably hairy cell variant leukaemia

Reference

1 Cessna, M.H., Hartung, L., Tripp, S., Perkins, S.L. & Bahler, D.W. (2005) Hairy cell leukemia variant: fact or fiction. *American Journal of Clinical Pathology*, **123** (1), 132–138. PubMed PMID: 15762289.

40

Case 40

An 83-year-old woman with a working diagnosis of Waldenström macroglobulinaemia (WM) presented to another hospital with symptoms of hyperviscosity and an IgM paraprotein level of 40 g/L. The available history was incomplete. She was noted to have had a peripheral blood lymphocytosis with some of the cells showing cytoplasmic villous projections and so was fully re-assessed for consideration of management options.

Laboratory results

FBC: Hb 108 g/L, WBC 9 × 10^9/L (neutrophils 3.6 × 10^9/L, lymphocytes 2.3 × 10^9/L, 'monocytes' 3.3 × 10^9/L) and platelets 113 × 10^9/L.

U&Es, LFTs and LDH were all normal.

Blood film

The peripheral blood lymphoid cells showed a variety of morphological characteristics. Some were small with minimal basophilic cytoplasm (Figure 40.1), some showed plasmacytoid features (Figure 40.2) and some larger cells had nuclear convolutions and were approaching the size of monocytes (Figures 40.3 and 40.4). The true lymphocyte count was likely higher than that indicated by the analyser. Some of the larger cells were encroaching on the monocyte zone.

Flow cytometry (peripheral blood)

Using a CD2 versus CD19 analysis almost 50% of leucocytes were B cells. Only 5% were T cells. The B cells were monoclonal (strong kappa expression) and expressed CD20^{bright},

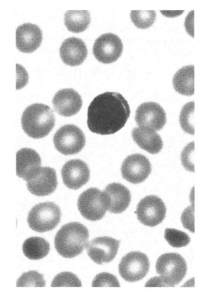

Figure 40.1 MGG, ×1000.

FMC7, CD23, CD22 and CD79b. CD38 was expressed in only 3.6% of cells. CD11c, CD25, CD103 and CD123 were not expressed. The morphology and immunophenotype did not generate a specific diagnosis but lymphoplasmacytic lymphoma or splenic marginal zone lymphoma was considered most likely.

Histopathology

Bone marrow trephine biopsy

There were scattered small clusters of small to medium sized lymphoid cells (Figure 40.5) and occasional Dutcher

Practical Flow Cytometry in Haematology: 100 Worked Examples, First Edition. Mike Leach, Mark Drummond, Allyson Doig, Pam McKay, Bob Jackson and Barbara J. Bain.
© 2015 John Wiley & Sons, Ltd. Published 2015 by John Wiley & Sons, Ltd.

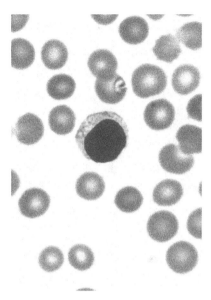

Figure 40.2 MGG, ×1000.

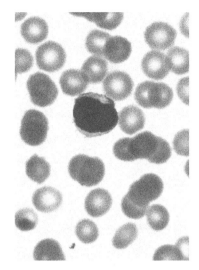

Figure 40.4 MGG, ×1000.

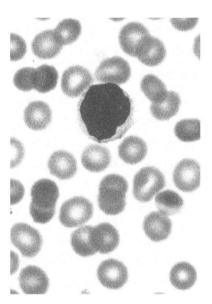

Figure 40.3 MGG, ×1000.

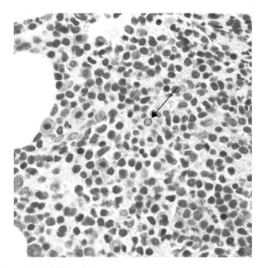

Figure 40.5 H&E, ×400.

bodies (intranuclear inclusions) within plasmacytoid cells were also seen (arrow, Figure 40.5,). Immunohistochemistry for CD20 (Figure 40.6) and CD79b showed the cells to be strongly positive and in addition highlighted an increase in interstitial B cells some of which had an intrasinusoidal pattern of spread. The plasmacytoid cells are highlighted using CD138 in Figure 40.7.

Note that Dutcher bodies are actually intranuclear invaginations of immunoglobulin-rich cytoplasm and are not true nuclear phenomena.

Imaging

A CT scan showed widespread small volume lymphadenopathy and 18 cm splenomegaly.

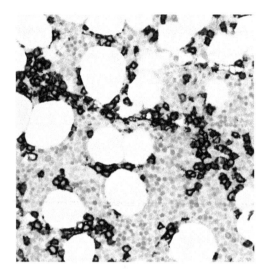

Figure 40.6 CD20, ×400.

Discussion

IgM paraproteins are seen in a number of lymphoproliferative disorders, namely chronic lymphocytic leukaemia (CLL), lymphoplasmacytic lymphoma (LPL) and marginal zone lymphoma (MZL). The differential diagnosis here lay between the latter two. There is morphological, immunophenotypic, histological and clinical overlap between these two entities and sometimes a definitive diagnosis is not possible. Marginal zone lymphomas often show lymphoplasmacytoid differentiation. In this case the pattern of sinusoidal spread seen in the trephine biopsy sections is somewhat more characteristic of SMZL although the presence of widespread lymphadenopathy and the prominent IgM paraprotein is more in keeping with LPL (Waldenström macroglobulinaemia). On balance a diagnosis of LPL was favoured. Attempts to achieve a specific diagnosis are justified as the treatment of these two entities can differ and the toxicity of planned therapy should be carefully considered in elderly patients.

Final diagnosis

Lymphoplasmacytic lymphoma with an associated IgM paraprotein (Waldenström macroglobulinaemia).

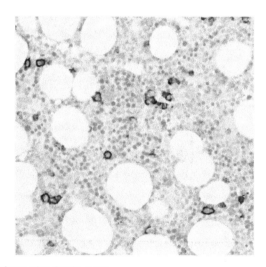

Figure 40.7 CD138, ×400.

41

Case 41

A 49-year-old female attended her GP complaining of a month long history of fatigue, weight loss, bruising and spontaneous nose bleeds. She had a prior history of Kikuchi disease (necrotising lymphadenitis) over 20 years previously but was on no recent medications. No lymphadenopathy or organomegaly was found on examination, although petechiae were noted over the lower limbs as well as small, scattered bruises. An FBC was taken.

Laboratory data

FBC: Hb 88 g/L, WBC 2.0×10^9/L, (neutrophils 0.1×10^9/L, lymphocytes 1.6×10^9/L, monocytes 0.1×10^9/L) and platelets 33×10^9/L.

U&Es, LFTs and bone profile: normal.

Blood film

Blood film analysis was initially performed at another centre and a provisional diagnosis of acute lymphoblastic leukaemia was made. A sample was sent to our centre for flow cytometry analysis. Blood film examination demonstrated a majority population of small lymphoid cells (Figures 41.1 and 41.2, Figure 41.3 (top cell)). Occasional cells had plentiful cytoplasm and small azurophilic granules (Figure 41.2). The chromatin in these cells had a mature appearance. A much smaller population of cells (<5%) was noted, comprising much larger forms with immature open chromatin and basophilic cytoplasm (Figure 41.3, bottom cell). Only a very occasional cytoplasmic granule was noted in the large cell population.

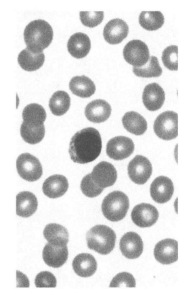

Figure 41.1 MGG, ×1000.

Bone marrow aspirate

Hypercellular particles and trails were noted. Over 90% of the cells were blasts, identical in appearance to the larger cells in the peripheral blood. Again, little maturation was evident, with only an occasional fine cytoplasmic granule observed. There was no evidence of a lymphoid population (Figure 4).

Flow cytometry (peripheral blood)

Flow cytometry was performed on both peripheral blood and marrow (peripheral blood results are shown in

Practical Flow Cytometry in Haematology: 100 Worked Examples, First Edition. Mike Leach, Mark Drummond, Allyson Doig, Pam McKay, Bob Jackson and Barbara J. Bain.
© 2015 John Wiley & Sons, Ltd. Published 2015 by John Wiley & Sons, Ltd.

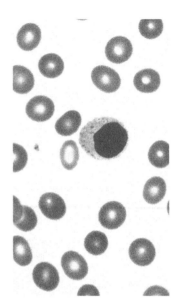

Figure 41.2 MGG, ×1000.

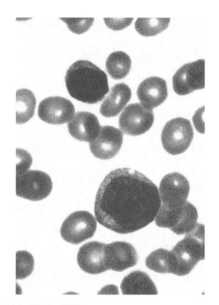

Figure 41.3 MGG, ×1000.

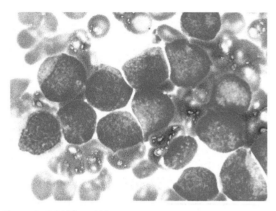

Figure 41.4 MGG, ×1000.

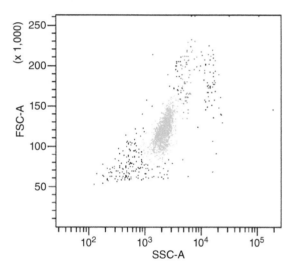

Figure 41.5 FSC/SSC.

Figures 41.5–41.7). The smaller cells (Figure 41.5, shown in green) comprised over 90% of total leucocytes and were CD45$^+$ and CD34$^-$. These were CD2$^+$, CD3$^+$, CD5$^+$ and CD7$^+$ mature T cells. The larger cells (shown in red and comprising less than 3% of leucocytes) were CD45^{dim}, CD34$^+$, CD117$^+$, MPO$^+$, HLA-DR$^+$, CD13$^+$, CD33$^+$ with aberrant expression of CD19 and CD7. Cytoplasmic CD3 and CD79a were not expressed.

Cytogenetic analysis

46,XX,r(18)(p11q21).

Molecular studies

FLT3 ITD and *NPM1* mutations were not identified.

Discussion

This patient presented with severe marrow failure; the predominant population in the peripheral blood (namely

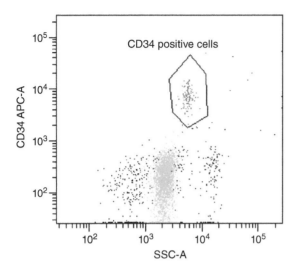

Figure 41.6 CD34/SSC.

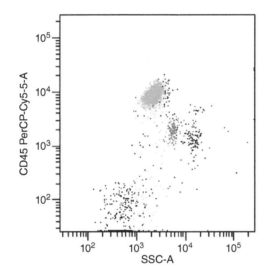

Figure 41.7 CD45/SSC.

mature reactive T cells) was initially assumed to be the pathological population, largely because of infrequent myeloblasts and the relative excess of lymphocytes, albeit in normal numbers. Overlooking rare malignant cells in blood films is an occupational hazard and must be guarded against by careful and thorough assessment. The myeloblasts in this case showed very little evidence of maturation. Although not the case here, lymphoid expansions (in particular T/NK) are reported in conjunction with haematological malignancies, in particular in MDS. Relative prominence of reactive large granular lymphocytes and NK cells is a fairly common finding in the peripheral blood of patients with a new presentation of a haematological malignancy.

The cytogenetic analysis of this case is of interest: ring chromosomes are rare in blood cancers, but have been reported in AML albeit usually in conjunction with a complex karyotype, reviewed in (1). They are formed when the two ends of a chromosome fuse to form a ring structure, with variable loss of genetic material.

The prognostic implications of such an event in isolation are unclear, due to the small number of reported cases in the literature. It would therefore seem prudent in such cases to screen for other genetic alterations of prognostic importance, such as *NPM1* mutations or *FLT3*-ITD, the results of which may help in directing appropriate therapy. This patient was treated on the UK AML17 Clinical Trial with intensive induction chemotherapy and entered morphological and cytogenetic CR after the first cycle of treatment. Treatment is now complete and the patient remains well on follow up.

Final diagnosis

Acute myeloid leukaemia without maturation and with ring chromosome 18.

Reference

1 Sivendran, S., Gruenstein, S., Malone, A.K., Najfeld, V. (2010) Ring chromosome 18 abnormality in acute myelogenous leukemia: the clinical dilemma. *Journal of Hematology & Oncology*, **3**, 25. PubMed PMID: 20649984.

42

Case 42

A previously well 20-year-old male student presented with a several week history of exertional dyspnoea and headache. He denied weight loss, night sweats or bleeding. There was no significant past medical history, no history of prescription or over-the-counter drug use and no substance abuse. On examination there was no hepatosplenomegaly or lymphadenopathy. Mild partial syndactyly of his toes was noted. Examination of skin and nails was normal.

Laboratory data

FBC: Hb 75 g/L, MCV 102 fl, WBC 2.7×10^9/L (neutrophils 0.4×10^9/L), platelets 20×10^9/L and reticulocytes 2×10^9/L.

U&Es, LFTs, LDH and thyroid function were all normal.
ANA negative.
Blood film: severe pancytopenia, no blast cells or dysplastic features.
HIV and hepatitis screen: negative.
Haematinics and serum copper: normal.
CXR and X-Ray hands and feet: normal.
Abdominal USS: normal.

Bone marrow aspirate

The marrow aspirate yielded an occasional particle but was profoundly hypocellular and there was initial concern that it might not be representative. Minor dyserythropoietic changes were noted. The apparent predominance of lymphocytes and plasma cells was noted to be due to the near absence of myeloid activity and scanty erythroid series. No obvious dysplasia was seen. Marrow cytogenetic analysis showed a normal male karyotype. Chromosome fragility studies gave a normal result and investigation for dyskeratosis congenita (including screening for known mutations in the *DKC1*, *TERC* and *TERT* genes) was negative.

Trephine biopsy

A good marrow trephine biopsy specimen (2 cm) confirmed profound hypocellularity in representative non-subcortical areas (Figures 42.1 and 42.2). Near empty marrow spaces contained occasional lymphocytes and plasma cells, with a very occasional erythroblast. No megakaryocytes were seen and there were no foci of blast cells.

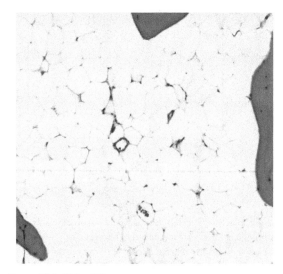

Figure 42.1 H&E, ×100.

Practical Flow Cytometry in Haematology: 100 Worked Examples, First Edition. Mike Leach, Mark Drummond, Allyson Doig, Pam McKay, Bob Jackson and Barbara J. Bain.
© 2015 John Wiley & Sons, Ltd. Published 2015 by John Wiley & Sons, Ltd.

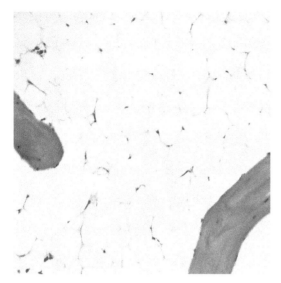

Figure 42.2 H&E, ×100.

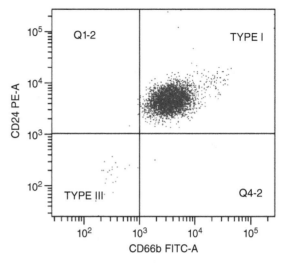

Figure 42.3 CD24/CD66b.

Flow cytometry

Flow cytometry of the marrow aspirate showed low event numbers despite prolonged analysis, run to collect a representative number of events (approaching 5000). The FSC/SSC plot showed little granulocytic maturation and the apparent 'excess' of lymphocytes was accounted for, simply by the fact that they represented the largest proportion of residual cells. These were mainly T cells with a normal CD4:CD8 ratio. B cells were mature and polyclonal with no haematogones noted. The CD34+ cells were 0.2% of total cells. Analysis of peripheral blood demonstrated a small type III PNH clone (0.4% of granulocytes) by FLAER/CD24/CD66b analysis (Figures 42.3 and 42.4). Note the tiny granulocyte PNH clone (red events) that was identified despite the severe peripheral blood neutropenia. Note that type I red cells are normal. It is the small type III population that is abnormal.

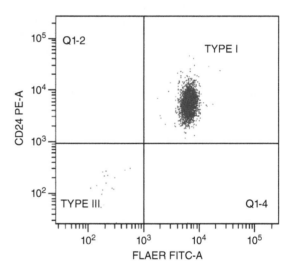

Figure 42.4 CD24/FLAER.

Discussion

This patient presented with a profound pancytopenia, for which the differential diagnosis is wide. Crucial in the work up of this laboratory picture is a good quality marrow aspirate and trephine biopsy (with differential diagnosis reviewed in (1)), and a diagnosis should not be assigned if diagnostic material is inadequate. Although hypocellular particles in a marrow aspirate may suggest the diagnosis

of a hypocellular marrow syndrome, the importance of a good trephine biopsy with which to gauge overall cellularity cannot be overestimated. Pancytopenia in the face of a normo- or hypercellular marrow leads to consideration of a very different diagnostic spectrum from that when the marrow is hypocellular. The former would include vitamin B_{12} and folate deficiency, copper deficiency, infiltration by a haematological or non-haematological neoplasm, myelodysplastic syndrome or hypersplenism. Infections (e.g. parvovirus B19) and autoimmune disease may cause mixed pictures.

A useful definition of marrow hypocellularity is trephine biopsy cellularity <30% (for <60 years of age) or <20% (for >60 years of age). The main differential diagnosis is between aplastic anaemia, hypoplastic MDS and a recent toxic marrow insult (e.g. chemotherapy, chemical exposure). A careful clinical history (to include a detailed drug and infection history) is critical, although management of severe aplastic anaemia (SAA) is generally the same whether a cause is identified or not. In a young person (usually defined as <40 years) appropriate investigations should be performed to determine whether the marrow failure is part of a genetic disorder, paying close attention to the family history (reviewed in (2)). These disorders comprise Fanconi anaemia and dyskeratosis congenita (DKC), detectable by chromosomal fragility studies and mutation analysis of telomere-maintenance components respectively. Investigation of the latter may be particularly challenging and involve careful clinical examination and organ screening (to look for cirrhosis, pulmonary fibrosis and skin and nail changes). The marrow aspirate and trephine biopsy, illustrated in Figures 42.5–42.8 and 42.9–42.11 respectively, is from a 20-year-old patient with short stature who presented with pancytopenia. Note the marked myeloid hypoplasia but importantly the erythroid dysplasia. Note the perivascular erythroid cluster and mitotic figure (arrow) in Figure 42.11. Morphological dysplasia of this degree is not generally seen in idiopathic aplastic anaemia and chromosome fragility studies and *FANCA* gene analysis indicated a diagnosis of Fanconi anaemia. This patient was treated by allogeneic transplantation.

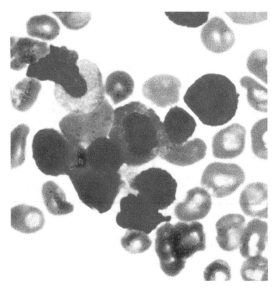

Figure 42.6 MGG, ×1000.

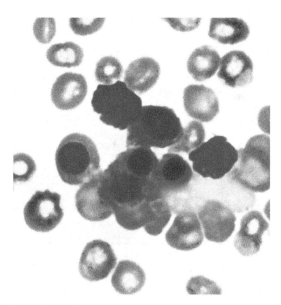

Figure 42.7 MGG, ×1000.

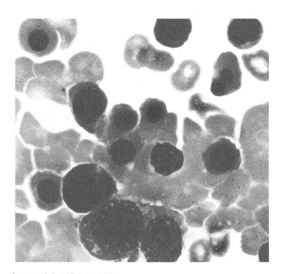

Figure 42.5 MGG, ×1000.

For a severely hypoplastic marrow, the differential diagnosis is usually between SAA and hypoplastic MDS. Consideration of all marrow results (aspirate cytology, trephine biopsy plus IHC for CD34 and CD42b, flow cytometry for CD34$^+$ cell populations and cytogenetic analysis) usually allows a distinction to be drawn although it can be difficult. The presence of MDS-associated cytogenetic

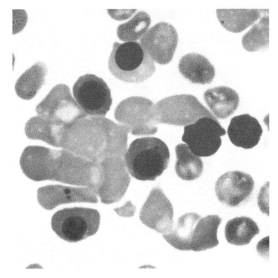

Figure 42.8 MGG, ×1000.

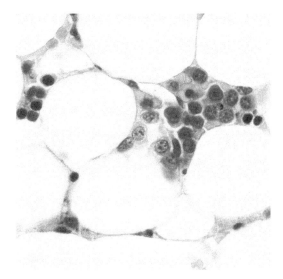

Figure 42.10 H&E, ×500.

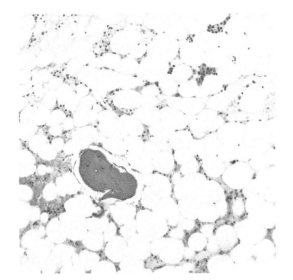

Figure 42.9 H&E, ×100.

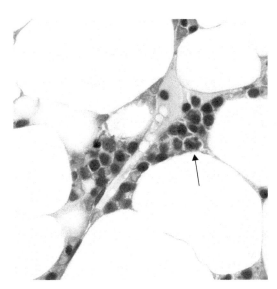

Figure 42.11 H&E, ×500.

abnormalities, significant dysplastic changes (in particular in megakaryocytes), >1% CD34$^+$ cells by flow (3) or eventual progression to MDS with excess blasts or AML is supportive of a diagnosis of hypoplastic MDS. This fits with what we know about the biology of these diseases, for example the cell-mediated immune attack on the stem cell compartment in SAA will result in a reduction in detectable CD34$^+$ cells.

Small PNH clones, as seen in this patient, may be found in both MDS and SAA, so rather than being discriminatory this

finding supports the presence of an underlying marrow disorder. The majority of patients with aplastic anaemia have small PNH clones detectable and approximately 30% of patients with clinically evident PNH have had preceding AA. Monitoring clonal size in such patients is useful.

Due to his young age this patient received an early allogeneic transplantation from an unrelated donor. One year later the patient is well with normal blood counts and 100% donor chimaerism.

Final diagnosis

Severe aplastic anaemia.

References

1 Weinzierl, E.P. & Arber, D.A. (2013) The differential diagnosis and bone marrow evaluation of new-onset pancytopenia. *American Journal of Clinical Pathology*, **139** (1), 9–29. PubMed PMID: 23270895.

2 Chirnomas, S.D. & Kupfer, G.M. (2013) The inherited bone marrow failure syndromes. *Pediatric Clinics of North America*, **60** (**6**), 1291–1310. PubMed PMID: 24237972.

3 Matsui, W.H., Brodsky, R.A., Smith, B.D., Borowitz, M.J. & Jones, R.J. (2006) Quantitative analysis of bone marrow CD34 cells in aplastic anemia and hypoplastic myelodysplastic syndromes. *Leukemia*; **20**(**3**), 458–62. PubMed PMID: 16437138.

Case 43

An 82-year-old man presented with abdominal fullness and fatigue. Physical examination identified splenomegaly but lymphadenopathy was not apparent.

Laboratory data

FBC: Hb 105 g/L, WBC 112 × 10⁹/L (neutrophils 3.5 × 10⁹/L, lymphocytes 105 × 10⁹/L) and platelets 151 × 10⁹/L.

U&Es, bone profile and LFTs were normal. Serum LDH was 300 U/L

Blood film

This revealed a population of medium sized lymphoid cells with round or ovoid nuclei with coarsely condensed chromatin, many having a single nucleolus (Figures 43.1–43.4). Most cells had a moderate amount of medium blue cytoplasm. Neutrophils were preserved and there were no significant red cell abnormalities.

Flow cytometry (peripheral blood)

This showed that there was a marked excess of B cells (89% of all events) with a mature kappa^{strong}, CD20⁺, FMC7^{dim}, HLA-DR⁺, CD79b⁺, CD22⁺, CD23⁻, CD5⁻, CD10⁻, CD11c⁻, CD25⁻, CD103⁻ and CD123⁻ phenotype. This is an example of a case of where immunophenotyping is only partially helpful; it confirms a mature B-cell disorder but there are no specific 'positive' characteristics. The morphology however is typical of B-cell prolymphocytic leukaemia

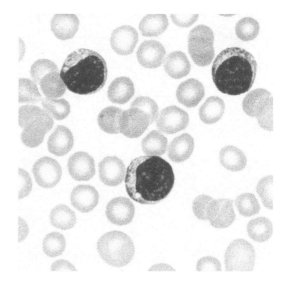

Figure 43.1 MGG, ×1000.

and this disorder typically has a pan-B phenotype. It differs from CLL in showing strong surface immunoglobulin, expression of FMC7 and CD79b and only occasionally expression of CD5 or CD23.

Histopathology

The trephine biopsy sections showed 60% cellularity with an interstitial and focally nodular infiltrate of medium sized lymphoid cells (Figure 43.5). These cells expressed CD20 (Figure 43.6) but not CD5, CD10, CD23, BCL6 or cyclin D1. Normal haemopoietic activity was reasonably preserved.

Practical Flow Cytometry in Haematology: 100 Worked Examples, First Edition. Mike Leach, Mark Drummond, Allyson Doig, Pam McKay, Bob Jackson and Barbara J. Bain.
© 2015 John Wiley & Sons, Ltd. Published 2015 by John Wiley & Sons, Ltd.

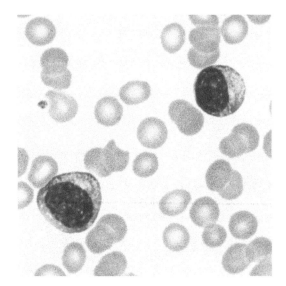

Figure 43.2 MGG, ×1000.

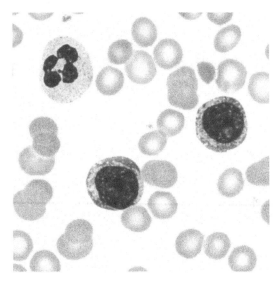

Figure 43.4 MGG, ×1000.

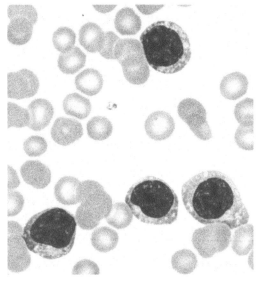

Figure 43.3 MGG, ×1000.

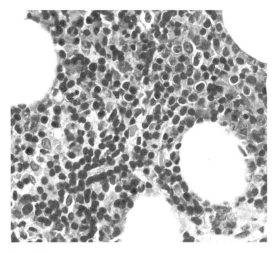

Figure 43.5 H&E, ×400.

Cytogenetic analysis

Standard metaphase preparations and FISH studies identified a 17p deletion in over 90% of cells. No other abnormality was identified.

Discussion

B-cell prolymphocytic leukaemia (B-PLL) is a rare disease most often affecting middle aged to elderly males. It normally presents with a moderate lymphocytosis, anaemia and variable thrombocytopenia with splenomegaly but no lymphadenopathy. It can be confused with leukaemic mantle cell lymphoma morphologically but cytogenetic

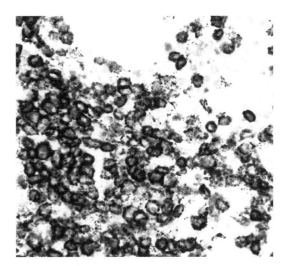

Figure 43.6 CD20, ×400.

studies, immunohistochemistry for cyclin D1 and t(11;14) FISH studies should discriminate between the two. B-PLL does not respond well to standard cytotoxic chemotherapy approaches as used for CLL or non-Hodgkin lymphoma, at least in part due to the frequent finding of 17p deletion indicative of loss of one allele of *TP53*. As the condition is often seen in elderly patients this needs to be recognised. The prognosis of B-PLL, unlike that of CLL, does not seem to be influenced by *IGH* gene mutation status, cytogenetic abnormalities other than del(17p) or expression of ZAP70 and CD38 (1). This condition arises *de novo* and should not be confused with advanced, atypical or 17p deletion CLL with increasing prolymphocytes, which has a very different presentation, immunophenotype and management algorithm.

Final diagnosis

B-cell prolymphocytic leukaemia.

Reference

1 Del Giudice, I., Davis, Z., Matutes, E. *et al.* (2006) IgVH genes mutation and usage, ZAP-70 and CD38 expression provide new insights on B-cell prolymphocytic leukemia (B-PLL). *Leukemia*, **20** (7), 1231–1237. PubMed PMID: 16642047.

Case 44

A 40-year-old man was referred to our centre from a regional hospital for consideration of plasma exchange with a working diagnosis of thrombotic thrombocytopenic purpura (TTP). He had presented with a recent history of weight loss, anorexia and back pain. On examination he looked unwell, was pale and jaundiced and was in obvious discomfort in moving from chair to bed. There were no other specific findings. He was afebrile and his vital signs were normal.

Laboratory investigations

FBC: Hb 57 g/L, MCV 93 fl, WBC 15.2 × 10⁹/L, and platelets 52×10^9/L.

Reticulocytes 250×10^9/L.

U&Es: Na 129 mmol/L, K⁺ 4.5 mmol/L, urea 90 mmol/L, creatinine 55 μmol/L.

LFTs/bone profile: albumin 32 g/L, calcium 2.3 mmol/L, phosphate 1.0 mmol/L, alkaline phosphatase 790 U/L, GGT 50 U/L, LDH 977 U/L.

Coagulation: PT 18 s, APTT 40 s, TT 17 s, fibrinogen 1.5 g/L, D-dimer 13,976 ng/mL.

Blood film

The blood film showed important features. Firstly, it showed significant red cell fragmentation, with spherocytes, microspherocytes and polychromasia (Figures 44.1 and 44.2). Secondly, it showed nucleated red cells and myeloid precursors (Figures 44.3 and 44.4). Leucoerythroblastosis can be a feature of severe bone marrow stress as a result of profound anaemia due to acute bleeding or haemolysis in critically ill patients. This patient, however, had a more chronic presentation so a leucoerythroblastic blood film as a result of bone marrow infiltration had to be considered.

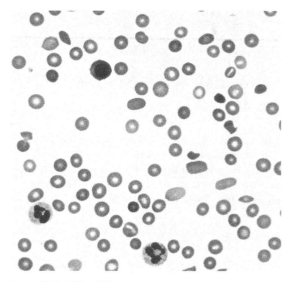

Figure 44.1 MGG, ×500.

In view of these findings a bone marrow aspiration and trephine biopsy were performed. The aspirate was grossly abnormal being hypocellular but containing clumps of likely non-haemopoietic cells, some with features approaching signet-ring morphology with expanded cytoplasm, sometimes a visible globule or globules and an eccentric displaced nucleus (Figures 44.5–44.7). These cytological features are typical of adenocarcinoma.

Flow cytometry

Flow cytometry studies on the marrow aspirate also indicated involvement by a CD45-negative non-haemopoietic tumour.

Practical Flow Cytometry in Haematology: 100 Worked Examples, First Edition. Mike Leach, Mark Drummond, Allyson Doig, Pam McKay, Bob Jackson and Barbara J. Bain.
© 2015 John Wiley & Sons, Ltd. Published 2015 by John Wiley & Sons, Ltd.

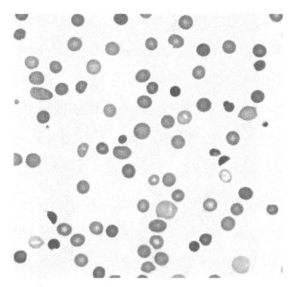

Figure 44.2 MGG, ×500.

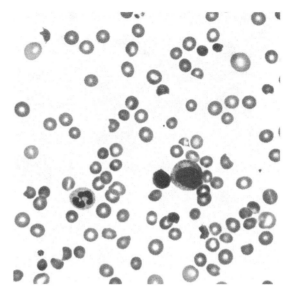

Figure 44.4 MGG, ×500.

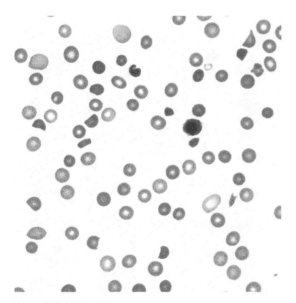

Figure 44.3 MGG, ×500.

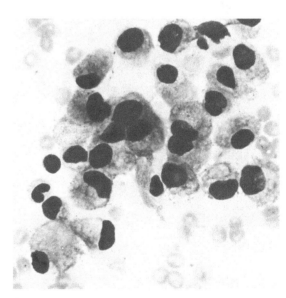

Figure 44.5 MGG, ×500.

Imaging

In view of the patient's back pain, and the bone marrow infiltration, a series of plain X-rays were undertaken but these were reported as normal. An MRI scan of the spine was more informative showing features of disseminated bone involvement by tumour (Figures 44.8 and 44.9).

The finding of bone marrow infiltration by a non-haemopoietic tumour suggested that the leucoerythroblastosis and disseminated intravascular coagulation (DIC) were the result of metastatic adenocarcinoma. The chronic DIC, with deposition of fibrin within the microvasculature, was responsible for the microangiopathic features of the blood film.

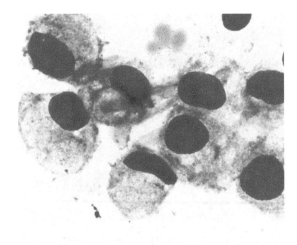

Figure 44.6 MGG, ×1000.

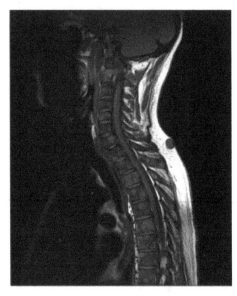

Figure 44.8 MRI.

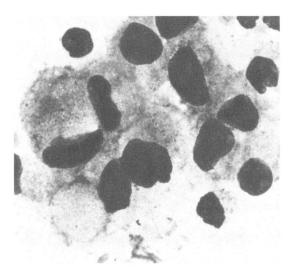

Figure 44.7 MGG, ×1000.

Histopathology

The bone marrow trephine biopsy specimen was hyper-cellular with a focal and interstitial infiltration by tumour (Figure 44.10); on higher magnification the infiltrating cells again showed signet ring type morphology (arrows, Figure 44.11). The same cells were highlighted using Cam5.2 (Figure 44.12) and were confirmed to be producing mucin using Alcian blue staining (Figure 44.13). The findings are those of bone marrow involvement by a mucinous adenocarcinoma.

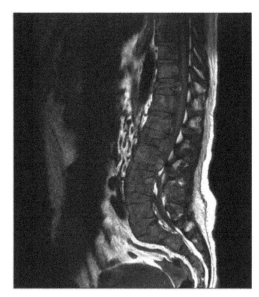

Figure 44.9 MRI.

A number of carcinomas are commonly responsible for inducing DIC, notably carcinomas arising from breast, lung, stomach, pancreas, colon and ovary. Mucin-secreting adenocarcinomas of the gastrointestinal tract are particularly implicated so we performed an upper GI endoscopy. This identified a small malignant ulcer in the lower oesophagus, which on histology was a mucin-secreting adenocarcinoma.

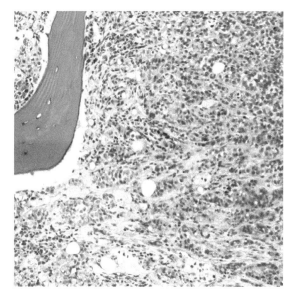

Figure 44.10 H&E, ×100.

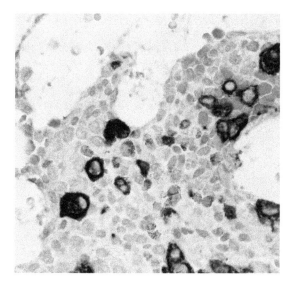

Figure 44.12 Cam5.2, ×400.

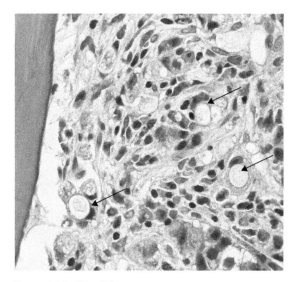

Figure 44.11 H&E, ×400.

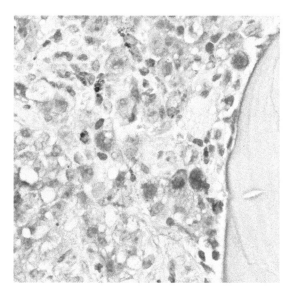

Figure 44.13 Alcian blue, ×400.

Discussion

This patient was referred to our centre with a working diagnosis of TTP but a number of features were not in keeping with this diagnosis. Classic TTP is an autoimmune disorder whereby platelets become activated in the presence of high molecular weight multimers of von Willebrand factor. These multimers are not normally present as von Willebrand factor is cleaved by an enzyme referred to as ADAMTS13 (a disintegrin and metalloproteinase with thrombospondin type activity). In the presence of autoantibodies to ADAMTS13 the level of the enzyme falls significantly allowing formation of these multimers with subsequent uncontrolled platelet aggregation and adherence of aggregates to microvascular endothelium. These platelet 'thrombi' are responsible for the red cell fragmentation syndrome that ensues. The vessels of the brain, myocardium and kidneys are particularly prone to involvement leading to neurological sequelae, cardiac dysfunction and renal failure. A pentad of features, specifically fever, microangiopathic haemolytic anaemia, thrombocytopenia, neurological symptoms and renal failure help to make a firm diagnosis together with the demonstration of ADAMTS13 levels below 10% normal (1) with specific ADAMTS13 autoantibodies. However, since early plasma exchange is crucial in management of TTP it is also necessary to recognise patients who do not have the complete pentad but do have a similarly reduced ADAMTS13 level. Activation of coagulation is not a feature of TTP where the coagulation profile and D-dimer level should be essentially normal. This patient, with widespread metastatic disease from a small, clinically silent adenocarcinoma of the lower oesophagus, presented with only two of the five features suggesting TTP and the reported additional symptoms of weight loss and back pain had to be explained. Furthermore, the laboratory investigations showed clear evidence of DIC, absence of overt renal failure and biochemical indices suggesting bone disease.

It is extremely important to carefully consider the clinical and laboratory features of any patient given a working diagnosis of TTP and alternative pathologies generating a microangiopathic haemolytic anaemia have to be excluded. Treatment with plasma exchange can be highly beneficial where the diagnosis is correct but is of no benefit to patients with DIC. Making this distinction is clinically urgent.

Final diagnosis

Mucinous adenocarcinoma of the oesophagus with secondary disseminated intravascular coagulation, bone marrow metastases and microangiopathic haemolytic anaemia.

Reference

1 Shah, N., Rutherford, C., Matevosyan, K., Shen, Y.-M. & Sarode, R. (2014) Role of ADAMTS13 in the management of thrombotic microangiopathies including thrombotic thrombocytopenic purpura (TTP). *British Journal of Haematology*, **163**, 514–519. PMID: 24111495.

45

Case 45

A 44-year-old man had undergone an unrelated donor allo-geneic stem cell transplant in first remission of a pro-B-cell acute lymphoblastic leukaemia. His clinical course had been relatively uncomplicated with prompt engraftment and easily manageable graft-versus-host disease affecting skin only. He underwent a scheduled day 100 bone marrow aspiration and a specimen was sent for flow cytometry analysis.

Laboratory data

FBC was normal.
U&Es, LFTs, bone profile and LDH were all normal.

Bone marrow aspirate

Morphologically the aspirate was of good cellularity with normal maturation of all lineages. No excess of blasts was identified.

Flow cytometry on marrow aspirate at diagnosis

This had shown a precursor-B ALL with a pro-B-cell pheno-type with aberrant myeloid antigen expression defined using the CD45^{dim} gate (percentage positive):

CD34 97%, CD79a 97%, CD19 99.8%, TdT 97%, HLA-DR 99%, CD10 0%, MPO 0.3%, CD19/CD15^{dim} 42% and CD19/CD13^{dim} 37.3%.

Cytogenetic profile at diagnosis

FISH studies had demonstrated trisomy 12 and tetrasomy 21 in 92% of cells, with 86% of cells showing, in addition, trisomy 9. No *MLL* gene rearrangement was had been identified.

Flow cytometry on marrow aspirate at day 100

The CD45 versus SSC analysis of the aspirate is shown in Figure 45.1. This shows a cellular specimen with a substan-tial population of CD45^{dim} cells (red events) accounting for 6.6% of cells. The phenotype of these cells (percentage posi-tive) was as follows:

CD34 6.9%, CD79a 92%, CD19 87.5%, TdT 6.4%, HLA-DR 73%, CD10 79%, CD20 29%, CD19/CD15 0.6%. There was no aberrant expression of myeloid antigens.

The CD10 versus CD20 analysis on the same CD45^{dim} population shows an important phenomenon (Figure 45.2). Here it can be seen that the CD45^{dim} cells are in fact made up of three distinct sub-populations with differing phenotypes according to the presence and intensity of expression of three antigens, CD34, CD10 and CD20. The phenotype of each subset was as follows:

Green events (8%): CD34$^+$, CD79a$^+$, CD19$^+$, TdT$^+$, HLA-DR$^+$, CD10^{bright}, CD20$^-$.

Purple events (71%): CD34$^-$, CD79a$^+$, CD19$^+$, TdT$^-$, HLA-DR$^+$, CD10$^+$, partial CD20$^+$.

Blue events (6%): CD34$^-$, CD79a$^+$, CD19$^+$, TdT$^-$, HLA-DR$^+$, CD10$^-$, CD20$^+$.

Practical Flow Cytometry in Haematology: 100 Worked Examples, First Edition. Mike Leach, Mark Drummond, Allyson Doig, Pam McKay, Bob Jackson and Barbara J. Bain.
© 2015 John Wiley & Sons, Ltd. Published 2015 by John Wiley & Sons, Ltd.

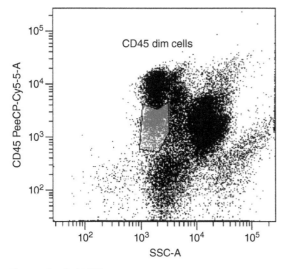

Figure 45.1 CD45/SSC.

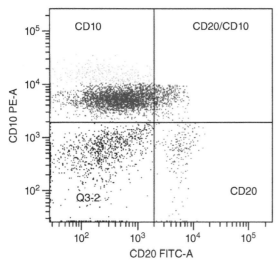

Figure 45.2 CD10/CD20.

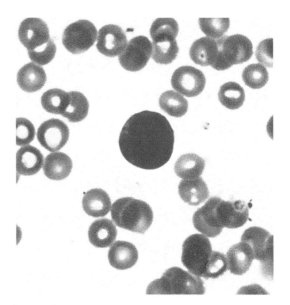

Figure 45.3 MGG, ×1000.

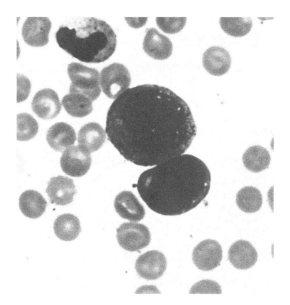

Figure 45.4 MGG, ×1000.

The three populations show typical phenotypic characteristics of haematogones type I (green), type II (purple) and type III (blue). Importantly, all three have an entirely different phenotype to the pro-B ALL at diagnosis.

Discussion

Haematogones are normal B-cell precursors found in healthy bone marrow. They are particularly prominent in children and in adult marrows recovering from chemotherapy or following stem cell transplantation. They have a characteristic profile, illustrated above, which differs according to maturity with type I cells having the most primitive and type III cells the most mature phenotype. Type II cells are normally the most prevalent as shown in this case.

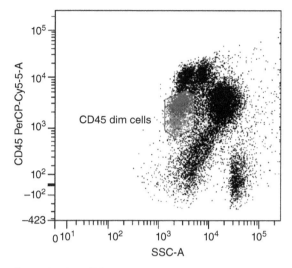

Figure 45.5 CD45/SSC.

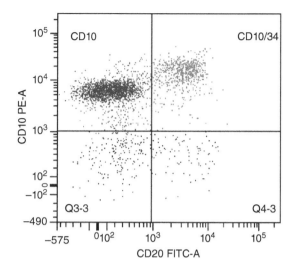

Figure 45.7 CD10/CD34.

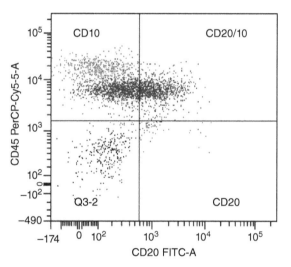

Figure 45.6 CD10/CD20.

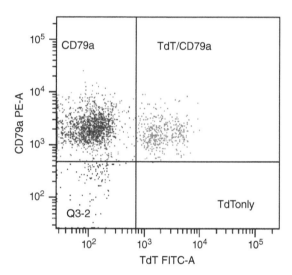

Figure 45.8 TdT/CD79a.

Haematogones must always be differentiated on flow studies from the blast cells of precursor-B ALL. This was easy in this case as pro-B ALL is CD10 negative and this patient's cells showed aberrant myeloid antigen expression. In common-B ALL the blasts can have a very similar morphology and phenotype to type I and II haematogones. In this situation it is important to have a diagnostic phenotype, with data on intensity of antigen expression, from the same flow cytometer. This data may not be readily available when patients are transferred between centres for transplantation.

Typical haematogone morphology is shown in Figure 45.3 and in Figure 45.4 adjacent to a promyelocyte.

This principle is illustrated in supplementary images showing plots from another patient with a history of previously treated common-B ALL (Figures 45.5–45.8). The CD45/SSC plot shows two populations with differing CD45 expression within the CD45^{dim} gate. The blue events are type II haematogones (CD10 positive, CD20 expression varying from negative to moderate, TdT and CD34 negative) whilst the red events are common ALL blasts showing bright CD10 and expression of CD34 and TdT, identical to findings at diagnosis. If the diagnostic phenotype had not been available the red events could have been attributed to type I haematogones though the size of this population was substantially larger than might normally be expected for such cells (25% of CD45^{dim} events).

Awareness of haematogones and their accurate differentiation from precursor-B ALL is absolutely essential in the safe and accurate analysis and reporting of bone marrow aspirate flow cytometry.

Final diagnosis

Prominent haematogones in a remission bone marrow following allogeneic transplant for pro-B acute lymphoblastic leukaemia.

46

Case 46

A 44-year-old man presented with left upper abdominal pain and was found to have 4-finger-breadth splenomegaly. He had been diagnosed with follicular lymphoma stage 4A some 8 years previously and had gone into complete remission following six cycles of chemotherapy (R-CVP). He had been well in the interim.

Laboratory results

FBC: Hb 151 g/L, WBC 35×10^9/L (neutrophils 4.1×10^9/L, lymphocytes 29.8×10^9/L) and platelets 122×10^9/L.

U&Es, LFTs and bone profile: normal.

Serum LDH was 300 U/L.

Blood film

This showed an increase in lymphoid cells comprising small to medium-sized cells with angulated nuclei, inconspicuous nucleoli and scanty cytoplasm (Figures 46.1–46.3). Some fine nuclear clefts were present. Prominent reactive large granular lymphocytes (Figures 46.2 and 46.3).

Flow cytometry (peripheral blood)

The majority of leucocytes (66.9%) were clonal, kappa-restricted B cells, positive for CD20, FMC7, CD10, CD79b and CD22. There was some CD23 expression but CD5 was negative.

Imaging

CT scan showed extensive lymphadenopathy, both peripheral and central.

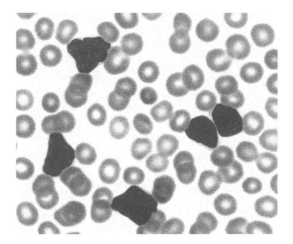

Figure 46.1 MGG, ×1000.

Bone marrow trephine biopsy

This showed a paratrabecular and heavy interstitial, bordering on diffuse, infiltrate of small to medium-sized lymphoid cells (Figures 46.4 and 46.5) with the immunophenotype being CD20$^+$ (Figures 46.6 and 46.7), CD79a$^+$, CD10$^+$, BCL6$^+$ and BCL2$^+$. The degree of marrow involvement was estimated at 70% of the total cellularity. The proliferation fraction (Ki-67) was low at 10%. The morphological features, together with the germinal centre marker profile (CD10$^+$ BCL6$^+$), are in keeping with a diagnosis of low-grade follicular lymphoma.

Discussion

Follicular lymphoma (FL) is a low-grade B-cell lymphoma that constitutes approximately 30% of all non-Hodgkin lym-

Practical Flow Cytometry in Haematology: 100 Worked Examples, First Edition. Mike Leach, Mark Drummond, Allyson Doig, Pam McKay, Bob Jackson and Barbara J. Bain.
© 2015 John Wiley & Sons, Ltd. Published 2015 by John Wiley & Sons, Ltd.

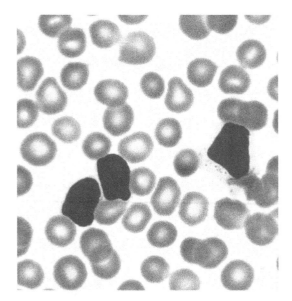

Figure 46.2 MGG, ×1000.

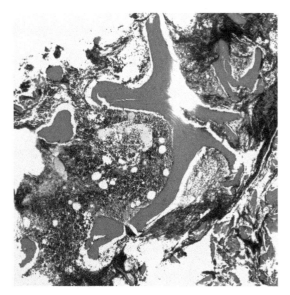

Figure 46.4 H&E, ×40.

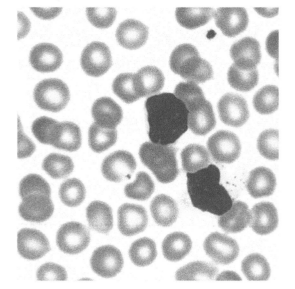

Figure 46.3 MGG, ×1000.

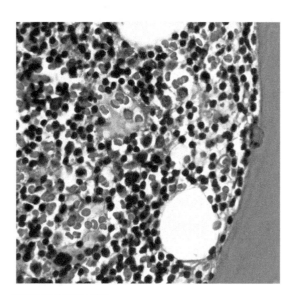

Figure 46.5 H&E, ×400.

phoma diagnoses. It commonly presents in an indolent fashion with painless lymphadenopathy or is found incidentally when patients are examined or imaged for other reasons. The genetic hallmark is the t(14;18)(q32;q21) translocation (or variant thereof) causing over-expression of BCL2, a regulator of apoptosis; this results in the loss of programmed cell death and accumulation of neoplastic cells.

This case demonstrates a late relapse of follicular lymphoma with typical advanced stage presentation. There was extensive bone marrow infiltration and overspill of lymphoid cells into the peripheral blood. The blood film morphology had typical features of a follicular lymphoma and the immunophenotype (mature B-cell disorder, CD10$^+$) was consistent with this diagnosis.

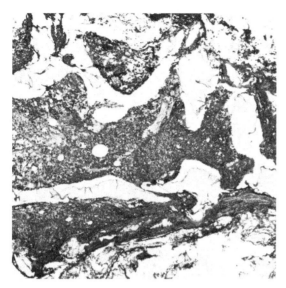

Figure 46.6 CD20, ×40.

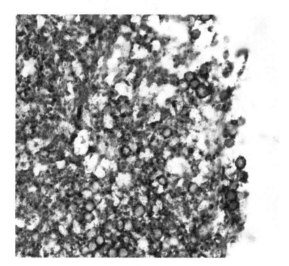

Figure 46.7 CD20, ×400.

Despite the long progression-free survival following first treatment in this patient there is some evidence that FL in leukaemic phase (1) predicts a poorer outcome with subsequent therapy. Escalated therapy using R-CHOP with a plan for a BEAM-conditioned autologous transplant in second complete remission (CR) is planned.

Final diagnosis

Relapsed follicular lymphoma in leukaemic phase.

Reference

1 Sarkozy, C., Baseggio, L., Feugier, P. *et al.* (2014) Peripheral blood involvement in patients with follicular lymphoma: a rare disease manifestation associated with poor prognosis. *British Journal of Haematology*, **164** (**5**), 659–667. PubMed PMID: 24274024.

Case 47

A 31-year-old female who had been treated for acute promyelocytic leukaemia (APL), 3 years previously, was seen for a routine follow up. Previous treatment incorporated an anthracycline/all-*trans*-retinoic acid (ATRA) regimen, with CR demonstrated after cycle 1. She complained of 7 weeks of sciatica-like symptoms and a shorter history of intermittent headache. No focal neurological signs were elicited.

Laboratory data

FBC: Hb 132 g/L, WBC 6.7×10^9/L and platelets 198×10^9/L.

Coagulation screen: PT 13 s, APTT 31 s, fibrinogen 3.1 g/L and D-dimers 290 ng/mL.

U&Es, LFTs and bone profile: normal.

Blood film normal.

Bone marrow aspirate morphology and flow cytometry studies were normal.

Imaging

MRI brain and spinal cord: no abnormality demonstrated.

CSF cytospin

The CSF specimen was hypercellular with a WBC of 0.66×10^9/L and protein of 2.3 g/L. Morphological appearances of the CSF cytospin are shown in Figures 47.1 and 47.2.

This demonstrated a population of medium-sized to large cells, with frequent granules and irregular bi- or multi-lobed nuclei. Auer rods were not easily seen and some nuclear

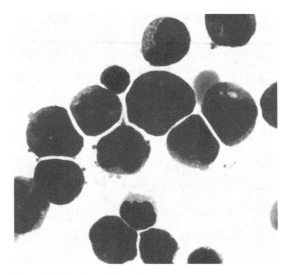

Figure 47.1 MGG, ×1000.

artefact was noted (note occasional multilobed cells). A background population of small mature lymphocytes was noted (seen in Figure 47.1) in keeping with a reactive process to the pathological cells.

Flow cytometry

Flow cytometry on CSF confirmed the presence of large numbers of neoplastic cells with high FSC and SSC (due to size and granularity respectively), which were CD117+, CD64+, CD33+, CD13+ and MPO+ but HLA-DR and CD34 negative, the typical immunophenotype of APL.

Practical Flow Cytometry in Haematology: 100 Worked Examples, First Edition. Mike Leach,
Mark Drummond, Allyson Doig, Pam McKay, Bob Jackson and Barbara J. Bain.
© 2015 John Wiley & Sons, Ltd. Published 2015 by John Wiley & Sons, Ltd.

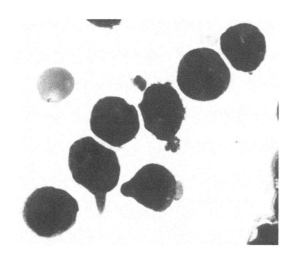

Figure 47.2 MGG, ×1000.

Genetic studies

FISH detected a *PML-RARA* fusion in a majority of cells in the CSF.

Discussion

This is an unusual case that demonstrates late CNS relapse of APL. The CNS is the commonest site of extramedullary disease in APL and approximately 10% of relapsed cases are complicated by CNS involvement (1). Peripheral blood counts were normal, although MRD analysis by quantitative RT-PCR demonstrated low-level *PML-RARA* transcripts, indicative of early marrow relapse. Although imaging is routinely performed in cases of suspected CNS relapse, the sensitivity of MRI scanning for leukaemic leptomeningeal disease is remarkably low: in a recent study the sensitivity was only 20% (the lowest for any tumour type), whereas it was 100% for CSF cytology (2) A lumbar puncture for CSF examination is therefore mandatory in any case of suspected CNS relapse. The importance of a well-prepared CSF cytospin is well illustrated here: cytomorphology is reasonably well preserved in this case, although some 'cloverleaf'-like nuclear morphological changes are noted; these are induced or accentuated by the cytospin process. Cell numbers were unusually high in this case, whereas in many disease states it is common to see relatively low pathological cell numbers, not infrequently 'diluted out'

with 'normal' reactive lymphoid cells. In this situation flow cytometry comes into its own in being able to separate out the pathological cells from the background noise of reactive cells and reduce false negative rates. Another pitfall is a 'blood tap' where malignant peripheral blood cells contaminate the CSF specimen and lead to false positive results. In this case there were no circulating leukaemic cells and contaminating red cells in the CSF were very few.

Careful handling of the CSF sample is important, with rapid (<4 h) processing and flow analysis being optimal. If sample timing or transport will incur a delay in flow cytometric analysis, cells may be placed directly into a cell-stabilising agent to preserve surface antigen integrity (3). It is also possible to deploy the full range of genetic techniques on a well-preserved and cellular sample such as this; FISH and RT-PCR are useful techniques to demonstrate disease-specific translocations. In this case FISH detected the *PML-RARA* fusion.

The patient was treated with repeated intrathecal cytarabine resulting in rapid clearance of leukaemic cells. Systemic treatment with arsenic trioxide was delivered simultaneously and MRD negativity was achieved. After stem cell harvesting she underwent a TBI autograft with apparent remission. Unfortunately, at time of writing, marrow MRD is once again detectable.

Final diagnosis

Acute promyelocytic leukaemia with CNS relapse.

References

1 Evans, G.D. & Grimwade, D.J. (1999) Extramedullary disease in acute promyelocytic leukemia. *Leukemia & Lymphoma*, **33**, 219–229.

2 Pauls, S., Fischer, A., Brambs, H., Fetscher, S., Höche, W. & Bommer, M. (2012) Use of magnetic resonance imaging to detect neoplastic meningitis: limited use in leukemia and lymphoma but convincing results in solid tumors. *European Journal of Radiology*, **81**, 974–978.

3 de Jongste, A.H., Kraan, J., van den Broek, P.D. *et al.* (2014) Use of TransFix™ cerebrospinal fluid storage tubes prevents cellular loss and enhances flow cytometric detection of malignant hematological cells after 18 hours of storage. *Cytometry Part B: Clinical Cytometry*, **86** (4), 272–279. PubMed 23674509.

Case 48

A 75-year-old male was admitted to the infectious diseases unit on account of confusion, dysuria and fever on a background of progressive night sweats and weight loss. He had a past history of atrial fibrillation, hypertension and type II diabetes mellitus. An initial assessment showed no clinical focus of infection and a CXR was normal. He was treated with broad-spectrum intravenous antibiotics but the fever persisted. Blood and urine cultures revealed no growth and screening tests for atypical infection were negative.

Laboratory data

Hb 95 g/L, MCV 89 fl, WBC 8.4×10^9/L, neutrophils 5.8×10^9/L, platelets 69×10^9/L. ESR 80 mm/hour.

U&Es: Na 128 mmol/L, K 5.5 mmol/L, urea 19 mmol/L, creatinine 126 μmol/L.

LFTs and bone profile: bilirubin 41 μmol/L, AST 167 U/L, ALT 57 U/L, GGT 49 U/L, ALP 1103 U/L, calcium 2.32 mmol/L, phosphate 1.98 mmol/L, albumin 22 g/L, globulins 34 g/L with no paraprotein detected.

Serum LDH: 4340 U/L, CRP 103 mg/L.

Coagulation screen: PT 16 s, APTT 33 s, TT 16.9 s, fibrinogen 2.33 g/L, D-dimer 3443 ng/mL.

A CT scan of chest, abdomen and pelvis was undertaken because of the possibility of an intra-abdominal abscess or occult tumour but apart from small volume para-aortic lymphadenopathy this was unremarkable. MRI of brain showed features of small vessel arterial disease but no evidence of tumour, abscess, subdural haematoma or venous sinus thrombosis. There were no serological features of a systemic vasculitis and no vegetations were seen on echocardiography. The patient continued to deteriorate but a diagnosis was elusive. In view of progressive anaemia and thrombocytopenia a haematology opinion was requested. There were no new specific clinical findings but the patient remained febrile and confused. The blood film showed no blasts or abnormal lymphoid cells but occasional nucleated red cells and myelocytes were seen. A bone marrow aspirate and a trephine specimen were taken.

Bone marrow aspirate

The bone marrow aspirate showed a population of very large pleomorphic lymphoid cells with a complex convoluted nucleus and multiple nucleoli (Figures 48.1–48.3). The cytoplasm was deep blue and some cells showed vacuolation but granules were not seen. The abnormal cells had a diameter two to three times greater than that of a neutrophil. Morphologically, an aggressive B-cell lymphoma or anaplastic large cell lymphoma seemed possible diagnoses.

Flow cytometry

Flow cytometry studies were performed and a high blast gate was selected on the FSC/SSC profile in order to characterise the large abnormal cells, Figure 48.4 (P1). This gating strategy was directed by the morphological review of the aspirate. A standard gating approach could easily have missed the cells of interest.

These largest cells were shown to express CD19, CD20 and HLA-DR. CD10 and surface immunoglobulin were not expressed but there was little doubt these cells were clonal and malignant.

Practical Flow Cytometry in Haematology: 100 Worked Examples, First Edition. Mike Leach, Mark Drummond, Allyson Doig, Pam McKay, Bob Jackson and Barbara J. Bain.
© 2015 John Wiley & Sons, Ltd. Published 2015 by John Wiley & Sons, Ltd.

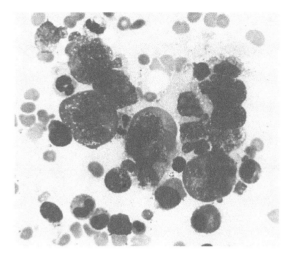

Figure 48.1 MGG, ×500.

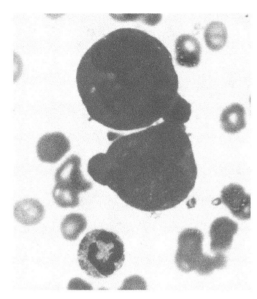

Figure 48.3 MGG, ×1000.

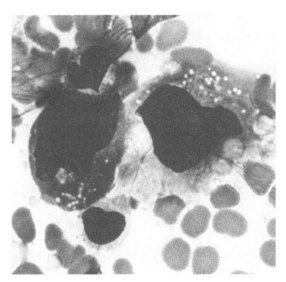

Figure 48.2 MGG, ×1000.

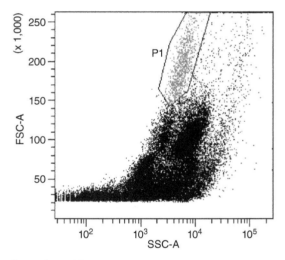

Figure 48.4 FSC/SSC.

Histopathology

The bone marrow trephine biopsy sections also showed important features. The marrow was hypercellular and clearly involved by the same large cell lymphoid population; these appeared to be primarily located within the blood vessels and marrow sinuses (arrows, Figures 48.5 and 48.6).

By using immunohistochemistry for CD20 this characteristic becomes even more apparent (Figures 48.7 and 48.8). Here again the extreme size of the lymphoma cells is

noted when compared to the residual normal haemopoietic marrow cells and non-neoplastic CD20+ interstitial small B cells.

The malignant cells expressed CD20 and MUM1 but were negative for CD5, CD10 and cyclin D1. These findings were indicative of an intravascular large B-cell lymphoma (IVL-BCL). In the interim, the condition of the patient had further deteriorated. He had suffered a fall and showed progressive confusion, bone marrow failure, capillary leak syndrome and

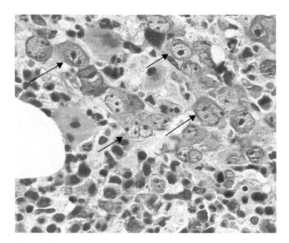

Figure 48.5 H&E, ×500.

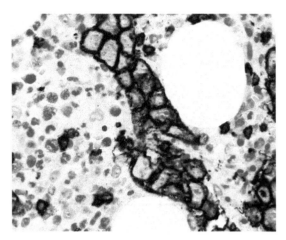

Figure 48.7 CD20, ×500.

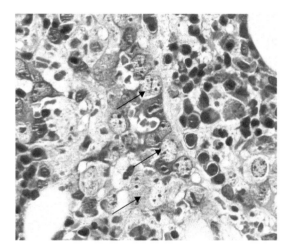

Figure 48.6 H&E, ×500.

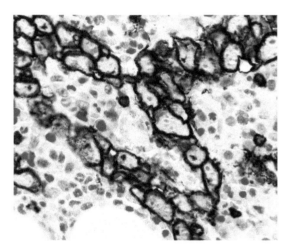

Figure 48.8 CD20, ×500.

respiratory failure. Despite the diagnosis his general condition was such that symptomatic care seemed most appropriate and he died shortly thereafter.

Another patient presented to the Neurology department with a fever, sweats, confusion and bilateral leg weakness. MRI did not show a specific focal spinal cord abnormality. He subsequently developed a nephrotic syndrome and a renal biopsy was performed. This showed abnormal hypertrophied glomeruli with interstitial expansion of the mesangium (Figure 48.9). CD20 staining identified a significant intravascular B-cell infiltrate in keeping with IVLBCL (Figure 48.10).

This second patient was treated with R-CHOP and a complete remission was achieved though the paraparesis did not

recover (likely ischaemic infarction of the spinal cord from lymphomatous occlusion of the spinal arterial vessels).

Discussion

Intravascular large B-cell lymphoma is a rare subtype of diffuse large B-cell lymphoma, diagnostically sub-classified into Asian and Western sub-types according to subtle variations in presentation and the presence of haemophagocytosis (1). The lymphoma cells have an affinity for blood vessels such that the classic features of lymphadenopathy and organomegaly are rarely apparent. Typical B symptoms with weight loss and night sweats are nearly always present and a

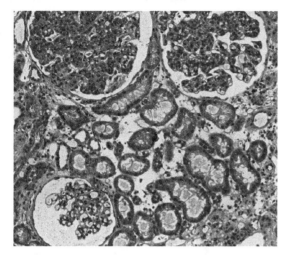

Figure 48.9 H&E, ×200.

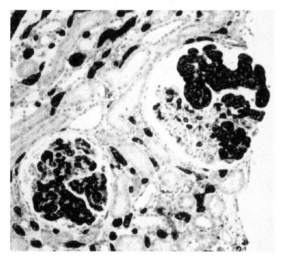

Figure 48.10 CD20, ×200.

fever and high serum LDH are common features. The other presenting symptoms are often vague but relate to vascular occlusion of the affected organ. Neurological symptoms due to cerebrovascular and spinal cord vessel involvement, skin rash due to dermal involvement and nephrotic syndrome from glomerular vessel disease are all seen.

Organomegaly and lymphadenopathy are not usually present in the Western type, so lymphoma is often not considered in the differential diagnosis. The diagnostic process is often protracted so patients can be severely debilitated when the diagnosis is finally made. Standard R-CHOP therapy can be effective in this condition (2) so it is important to consider this diagnosis in any patient with unexplained pyrexia, weight loss and night sweats with an elevated serum LDH.

Final diagnosis

Intravascular large B-cell lymphoma, Western sub-type.

See also Case 92, Asian sub-type intravascular B-cell lymphoma.

References

1 Ponzoni, M., Ferreri, A.J., Campo, E. *et al.* (2007) Definition, diagnosis, and management of intravascular large B-cell lymphoma: proposals and perspectives from an international consensus meeting. *Journal of Clinical Oncology*, **25** (**21**), 3168–3173. PubMed PMID: 17577023.

2 Hong, J.Y., Kim, H.J., Ko, Y.H. *et al.* (2014) Clinical features and treatment outcomes of intravascular large B-cell lymphoma: a single-center experience in Korea. *Acta haematologica*, **131** (**1**), 18–27. PubMed PMID: 24021554.

Case 49

A 64-year-old male had a full blood count taken whilst attending the hypertension clinic. He was clinically well. In particular he had no skin, joint or respiratory symptoms and had not noted weight loss or night sweats. On examination he appeared well and without lymphadenopathy but his spleen tip was just palpable. His medications comprised atenolol and captopril with satisfactory blood pressure control. No new medicines had recently been added and there was no history of recent travel abroad. He had no prior history of a connective tissue disorder but he was known to have nasal polyps and mild asthma.

Laboratory data

FBC: Hb 144 g/L, WBC 19×10^9/L (neutrophils 4.5×10^9/L, lymphocytes 3.1×10^9/L, eosinophils 10.5×10^9/L, monocytes 0.8×10^9/L) and platelets 256×10^9/L. ESR: 12 mm/h. Autoimmune serology, including cytoplasmic and perinuclear anti-neutrophil cytoplasmic antibodies (cANCA and pANCA), was negative.

U&Es: Na 135 mmol/L, K 4.6 mmol/L, urea 5 mmol/L, creatinine 95 μmol/L.

LFTs, bone profile, CRP and LDH: normal.

Blood film

There was marked eosinophilia and these forms were all mature. There was no myeloid left shift, blasts or excess of monocytes or basophils. Nucleated red cell precursors were not seen and there were no dysplastic features of red cells, leucocytes and platelets. The eosinophils showed only

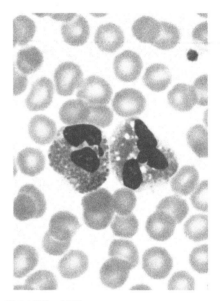

Figure 49.1 MGG, ×1000.

minor cytological abnormalities: hyperlobation, reduced numbers of granules, granules smaller than normal and some vacuolation (Figures 49.1–49.3).

Imaging

A CXR is an important investigation in any patient presenting with eosinophilia, even in the absence of respiratory symptoms. The finding of pulmonary infiltrates, lung nodules or mediastinal masses can all be informative and

Practical Flow Cytometry in Haematology: 100 Worked Examples, First Edition. Mike Leach,
Mark Drummond, Allyson Doig, Pam McKay, Bob Jackson and Barbara J. Bain.
© 2015 John Wiley & Sons, Ltd. Published 2015 by John Wiley & Sons, Ltd.

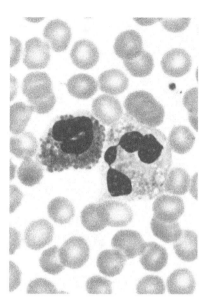

Figure 49.2 MGG, ×1000.

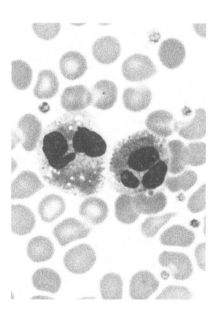

Figure 49.3 MGG, ×1000.

guide further investigations. The CXR was normal in this case. CT imaging was also performed for more detailed assessment of the lungs and mediastinum but also to image the abdomen for deep lymphadenopathy and organomegaly. The spleen was enlarged at 16 cm but no other abnormality was seen.

Flow cytometry (peripheral blood and bone marrow)

When investigating eosinophilia the blood and bone marrow morphological assessment forms an important starting point. Eosinophils can be assessed by flow cytometry but our current understanding is such that there are no reliable markers to differentiate clonal from reactive proliferations. Similarly the actual eosinophil morphology is rarely useful in the identification of the underlying pathology. Significant changes in cell size, granulation and nuclear lobulation can all be seen in reactive and neoplastic proliferations alike. What is vitally important is the assessment of any other abnormal cells that accompany the eosinophils. It is worthwhile making a careful search of peripheral blood and marrow for myeloid and lymphoid blasts, mast cells, monocytes and plasma cells. Bone marrow biopsy specimens may show lymphoma, systemic mastocytosis or a non-haemopoietic tumour. Appropriate flow cytometry studies can then be performed according to the cell type and lineage in question.

In this case the marrow aspirate showed excess eosinophils and their precursors but no other abnormal population (Figures 49.4 and 49.5).

The trephine biopsy specimen was moderately hypercellular with an interstitium expanded by eosinophils and their precursors (Figures 49.6–49.8). Charcot–Leyden crystals were not present. No abnormal infiltrate was identified and the reticulin stain was normal. There was a mild increase in

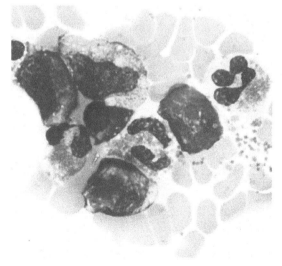

Figure 49.4 MGG, ×1000.

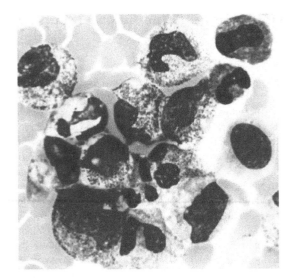

Figure 49.5 MGG, ×1000.

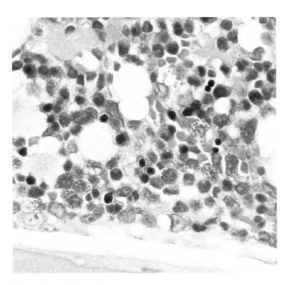

Figure 49.7 H&E, ×500.

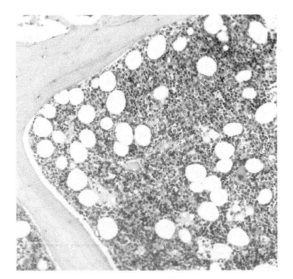

Figure 49.6 H&E, ×100.

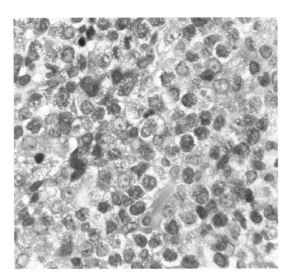

Figure 49.8 H&E, ×500.

cytologically normal interstitial mast cells, some of which were spindle shaped (Figure 49.9).

Cytogenetics

Standard metaphase cytogenetics showed a normal 46,XY. There was no t(9;22)(q32;q12) or apparent chromosome

rearrangement at 4q12 (*PDGFRA*), 5q31-33 (*PDGRFB*) or 8p11 (*FGFR1*).

Molecular

In view of the clinical presentation with a persistent marked eosinophilia and without having identified an underlying disorder indicating a reactive cause, a *FIP1L1-PDGRFA*

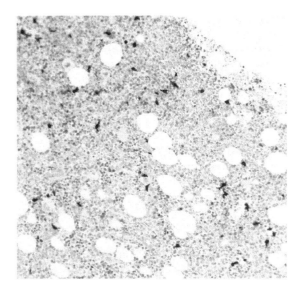

Figure 49.9 Mast cell tryptase, ×100.

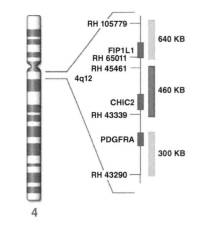

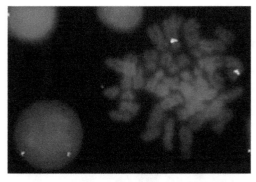

Normal profile, *CHIC2* present (green-red-green)

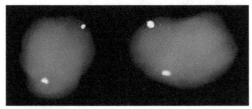

Normal profile, *CHIC2* present (green-red-green)

Figure 49.10 *CHIC2* FISH studies.

fusion was suspected and subsequently identified using RT-PCR. It should be noted that the greater sensitivity of nested RT-PCR may be needed for recognition of this fusion gene.

FISH studies utilising a *CHIC2* probe (Figure 49.10) showed a loss of signal due to the interstitial deletion at 4q12, indicating the presence of a *FIP1L1-PDGRFA* fusion gene. This fusion gene encodes a novel tyrosine kinase, which is constitutively activated and leads to eosinophil proliferation.

Abnormal profile, *CHIC2* absent in one chromosome of each cell with *FIP1L1-PDGRFA* fusion signal present (pure green) plus one normal green-red-green signal.

Discussion

Peripheral blood eosinophilia is a regular consequence of a variety of medical conditions including asthma, eczema, drug reactions, food intolerance, collagen vascular disorders, vasculitides, pulmonary eosinophilia and helminth infections. It can be seen as a reaction to solid tumours affecting the lung, thyroid, GI tract and cervix. It may be a product of a variety of haematological disorders including acute myeloid leukaemia (AML), T-lymphoblastic leukaemia/lymphoma (T-LBL), B lymphoblastic leukaemia/lymphoma, myelodysplastic syndromes, myeloproliferative neoplasms (including chronic myeloid leukaemia), myelodysplastic/myeloproliferative neoplasms (including chronic myelomonocytic leukaemia), systemic mastocytosis, T-cell non-Hodgkin lymphoma,

Hodgkin lymphoma and multiple myeloma (1). Figures 49.11 and 49.12 illustrate a case of marked reactive peripheral blood eosinophilia as a response to a T-lymphoblastic leukaemia and probable interleukin-5 release. Note the relatively few blasts in peripheral blood, but of course the marrow was heavily involved.

Once all the above have been effectively excluded there remains a proportion of patients with persistent eosinophil proliferations as described in this case. Importantly, the persistence of blood and tissue eosinophilia is capable of causing significant organ damage through release of cytokines and

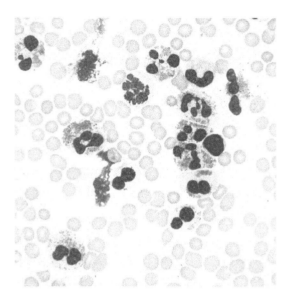

Figure 49.11 MGG, ×500.

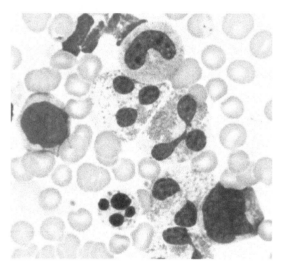

Figure 49.12 MGG, ×1000.

humoral factors derived from the eosinophil granules. Patients often develop fatigue, fever, rash, angioedema, erythroderma, myalgia, weight loss and diarrhoea. The risk of venous thrombosis is increased. With time the eosinophilia is capable of inducing pulmonary infiltrates, peripheral neuropathy and a wasting syndrome from chronic malabsorption. Perhaps most seriously a restrictive cardiomyopathy (due to endomyocardial fibrosis), heart valve deformity and embolism of intracardiac thrombi can all occur. Many of these cases were previously referred to as the hypereosinophilic syndrome (HES) in the absence of a specific cytogenetic or molecular marker.

With the improved understanding of these eosinophilic proliferations and the development in molecular diagnostics it is now possible to show that many of these cases are in fact clonal and the *FIP1L1-PDGRFA* fusion gene due to a cryptic deletion at 4q12 will be present in many of the previously categorised HES cases. The presentation is typically with an eosinophilic leukaemia but transformed cases with AML, T LBL or both, have all been reported. The disease usually affects middle-aged males. It is an important entity to recognise as the fusion gene generates a tyrosine kinase that is very effectively blocked by imatinib.

The patient was commenced on imatinib under steroid cover, as there are reports of worsening tissue damage during the initial exposure. The drug has been well tolerated and remarkably effective at just 100 mg daily. The eosinophilia resolved completely within 4 weeks, he has suffered no known organ damage and remains entirely well on follow up.

It is of interest that the cytological abnormalities in eosinophils were greater in the patient illustrated with a reactive eosinophilia than in the patient with chronic eosinophilic leukaemia resulting from *FIP1L1-PDGFRA*, emphasising that the presence or absence of cytological abnormalities is not very useful in recognising a clonal eosinophil proliferation. It should also be noted that the presence of an increase of interstitial mast cells, sometimes spindle shaped, as seen in this patient, is a fairly frequent observation in *FIP1L1-PDGFRA*-associated chronic eosinophilic leukaemia and sometimes a diagnostic suspicion of mastocytosis is raised. Making this distinction is important since the great majority of cases of systemic mastocytosis are not responsive to imatinib.

Final diagnosis

FIP1L1-PDGFRA-associated chronic eosinophilic leukaemia.

Reference

1 Bain, B.J. (2010) Myeloid and lymphoid neoplasms with eosinophilia and abnormalities of *PDGFRA*, *PDGFRB* or *FGFR1*. *Haematologica*, **95** (**5**), 696–698. PubMed PMID: 20442440.

Case 50

A 22-year-old male presented to the emergency department with a few hours history of feeling non-specifically unwell with episodes of diarrhoea, which he felt might have resulted from eating at a fast food outlet the night before. There was no personal past history of note but his younger brother and a male cousin both had a history of meningococcal septicaemia. On initial assessment the patient was febrile but had no clear focus of infection and physical examination was unremarkable. Cultures were taken and intravenous fluid therapy was commenced. He was admitted to a medical ward for observation.

Initial laboratory data

FBC: Hb 159 g/L, WBC 4.4×10^9/L, neutrophils 4.2×10^9/L, platelets 83×10^9/L.

Coagulation screen: PT 24 s, APTT 56 s, TT 15 s, fibrinogen 1.75 g/L.

U&Es, LFTs: normal. CRP was 80 mg/L.

Subsequent course

Within a few hours of admission the patient became acutely unwell with a rapid onset of hypotension and hypoxia requiring intubation, intravenous inotropes and transfer to the intensive care unit. Broad-spectrum intravenous antibiotics were commenced. He was now noted to have a rapidly developing purpuric rash over his torso whilst his peripheries were grossly discoloured, cyanosed and poorly perfused.

Repeat laboratory data

FBC: Hb 109×10^9/L, WBC 1.0×10^9/L, neutrophils 0.51×10^9/L and platelets 13×10^9/L.

Coagulation screen: PT 36 s, APTT 132 s, TT 21 s, fibrinogen 0.49 g/L, D-dimer 12,000 ng/mL.

U&Es: Na 130 mmol/L, K^+ 5.5 mmol/L, urea 9 mmol/L, creatinine 229 μmol/L and CRP 300 mg/L.

The working diagnosis was of a fulminant septicaemic illness but in view of the profound pancytopenia and coagulopathy a haematology opinion was requested. An overwhelming infection superimposed on acute leukaemia (particularly acute promyelocytic leukaemia) had to be considered and excluded.

Blood film

The peripheral blood film (Figures 50.1 and 50.2) showed neutrophils with marked toxic granulation and prominent cytoplasmic vacuolation. There was minimal myeloid left shift and no blasts or promyelocytes were seen. Red cell fragments were infrequent and the severe thrombocytopenia was confirmed.

Subsequently, on further scrutiny some neutrophils were noted to have diplococci within their cytoplasm (arrows, Figures 50.3 and 50.4) and some neutrophils were undergoing apoptosis (Figure 50.4). These findings were all in keeping with a diagnosis of meningococcal septicaemia. There were no findings to suggest the presence of a coexistent acute leukaemia and the full blood count parameters on admission were reasonably preserved apart from thrombocytopenia associated with disseminated intravascular coagulation (apparent on the admission coagulation screen). The pancytopenia was due to overwhelming sepsis.

A diagnosis of meningococcal septicaemia was subsequently confirmed when group W135 meningococcal DNA was detected in blood using PCR studies. No other organism was identified using PCR or culture. The patient survived the infection but has chronic renal impairment and has suffered loss of fingers and toes. His rehabilitation is ongoing.

Practical Flow Cytometry in Haematology: 100 Worked Examples, First Edition. Mike Leach, Mark Drummond, Allyson Doig, Pam McKay, Bob Jackson and Barbara J. Bain. © 2015 John Wiley & Sons, Ltd. Published 2015 by John Wiley & Sons, Ltd.

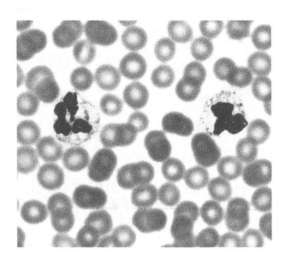

Figure 50.1 MGG, ×500.

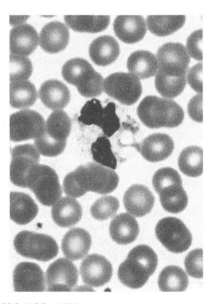

Figure 50.2 MGG, ×1000.

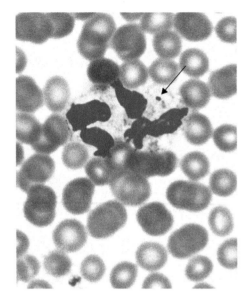

Figure 50.3 MGG, ×1000.

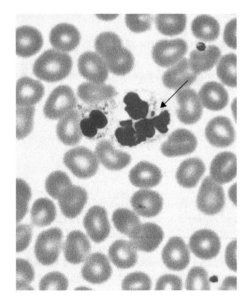

Figure 50.4 MGG, ×1000.

Meningococcal septicaemia is a devastating illness that can affect young immunocompetent patients. This patient had no prior medical history of note and no previous significant bacterial infections but the history of the same infection in close relatives should generate further thought. Although most cases of meningococcal septicaemia occur in immunocompetent individuals, some inherited immunodeficiencies involving abnormalities of the classical and alternate complement pathways, do significantly predispose to infection by this organism. Normal complement activity

is particularly important in clearing meningococci. Both quantitative and functional complement defects have been implicated but properdin deficiency, a component of the alternate pathway, increases the risk up to 7,000 fold and atypical meningococcal strains are often implicated. Subsequent investigations have shown normal CH100 classical pathway activity, normal AP100 alternate pathway activity, normal levels of C2, C3 and C4 and normal immunoglobulin levels. A normal AP100 does not exclude properdin deficiency but unfortunately properdin assays are not currently available in the UK.

Flow cytometry

Subsequent studies on the patient's neutrophils showed normal counts and morphology and normal expression of CD11, CD15 and CD18 (absent in leucocyte adhesion disorders). Lymphocyte subset studies and serum immunoglobulins were normal.

In view of the family history, the atypical meningococcal isolate and the fact that an inherited complement disorder has not been excluded the patient and his two siblings and cousins have been vaccinated with the tetravalent meningococcal A, C, Y and W135 serotype vaccine. There is evidence, that even in the presence of an inherited complement disorder, such vaccines can still be effective. The family will also be vaccinated with the meningococcal B serotype vaccine when it becomes available in the UK.

Discussion

Meningococcal septicaemia is a devastating systemic infection causing septic shock, meningitis, adrenal necrosis, DIC, acute renal failure and tissue necrosis. The mortality is as high as 50% in some series. Prompt treatment is essential but the initial symptoms are often vague and non-specific. An acute onset purpuric rash, due to thrombocytopenia and DIC, is an early highly suggestive sign that should always be recognised and should prompt early antibiotic therapy.

The haematological consequences of this infection are illustrated in this case with the rapid onset cytopenias, coagulopathy and toxic neutrophil changes in the blood film. The finding of diplococci within the neutrophils in this case was fortuitous and was only evident after rescrutinising the film some time afterwards: it did not inform decision making on the day but there was already overwhelming clinical and laboratory evidence of the later confirmed diagnosis. In other patients we have seen, identification of diplococci within neutrophils on presentation was diagnostic (1). The family history of meningococcal infection also makes this case unusual. A familial complement disorder is possible but our understanding of complement function and how it is best studied through quantitative and qualitative assays is still far from complete.

Final diagnosis

Meningococcal septicaemia with disseminated intravascular coagulation.

Possible familial properdin deficiency.

Reference

1 Uprichard, J. & Bain, B. (2008) A young woman with sudden onset of a severe coagulation abnormality. *American Journal of Hematology*, **83** (**8**), 672. PubMed PMID: 18553562.

Case 51

An 82-year-old woman presented with profound fatigue and bruising. She had no prior medical history of note and had been happily independent until two weeks prior to this medical presentation.

Laboratory data

FBC: Hb 77 g/L, WBC 1.8×10^9/L (neutrophils 0.28×10^9/L) and platelets 26×10^9/L.

U&Es, LFTs, bone profile and LDH were normal.

Blood film

Peripheral blood examination revealed a number of medium sized to large undifferentiated lymphoid cells with occasional nucleoli and a high nuclear to cytoplasmic ratio (Figures 51.1 and 51.2). The residual circulating neutrophils had normal morphology. A few nucleated red blood cells were seen.

Bone marrow aspirate

Attempts to obtain a bone marrow aspirate were unsuccessful due to a dry tap.

Flow cytometry (peripheral blood)

Peripheral blood analysis identified a CD45-negative population (red events, annotated CD45 dim) alongside normal

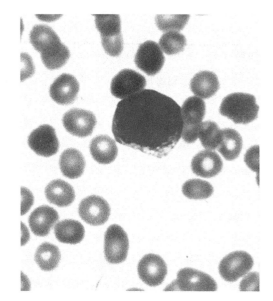

Figure 51.1 MGG, ×1000.

lymphocytes and neutrophils (Figure 51.3); the former had heterogeneous characteristics on FSC/SSC analysis (Figure 51.4). A true CD45^{dim} population was not readily apparent. The CD45$^-$ cells expressed cytoplasmic CD79a, TdT, CD19, HLA-DR, CD10 and CD20 indicating a diagnosis of common-B-cell acute lymphoblastic leukaemia (ALL).

Cytogenetic analysis

Failed chromosome analysis; isochromosome 9q and an extra copy of part of 5p detected by FISH.

Practical Flow Cytometry in Haematology: 100 Worked Examples, First Edition. Mike Leach, Mark Drummond, Allyson Doig, Pam McKay, Bob Jackson and Barbara J. Bain.
© 2015 John Wiley & Sons, Ltd. Published 2015 by John Wiley & Sons, Ltd.

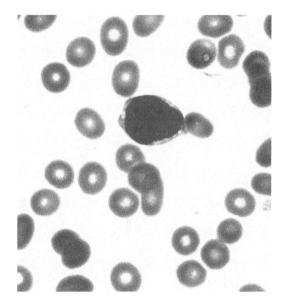

Figure 51.2 MGG, ×1000.

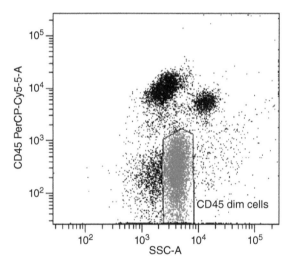

Figure 51.3 CD45/SSC.

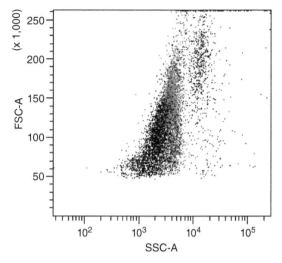

Figure 51.4 FSC/SSC.

Discussion

The identification of acute lymphoblastic leukaemia (ALL) in a patient of over 80 years is clearly a poor prognostic finding. The treatment approach needs very careful consideration in patients with ALL at this age. Induction therapy with steroids and vincristine and attenuated anthracyclines can induce remission and this can be maintained in our experience using a direct transfer to maintenance therapy with mercaptopurine and methotrexate. It is important to exclude *BCR-ABL1*-positive cases since very elderly patients who fall into this group can have useful responses to corticosteroids plus imatinib (1).

The immunophenotype in this case was interesting in that the lymphoid blasts were CD45 negative, an attribute normally associated with erythroid precursors, plasma cells and non-haematopoietic proliferations. CD45 negativity in ALL might be expected to incur an adverse prognosis as this feature suggests a very primitive derivation well removed from normal lymphoid maturation. In fact the opposite conclusion appears nearer to the truth particularly in paediatric practice where CD45 negativity in ALL appears to carry a more favourable prognosis in studies paying particular attention to this feature (2, 3). The lymphoblasts in this case also expressed CD20. This is normally associated with a more mature phenotype ALL and is commonly seen in paediatric practice and as an independent marker does not appear to carry prognostic significance (4). It remains to be seen whether the introduction of rituximab to treatment of CD20+ B-cell precursor ALL improves clinical response and long-term outcome.

An isochromosome is formed by the duplication of the two short arms or the two long arms of a chromosome hinged at the centromere. Several isochromosomes are recurrent abnormalities in ALL including i(6p), i(7q), i(9q) and i(17q). Isochromosome (9q) is most frequently seen and may be the sole anomaly or in combination with other abnormalities. In isolation it appears to be a favourable prognostic finding in children but substantive data is lacking in adults.

Final diagnosis

B lymphoblastic leukaemia/lymphoma – common ALL type.

References

1 Vignetti, M,, Fazi, P., Cimino, G. *et al.* (2007) Imatinib plus steroids induces complete remissions and prolonged survival in elderly Philadelphia chromosome-positive patients with acute lymphoblastic leukemia without additional chemotherapy: results of the Gruppo Italiano Malattie Ematologiche dell'Adulto (GIMEMA) LAL0201-B protocol. *Blood,* **109** (**9**), 3676–3678. PubMed PMID: 17213285.

2 Borowitz, M.J., Shuster, J., Carroll, A.J. *et al.* (1997) Prognostic significance of fluorescence intensity of surface marker expression in childhood B-precursor acute lymphoblastic leukemia. A Pediatric Oncology Group Study. *Blood,* **89** (**11**), 3960–3966. PubMed PMID: 9166833.

3 Behm, F.G., Raimondi, S.C., Schell, M.J. *et al.* (1992) Lack of CD45 antigen on blast cells in childhood acute lymphoblastic leukemia is associated with chromosomal hyperdiploidy and other favorable prognostic features. *Blood,* **79** (**4**), 1011–1016. PubMed PMID: 1531305.

4 Naithani, R., Asim, M., Abdelhaleem, M. *et al.* (2012) CD20 has no prognostic significance in children with precursor B-cell acute lymphoblastic leukemia. *Haematologica,* **97** (**9**), e31–e32. PubMed PMID: 22952332.

Case 52

A 71-year-old man was admitted to the acute receiving unit with diarrhoea. This was presumed to be viral in origin and settled spontaneously. He was noted to have a lymphocytosis. He gave no history of night sweats or weight loss and there was no evidence of lymphadenopathy or splenomegaly on examination.

Laboratory data

FBC: Hb 124 g/L, WBC 27×10^9/L (neutrophils 4.5×10^9/L, lymphocytes 22×10^9/L) and platelets 142×10^9/L.

Reticulocyte count was normal and direct Coombs test was negative.

U&Es, LFTs, bone profile: normal. LDH was normal.

Immunoglobulins and electrophoresis identified an IgA kappa paraprotein quantified at 33.3 g/L. IgG and IgM levels were low.

Blood film

This showed a moderate lymphocytosis of mature cells with condensed chromatin; smear cells were present (not shown).

Flow cytometry (peripheral blood)

B cells accounted for the majority of cells in the lymphoid gate. These had a CD19+, CD20dim, CD5+, CD23+, CD22dim, FMC7−, CD79b−, kappadim phenotype. These results were entirely in keeping with B-cell chronic lymphocytic leukaemia (CLL score 5/5). The high concentration

IgA kappa paraprotein was considered somewhat unusual in CLL so a bone marrow biopsy was taken.

Bone marrow aspirate

There was a reduction in normal haemopoiesis with an infiltrate of small to medium sized lymphoid cells with condensed chromatin and relatively little cytoplasm accounting for approximately 35% of nucleated cells. In addition there was a plasma cell population (37%) with more prominent cytoplasm with some of the cells showing prominent nucleoli (Figures 52.1 and 52.2).

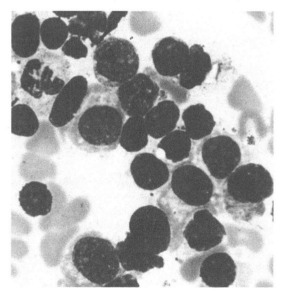

Figure 52.1 MGG, ×1000.

Practical Flow Cytometry in Haematology: 100 Worked Examples, First Edition. Mike Leach, Mark Drummond, Allyson Doig, Pam McKay, Bob Jackson and Barbara J. Bain.
© 2015 John Wiley & Sons, Ltd. Published 2015 by John Wiley & Sons, Ltd.

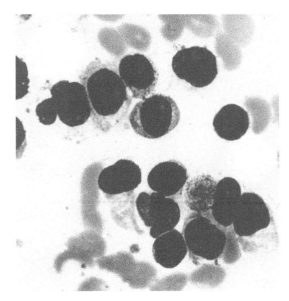

Figure 52.2 MGG, ×1000.

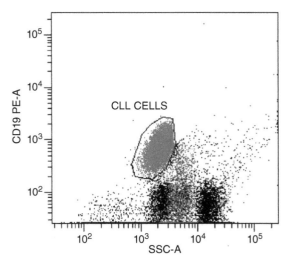

Figure 52.3 CD19/SSC.

Flow cytometry (bone marrow)

In addition to confirming bone marrow involvement by CLL, a malignant plasma cell population was also identified. A CD19$^+$ gate was used to define the CLL cells (Figure 52.3) which had a typical phenotype noted above. CD138 was used to isolate the plasma cells (Figure 52.4), which showed a neoplastic CD45$^-$, CD19$^-$, CD38$^+$, CD56$^+$ phenotype. The FSC/SSC back-gating plot shows the respective locations of the two populations (Figure 52.5).

Bone marrow trephine biopsy

The specimen was hypercellular with numerous non-paratrabecular lymphoid nodules together with a diffuse plasma cell infiltrate (70% by CD138 staining). Note the nodule of CLL cells (arrow) in Figure 52.6 surrounded by a diffuse plasma cell infiltrate. The condensed nuclei of the CLL cells are contrasted with the more open nuclei of the plasma cells in Figure 52.7 and the latter are clearly identified using CD138 in Figure 52.8.

Skeletal survey/MRI

A skeletal survey showed degenerative change but no definite features of myelomatous bone damage.

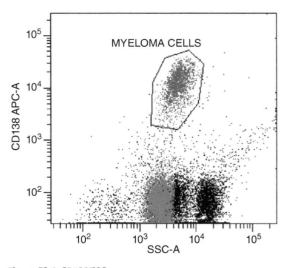

Figure 52.4 CD138/SSC.

Discussion

CLL is commonly found as an incidental finding when patients are admitted to hospital for other reasons. Monoclonal immunoglobulins can occur in patients with lymphoproliferative disorders including CLL, lymphoplasmacytic lymphoma (LPL) and marginal zone lymphoma (MZL). Low concentration paraproteins of IgM class are commonly found in CLL: they are rarely implicated in patient symptomatology. The level and nature of the paraprotein in this patient prompted further investigation to

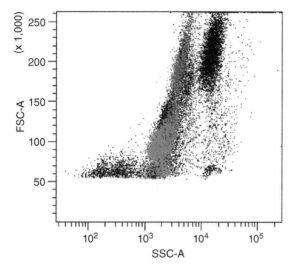

Figure 52.5 FSC/SSC.

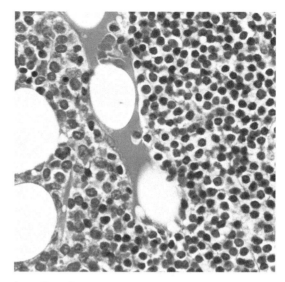

Figure 52.7 H&E, ×400.

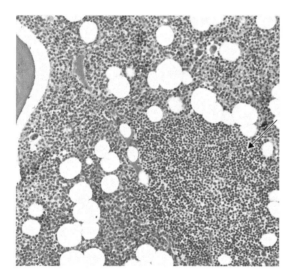

Figure 52.6 H&E, ×100.

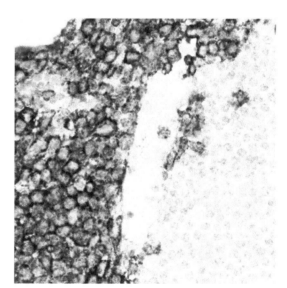

Figure 52.8 CD138, ×400.

exclude a co-existent plasma cell neoplasm even in the absence of associated bone symptoms, anaemia or renal dysfunction. Careful morphological examination of the bone marrow aspirate revealed the two malignant cell populations, and flow cytometry was able to define the CD19$^+$ and CD138$^+$ populations. This was further supported by the bone marrow trephine biopsy findings where the nodular CLL population contrasted with the diffuse plasma cell infiltrate. The two diagnoses are not connected but their

co-existence should lead to careful consideration of the optimal management plan.

Final diagnoses

1. B-cell chronic lymphocytic leukaemia
2. IgA multiple myeloma

Case 53

A 49-year-old female presented with a few months, history of fatigue. Her weight was steady and she did not report night sweats. Clinical examination revealed splenomegaly but no lymphadenopathy.

Laboratory results

FBC: Hb 105 g/L, WBC 27.9 × 10^9/L (neutrophils 2.37 × 10^9/L, lymphocytes 24.9 × 10^9/L) and platelets 123 × 10^9/L.

U&Es, LFTs and serum LDH were normal.

A low concentration IgG kappa paraprotein was identified (2.7 g/L) but without immune paresis.

Blood film

The film showed a lymphocytosis due to a population of medium sized lymphoid cells with condensed chromatin and without nucleoli. A notable feature was the presence of cytoplasmic irregularities and villi with some cells showing this in a bipolar orientation (Figures 53.1–53.3). Some cells had small cytoplasmic vacuoles (Figure 53.3).

Flow cytometry

A monoclonal (kappa restricted) B-cell lymphoid population was identified which showed strong CD20 expression together with FMC7, HLA-DR, CD79b and CD22. These cells were negative for CD5, CD10 and CD23 whilst a secondary panel showed negativity for CD11c, CD25, CD103 and CD123 (hairy cell score 0/4). A diagnosis of splenic marginal zone lymphoma (SMZL) appeared likely.

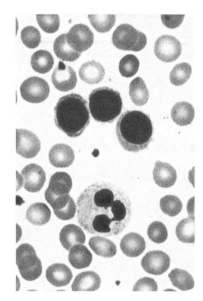

Figure 53.1 MGG, ×500.

Imaging

A CT scan showed small volume lymphadenopathy in the abdomen in addition to a homogenous enlarged spleen (18.5 cm). There was no significant lymphadenopathy.

Bone marrow aspirate and trephine biopsy

The bone marrow aspirate identified similar cells to those seen in peripheral blood. The trephine biopsy sections showed subtle involvement by a low-grade lymphopro-

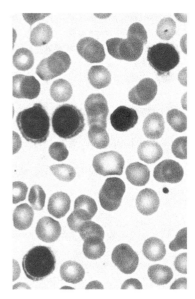

Figure 53.2 MGG, ×500.

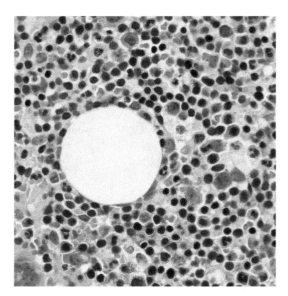

Figure 53.4 H&E, ×400.

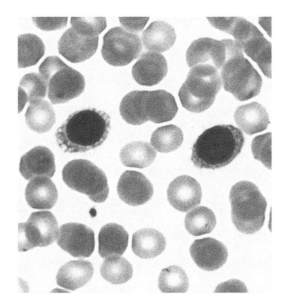

Figure 53.3 MGG, ×1000.

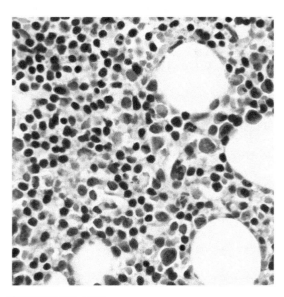

Figure 53.5 H&E, ×400.

liferative disorder but with good haemopoietic reserve (Figures 53.4 and 53.5). The infiltrate was clearly involving the bone marrow sinuses but this was only readily apparent when immunostaining for CD20 was carried out (Figure 53.6).

Discussion

The clinical finding of splenomegaly with minimal lymphadenopathy, the lymphocyte morphology and immunophenotyping results with hairy cell score of 0/4, together with the pattern of bone marrow involvement (particularly the sinusoidal infiltration) and presence of a

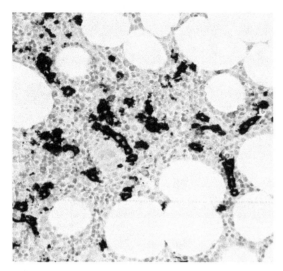

Figure 53.6 CD20, ×200.

paraprotein, were all in keeping with a diagnosis of SMZL. The diagnostically important sinusoidal infiltration can also be highlighted by immunohistochemistry to identify CD34-positive endothelial cells. The abnormal lymphocytes in SMZL typically show strong expression of CD20 in the region of 10 times the intensity normally seen in chronic lymphocytic leukaemia. This renders this condition a suitable target for rituximab therapy and use of this antibody as a single agent has now replaced splenectomy as the first line standard of care (1, 2).

Final diagnosis

Splenic marginal zone lymphoma.

References

1 Kalpadakis, C., Pangalis, G.A., Angelopoulou, M.K. *et al.* (2013) Treatment of splenic marginal zone lymphoma with rituximab monotherapy: progress report and comparison with splenectomy. *The Oncologist,* **18** (2), 190–197. PubMed PMID: 23345547. Pubmed Central PMCID: 3579603.
2 Else, M., Marin-Niebla, A., de la Cruz, F. *et al.* (2012) Rituximab, used alone or in combination, is superior to other treatment modalities in splenic marginal zone lymphoma. *British Journal of Haematology,* **159** (3), 322–328.

Case 54

A 64-year-old female presented to her GP with a short history of fatigue and pallor. Her past medical history comprised controlled hypertension only. An FBC was taken.

Laboratory data

FBC: Hb 59 g/L, WBC 31 × 10^9/L (nucleated red blood cells 2.4 × 10^9/L) and platelets 185 × 10^9/L.

U&Es, bone profile, LFTs were normal with a serum LDH 1100 U/L.

Blood film

This showed gross erythroid dysplasia with numerous circulating dysplastic erythroblasts at various stages of maturation. The myeloid series was left shifted and large blasts were also noted, many with monoblastic characteristics (not shown).

Bone marrow aspirate

A particulate, hypercellular specimen was obtained. The majority of the cells were blast cells. Two populations were present (Figures 54.1–54.5). A larger population exhibited basophilic cytoplasm, round nuclei with very open 'sieve-like' chromatin and occasional prominent Golgi zones (best seen Figures 54.1–54.4). A second population had plentiful grey-blue cytoplasm with frequent folded nuclei and immature chromatin (best seen in Figure 54.5). A very occasional late normoblast was noted, and there were prominent dysplastic changes in the few remaining myeloid precursors (Figures 54.3 and 54.4). A proportion of early

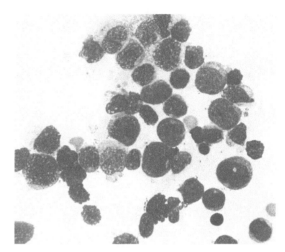

Figure 54.1 MGG, ×500.

precursors had intermediate morphological features, which made it difficult to determine if they were proerythroblasts or monoblasts (Figure 54.3).

Flow cytometry

Two blast populations were confirmed:
CD45$^+$, CD38$^+$, CD15^{bright}, CD33$^+$, CD13$^+$, HLA-DR$^+$, CD64^{bright}, CD14^{dim}, MPO$^+$.
CD45$^-$, CD34$^+$, glycophorin A (CD235a)$^{++}$.

Marrow trephine biopsy

Maximal marrow cellularity was noted (Figure 54.6), due to a diffuse and extensive blast cell infiltrate (Figures 54.7

Practical Flow Cytometry in Haematology: 100 Worked Examples, First Edition. Mike Leach,
Mark Drummond, Allyson Doig, Pam McKay, Bob Jackson and Barbara J. Bain.
© 2015 John Wiley & Sons, Ltd. Published 2015 by John Wiley & Sons, Ltd.

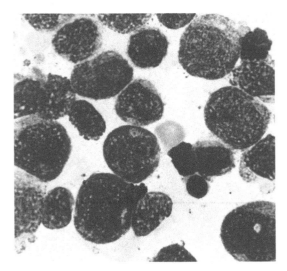

Figure 54.2 MGG, ×1000.

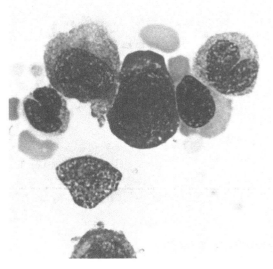

Figure 54.4 MGG, ×1000.

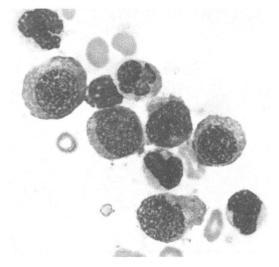

Figure 54.3 MGG, ×1000.

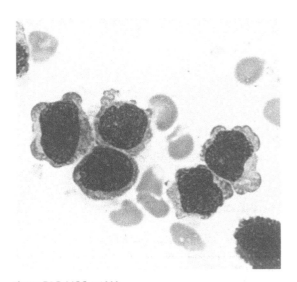

Figure 54.5 MGG, ×1000.

and 54.8). Nucleoli were prominent, and some blast cells exhibited nuclear indentations or even folding. Late erythroblasts were present but little mature myeloid activity was noted (Figure 54.8). In keeping with flow results, CD117 was present on <10% of cells (Figure 54.9 – normal mast cells are strongly immunoreactive whilst some early erythroid precursors show weak positivity) but CD11c, CD15 and CD33 were positive (Figures 54.10–54.12). Glycophorin C (CD236R) was positive in >50% of cells (Figure 54.13), in particular the larger precursors.

Cytogenetics

46, XX in all cells.

Discussion

This case is a good example of the merits of combining morphology, flow cytometry and IHC to arrive at a diagnosis.

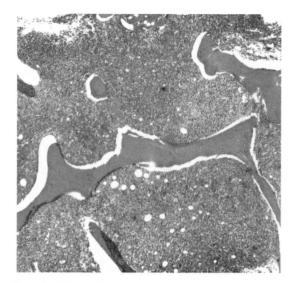

Figure 54.6 H&E, ×40.

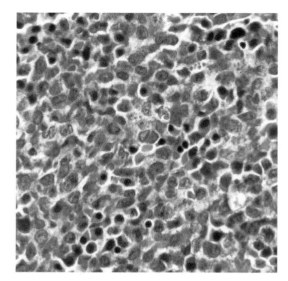

Figure 54.8 H&E, ×400.

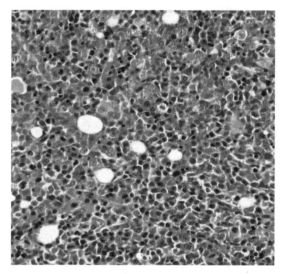

Figure 54.7 H&E, ×200.

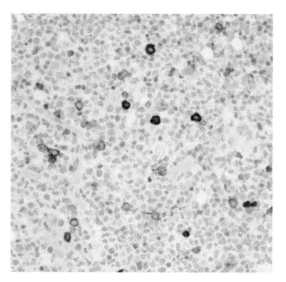

Figure 54.9 CD117, ×200.

The cytological assessment revealed two distinct blast populations: a larger erythroblast and a smaller monoblast population. Flow cytometry confirmed these findings, with the CD45$^-$ glycophorin A$^+$ erythroblast and the CD45$^+$, CD14$^+$ CD64^{++} monoblast populations easily separated. These antigen profiles were confirmed using IHC where CD15 was present on almost 100% of marrow blast cells indicating expression on both monoblasts and erythroblasts, which is well recognised (1). The relative proportions of the blast cell types are of importance here with regards to classification. A marrow differential indicated that 60% of cells were erythroblasts, with the bulk of the remainder (35%) monoblasts or promonocytes in keeping with a diagnosis of erythroleukaemia (≥50% erythroblasts and ≥20% blast cells or equivalents in the non-erythroid compartment). The unusual aspect of the case is the monoblastic lineage of the non-erythroid blast component. These features distinguish this entity from the much rarer pure erythroid

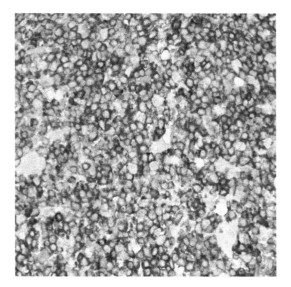

Figure 54.10 CD33, ×200.

Figure 54.12 CD15, ×200.

Figure 54.11 CD11c, ×200.

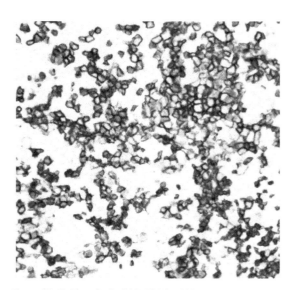

Figure 54.13 Glycophorin C (CD236R), ×200.

leukaemia, where ≥80% of cells are of erythroid lineage and no additional myeloid component is present.

Final diagnosis

Acute erythroid leukaemia (erythroleukaemia) with monoblastic myeloid component.

Reference

1 Davey, F.R., Abraham, N. Jr.,, Brunetto, V.L. *et al.* (1995) Morphologic characteristics of erythroleukemia (acute myeloid leukemia; FAB-M6): a CALGB study. *American Journal of Hematology*, **49**, 29–38.

Case 55

A 60-year-old man had received a cadaveric renal transplant some 3 years earlier for end stage renal failure due to chronic glomerulonephritis. He had developed a progressive anaemia requiring blood transfusion despite adequate graft function. His medication consisted of prednisolone and tacrolimus. There was no significant improvement in the anaemia despite the re-introduction of erythropoietin therapy and intravenous iron infusions.

Laboratory data

FBC: Hb 60 g/L, WBC 10×10^9/L (neutrophils 4.5×10^9/L, lymphocytes 4.5×10^9/L, monocytes 0.8×10^9/L) and platelets 225×10^9/L.

    Haematinics: normal.

    ESR: 10 mm/h. Reticulocytes 2×10^9/L.

    U&Es: Na 135 mmol/L, K 4.6 mmol/L, urea 10 mmol/L, creatinine 120 µmol/L.

    LFTs and bone profile: normal.

Blood film

The blood film showed prominent large granular lymphocytes with notable nuclear pleomorphism and prominent clefts and lobulation. There was not a significant lymphocytosis in absolute terms but these cells seemed prominent and worthy of further investigation (Figures 55.1 – 55.4).

Flow cytometry (peripheral blood)

A lymphoid gating strategy was applied. This identified a prominent T-lymphoid population (T cells 98%, B cells 2%);

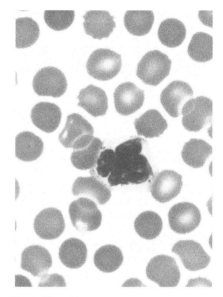

Figure 55.1 MGG, ×1000.

the T-cell population showed a subset with a CD2$^+$, CD3$^+$, CD8$^+$, CD5$^-$, CD7$^-$, CD26$^-$, CD57$^+$, CD16$^-$ phenotype. Reactive and polyclonal T-cell proliferations are frequently encountered in immunosuppressed patients following organ transplantation but the phenotype of the cells in this patient suggested a clonal disorder.

Molecular studies

Polymerase chain reaction-based T-cell receptor gene rearrangement studies identified a monoclonal peak in keeping with a clonal T-cell disorder.

Practical Flow Cytometry in Haematology: 100 Worked Examples, First Edition. Mike Leach, Mark Drummond, Allyson Doig, Pam McKay, Bob Jackson and Barbara J. Bain.
© 2015 John Wiley & Sons, Ltd. Published 2015 by John Wiley & Sons, Ltd.

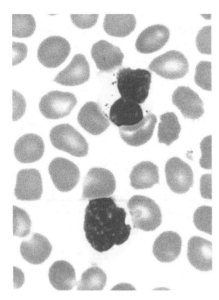

Figure 55.2 MGG, ×1000.

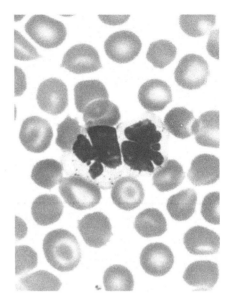

Figure 55.4 MGG, ×1000.

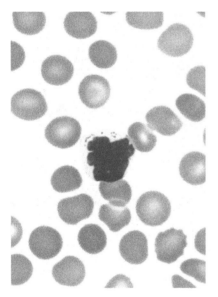

Figure 55.3 MGG, ×1000.

Imaging

CT imaging did not identify lymphadenopathy or splenomegaly. The transplant kidney was located in the right iliac fossa and appeared well perfused with normal anatomy.

Bone marrow aspirate

A bone marrow aspirate showed complete absence of erythroid precursors. The myeloid and megakaryocyte lineages appeared normal and there was no abnormal infiltrate. A trephine biopsy was not undertaken.

Discussion

Acquired pure red cell aplasia (PRCA) is a serious condition characterised by the complete loss of bone marrow erythroid precursors with an associated severe reticulocytopenia and anaemia requiring blood transfusion. It can develop in relation to drug therapy, autoimmune disorders and lymphoproliferative disorders. In the context of renal disease it can be seen as a rare consequence of erythropoietin therapy in patients who develop anti-erythropoietin antibodies. The latter were not detected in this case and the patient had not been exposed to erythropoietin treatment after the successful renal transplant. The large granular lymphocyte clone detected in this patient was not coincidental. Such proliferations are a rare but well recognised subset of post-transplant lymphoproliferative disorders (1). They are often indolent and do not commonly cause symptoms unless they happen to induce PRCA, neutropenia or auto-immune haemolytic anaemia.

On recognising this clone and without an alternative explanation for the PRCA the patient underwent a trial of oral cyclophosphamide therapy. Within a few weeks the reticulocytopenia resolved, the haemoglobin concentration gradually rose back to normal and blood transfusion support was stopped. The peripheral blood LGL population gradually regressed such that the cyclophosphamide could eventually be withdrawn.

Final diagnosis

T-LGL leukaemia with acquired pure red cell aplasia occurring as a post-transplant lymphoproliferative disorder following renal transplant.

Reference

1 Swerdlow, S.H. (2007) T-cell and NK-cell posttransplantation lymphoproliferative disorders. *American Journal of Clinical Pathology,* **127** (**6**), 887–895. PubMed PMID: 17509986.

Case 56

A 62-year-old man presented with a year's history of an itchy erythematous rash. A skin biopsy showed features in keeping with vasculitis/panniculitis. He then developed symptoms including weight loss, night sweats, chest pain and shortness of breath.

Laboratory results

FBC: Hb 138 g/L, WBC 3.1×10^9/L (neutrophils 1.19×10^9/L, lymphocytes 0.8×10^9/L), platelets 142×10^9/L.

U&Es: normal

LFTs: bilirubin 22 µmol/L, ALT 171 U/L, AST 122 U/L, GGT 88 U/L, alkaline phosphatase 236 U/L, albumin 30 g/L.

LDH: 1709 U/L.

Imaging

CT scan of thorax, abdomen and pelvis showed abnormal lymph nodes in the aortopulmonary window, small bowel mesentery and left iliac region. In addition, there was a large, infiltrative retroperitoneal mass.

Histopathology

CT-guided biopsy of the retroperitoneal mass showed infiltration of skeletal muscle by a diffuse highly pleomorphic large cell infiltrate. The cells had hyperchromatic pleomorphic nuclei, occasionally polylobulated. There was prominent apoptosis and brisk mitotic activity with focal necrosis (Figures 56.1 and 56.2).

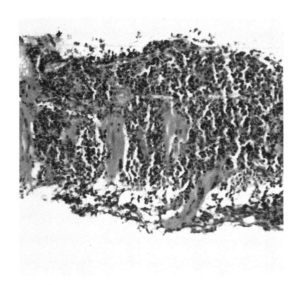

Figure 56.1 H&E, ×100.

The immunophenotype was as follows:

Positive – CD45, CD2, CD3 (Figure 56.3), CD4 (Figure 56.4) and MUM1

Negative – CD20, CD5 (Figure 56.5, positive staining cells are normal residual T cells), CD8, CD7, CD79a, BF1, TdT, CD10, BCL6, CD30, CD56, ALK1 and cyclin D1. *In situ* hybridisation for EBV was negative and the proliferation fraction was 90% (Figure 56.6).

This was a mature CD4+ T-cell lymphoma with high proliferative activity showing multiple antigen loss (CD5 and CD7) presenting as a retroperitoneal nodal mass. The bone marrow aspirate and trephine biopsy were not involved by tumour though a degree of reactive haemophagocytosis was seen, probably accounting for the peripheral blood

Practical Flow Cytometry in Haematology: 100 Worked Examples, First Edition. Mike Leach, Mark Drummond, Allyson Doig, Pam McKay, Bob Jackson and Barbara J. Bain.
© 2015 John Wiley & Sons, Ltd. Published 2015 by John Wiley & Sons, Ltd.

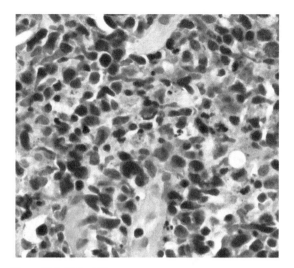

Figure 56.2 H&E, ×400.

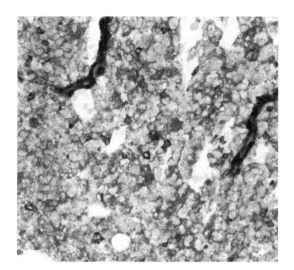

Figure 56.4 CD4, ×200.

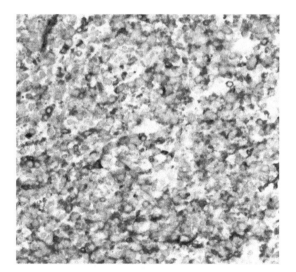

Figure 56.3 CD3, ×200.

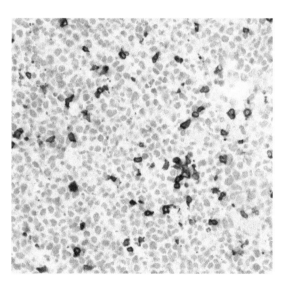

Figure 56.5 CD5, ×200.

cytopenias. The results were therefore in keeping with a diagnosis of peripheral T-cell lymphoma, not otherwise specified (PTCL-NOS).

Clinical course

He was treated with multi-agent CHOP chemotherapy and achieved a complete remission with resolution of all symp-

toms. In view of the adverse prognosis of these high-grade T-cell lymphomas, this was consolidated using an autologous stem cell transplant (BEAM conditioning).

Two months post-transplant, he complained of malaise, weight loss and breathlessness on minimal exertion. Clinical examination was unremarkable but a full blood count now showed pancytopenia with profound thrombocytopenia (platelets 28×10^9/L). The serum LDH was again markedly

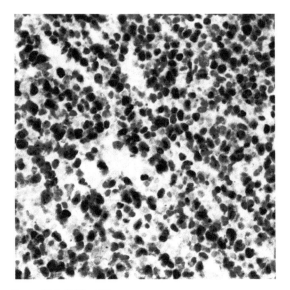

Figure 56.6 Ki-67, ×200.

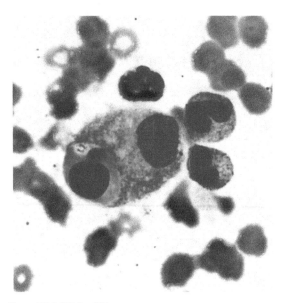

Figure 56.8 MGG, ×500.

elevated at 1419 U/L. A bone marrow aspirate and trephine biopsy were taken.

Bone marrow aspirate

The first feature in the aspirate was the presence of haemophagocytosis (Figures 56.7 and 56.8). In addition, a population of large undifferentiated lymphoid cells was noted (Figures 56.9 and 56.10).

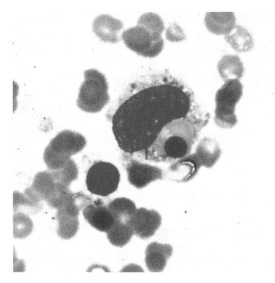

Figure 56.7 MGG, ×500.

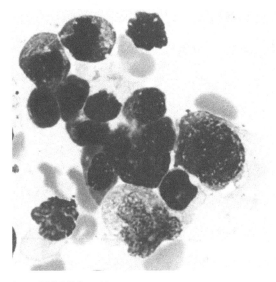

Figure 56.9 MGG, ×500.

Bone marrow trephine biopsy

The trephine biopsy specimen was diffusely involved by T-cell lymphoma (Figure 56.11) now showing partial loss of CD3 expression (Figure 56.12).

Flow cytometry

In order to achieve a rapid diagnosis and exclude another treatment-related pathology the bone marrow aspirate was

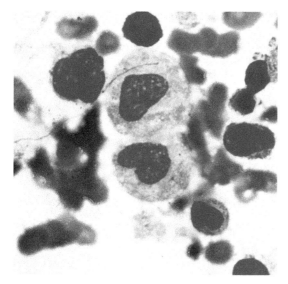

Figure 56.10 MGG, ×500.

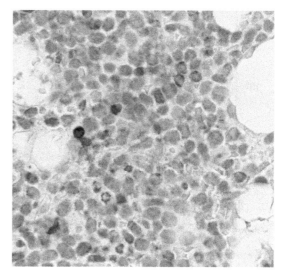

Figure 56.12 CD3, ×400.

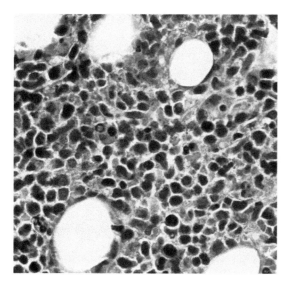

Figure 56.11 H&E, ×400.

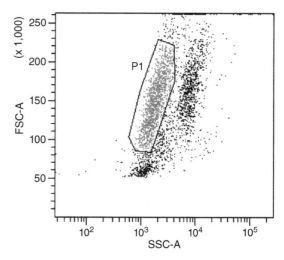

Figure 56.13 FSC/SSC.

examined. A large cell population, corresponding to that seen morphologically was occupying the blast gate on FSC versus SSC analysis (population P1, Figure 56.13) and was expressing HLA-DR with the majority showing loss of CD3 (red events, Figure 56.14, noting the residual activated reactive T cells, black events). CD2, CD4 and MUM1 were preserved with uniform strong expression of CD26 (Figure 56.15).

Discussion

This case illustrates the frequently observed aggressive clinical behaviour of high-grade mature T-cell lymphomas categorised as PTCL-NOS. There is still biological heterogeneity within this group comprised of the cases remaining when those T-cell lymphomas satisfying specific criteria

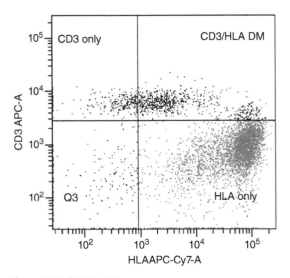

Figure 56.14 CD3/HLA-DR.

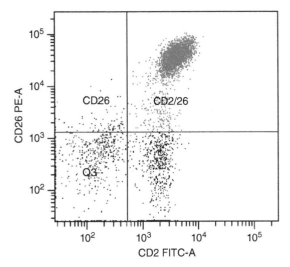

Figure 56.15 CD2/CD26.

for a precise classification, for example, anaplastic large-cell lymphoma, enteropathy-associated T-cell lymphoma, angio-immunoblastic T-cell lymphoma and NK/T-cell lymphoma, are excluded. They do, however share common clinical characteristics, are difficult to treat and often relapse. This patient suffered an early relapse with rapid onset of B symptoms and peripheral blood cytopenias due to marrow involvement with associated haemophagocytosis.

Final diagnosis

Relapsed peripheral T-cell lymphoma (PTCL-NOS) with bone marrow infiltration and haemophagocytosis.

57

Case 57

A 64-year-old man presented to the dermatology department with a relatively short history of multiple haemorrhagic purple plaques and nodules on his trunk (Figures 57.1 and 57.2) and face. These were not painful but he experienced some itch particularly if the lesions were rubbed or traumatised. He was a non-smoker and had no past medical history of note.

Clinical images

Laboratory data

FBC: Hb 147 g/L, WBC 12.5×10^9/L (neutrophils 8.3×10^9/L, lymphocytes 2.3×10^9/L, monocytes 1.7×10^9/L, eosinophils 0.2×10^9/L) and platelets 209×10^9/L.

U&Es, LFTs, bone profile and LDH were normal.

Blood film

The blood film was normal apart from a mild monocytosis without atypical features. No blasts were identified.

Histopathology

The skin biopsy showed a diffuse infiltrate of intermediate sized mononuclear cells involving the full thickness of the dermis extending into subcutaneous tissue with sparing of the epidermis (Figure 57.3). These cells had irregular elongated nuclei with inconspicuous nucleoli and abundant non-granular cytoplasm (Figure 57.4). Mitotic activity was brisk. The infiltrate showed the following phenotype:
- Positive: CD43, CD123 (Figure 57.5), CD56 (Figure 57.6), CD33 (Figure 57.7) and CD4 (Figure 57.8).

- Negative: CD20, PAX5, CD10, CD3, CD2, CD5, CD7, MUM1, TdT, CD34, Cyclin D1, CD30, myeloperoxidase and granzyme B.

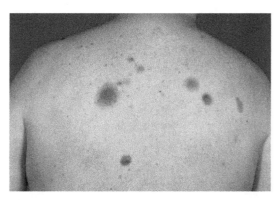

Figure 57.1

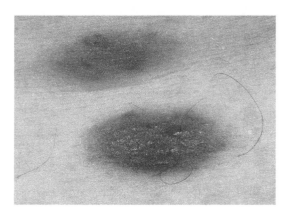

Figure 57.2

Practical Flow Cytometry in Haematology: 100 Worked Examples, First Edition. Mike Leach, Mark Drummond, Allyson Doig, Pam McKay, Bob Jackson and Barbara J. Bain.
© 2015 John Wiley & Sons, Ltd. Published 2015 by John Wiley & Sons, Ltd.

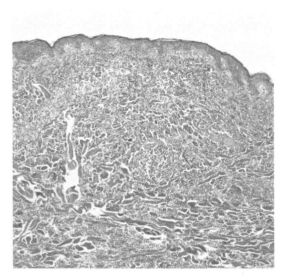

Figure 57.3 H&E, ×40.

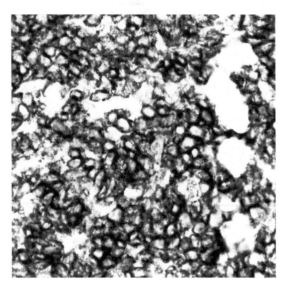

Figure 57.5 CD123, ×400.

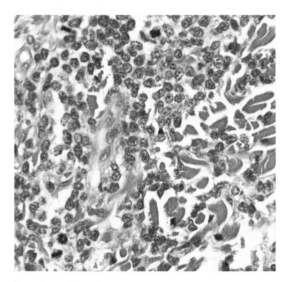

Figure 57.4 H&E, ×400.

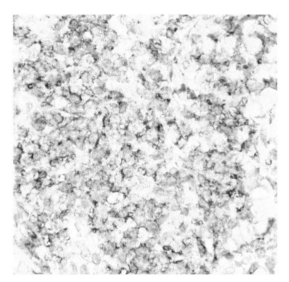

Figure 57.6 CD56, ×400.

The clinical presentation and immunophenotype in this case were in keeping with a diagnosis of blastic plasmacytoid dendritic cell neoplasm.

In the light of this working diagnosis a bone marrow aspirate was taken for morphology and flow cytometry studies.

Bone marrow aspirate

The aspirate was hypercellular with myeloid hyperplasia (Figure 57.9). There were mild dysplastic features in the

erythroid precursors but megakaryocytes were normal. A small population of medium sized blastoid cells was noted but these accounted for less than 2% of the overall cellularity (Figures 57.10 and 57.11).

Flow cytometry

This technique is the ideal tool for delineating small populations of abnormal cells. We had the benefit of knowing

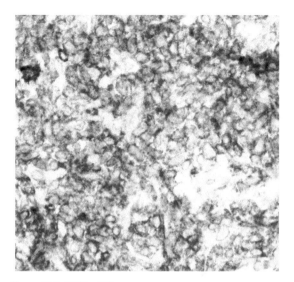

Figure 57.7 CD33, ×400.

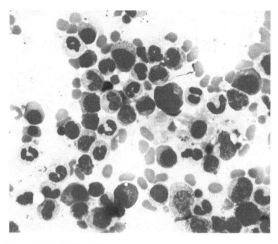

Figure 57.9 MGG, ×500.

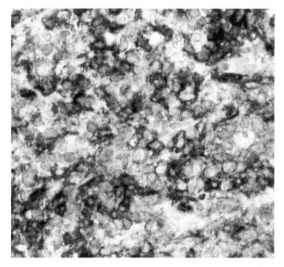

Figure 57.8 CD4, ×400.

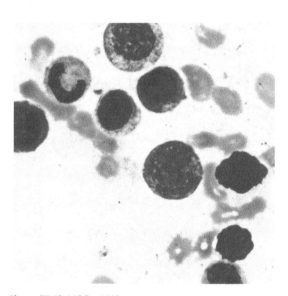

Figure 57.10 MGG, ×1000.

the working diagnosis from the skin biopsy so our approach could be tailored accordingly. As the disease cell population has a unique phenotype a broader spectrum of antibodies and fluorochromes than usual was employed to show the characteristic antigen co-expression. We started by using an acute leukaemia panel because this entity can closely resemble leukaemia cutis in skin biopsies. No distinct blast population could be identified using a FSC/SSC or CD45/SSC approach but by using CD123 versus SSC an aberrant cell

population could be shown (Figure 57.12). Using back gating the position of these cells in the FSC/SSC and CD45/SSC plots could now be seen (Figures 57.13 and 57.14).

The cells are of intermediate size and show minimal granularity (FSC/SSC) and heterogeneous but dim CD45 expression. The CD123 positive cells had the following phenotype:

- Positive: CD45^{dim}, CD56, CD33, HLA-DR and CD4^{dim}.
- Negative: CD34, CD117, MPO, CD14, CD64, CD15, CD7, cCD3, CD19, cCD79a, CD10 and CD20.

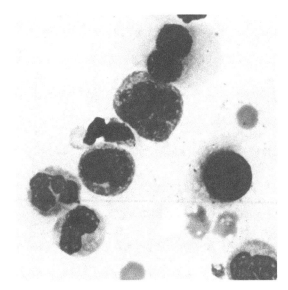

Figure 57.11 MGG, ×1000.

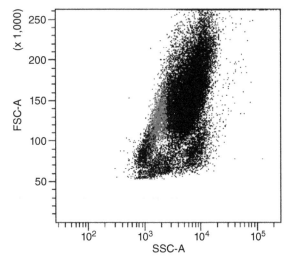

Figure 57.13 FSC/SSC.

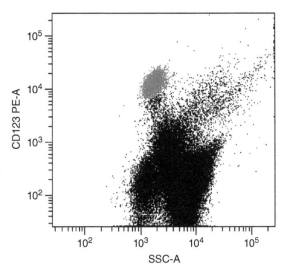

Figure 57.12 CD123/SSC.

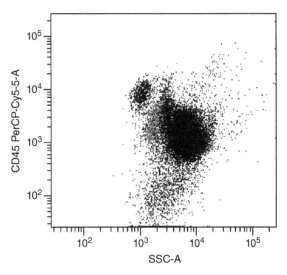

Figure 57.14 CD45/SSC.

Note that the granulocyte series showed rather dim CD45 expression in this case (large cloud of black events with extreme SSC) in Figure 57.14.

Discussion

Blastic plasmacytoid dendritic cell neoplasm (BPDCN), previously known as CD4⁺CD56⁺ haematodermic neoplasm or blastic NK cell lymphoma, is believed to originate from plasmacytoid dendritic cells (or plasmacytoid monocytes) (1, 2). This rare tumour frequently presents with nodular skin lesions often followed by progressive bone marrow infiltration and progressive cytopenias. Cases with a frankly leukaemic presentation have been described. It can present at any age though it typically affects elderly males.

Though rare, this condition is important to recognise and must be differentiated from leukaemia cutis, particularly skin involvement by the monocytic leukaemias which can express CD56 alongside HLA-DR and CD4 (3). Importantly,

BPDCN may show myeloid antigen expression but does not express MPO, CD11c or CD14 whilst leukaemia cutis will express MPO or monocytic lineage markers (CD14, CD64, CD11c) in the majority of cases and CD123 expression is unusual. The tumour infiltrates in BPDCN typically involve the dermis with extension into subcutaneous fat but typically spare the epidermis. Early bone marrow involvement may only be detectable using flow cytometry as in this case and it seems possible (though not proven) that treatment at this point, prior to evolution to bone marrow failure, would lead to a better outcome. Interestingly, the residual haemopoietic series may show dysplastic features (1), as seen in this case where dyserythropoiesis was detected. There is no specific cytogenetic or molecular aberration associated with BPDCN but complex karyotypes with partial or complete chromosome losses are frequent with deletions at 9p21 (*CKND2A/CDKN2B*) being most commonly reported in one series (4).

The optimal approach to flow cytometry assessment of such cases is still open to debate. Bone marrow involvement is often subclinical in early cases and standard gating strategies using CD34/SSC, CD45/SSC and the blast gate on FSC/SSC may not reveal the neoplastic population. By using CD123/SSC we were able to detect these cells, clarify other relevant antigen co-expression and exclude an early monocytic lineage leukaemia with skin involvement.

The optimal treatment for this condition is far from clear. Typically responses to acute leukaemia therapies (both myeloid and lymphoid) have been short lived and survival has generally been reported to be poor (5). The use of intensive high-grade lymphoma type therapies can induce complete responses in up to 70% of cases but autologous or allogeneic transplant appears necessary if such responses are to be maintained (6). The authors have had a successful outcome using CODOX M/IVAC therapy and autologous stem cell transplantation in first CR for a 58-year-old male with typical skin and marrow involvement. The rarity of this condition, unfortunately, precludes any potential future study of novel treatment approaches using randomised clinical trials.

Final diagnosis

Blastic plasmacytoid dendritic cell neoplasm.

References

1 Petrella, T., Comeau, M.R., Maynadie, M. *et al.* (2002) Agranular CD4+ CD56+ hematodermic neoplasm' (blastic NK-cell lymphoma) originates from a population of CD56+ precursor cells related to plasmacytoid monocytes. *The American Journal of Surgical Pathology*, **26** (7), 852–862. PubMed PMID: 12131152.

2 Herling, M. & Jones, D. (2007) CD4+/CD56+ hematodermic tumor: the features of an evolving entity and its relationship to dendritic cells. *American Journal of Clinical Pathology*, **127** (5), 687–700. PubMed PMID: 17439829.

3 Cronin, D.M., George, T.I., Reichard, K.K. & Sundram, U.N. (2012) Immunophenotypic analysis of myeloperoxidase-negative leukemia cutis and blastic plasmacytoid dendritic cell neoplasm. *American Journal of Clinical Pathology*, **137** (3), 367–376. PubMed PMID: 22338048.

4 Lucioni, M., Novara, F., Fiandrino, G. *et al.* (2011) Twenty-one cases of blastic plasmacytoid dendritic cell neoplasm: focus on biallelic locus 9p21.3 deletion. *Blood*, **118** (17), 4591–4594. PubMed PMID: 21900200.

5 Pagano, L., Valentini, C.G., Pulsoni, A. *et al.* (2013) Blastic plasmacytoid dendritic cell neoplasm with leukemic presentation: an Italian multicenter study. *Haematologica*, **98** (2), 239–246. PubMed PMID: 23065521.

6 Reimer, P., Rudiger, T., Kraemer, D. *et al.* (2003) What is CD4+CD56+ malignancy and how should it be treated? *Bone Marrow Transplantation*, **32** (7), 637–646. PubMed PMID: 13130309.

58

Case 58

A 68-year-old man with a history of mycosis fungoides (MF) presented with the recent onset of marked leucocytosis and lymphadenopathy. His skin plaques and nodules remained problematic but no new changes were apparent.

Laboratory results

FBC: Hb 115 g/L, WBC 16.1 × 10⁹/L (neutrophils 7.03 × 10⁹/L, lymphocytes 5.03 × 10⁹/L, eosinophils 1.55 × 10⁹/L) and platelets 440 × 10⁹/L.

   U&Es and liver function profile was normal.

   Serum LDH was 350 U/L.

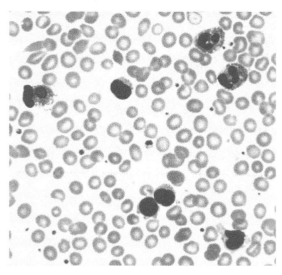

Figure 58.1 MGG, ×500.

Peripheral blood morphology

The film showed notable pleomorphic, medium sized lymphoid cells, often with prominent bi-lobed nuclei, together with marked eosinophilia (Figures 58.1 – 58.3). These two cell types accounted for the leucocytosis.

   Using a CD2 versus CD19 strategy the abnormal cells were noted to be T-lymphoid expressing CD2, CD3, weak HLA-DR, CD5 and uniform CD26 (Figures 58.4 and 58.5). There was loss of CD7 and, importantly, both CD4 and CD8 (Figures 58.6 and 58.7). A significant proportion of these cells co-expressed CD30.

Skin biopsy

There was a band-like lymphoid infiltrate within the upper dermis (arrows, Figures 58.8 and 58.9) with cells

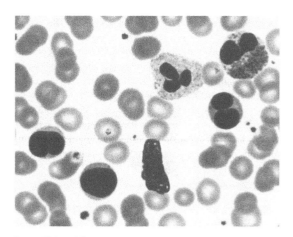

Figure 58.2 MGG, ×1000.

Practical Flow Cytometry in Haematology: 100 Worked Examples, First Edition. Mike Leach, Mark Drummond, Allyson Doig, Pam McKay, Bob Jackson and Barbara J. Bain.
© 2015 John Wiley & Sons, Ltd. Published 2015 by John Wiley & Sons, Ltd.

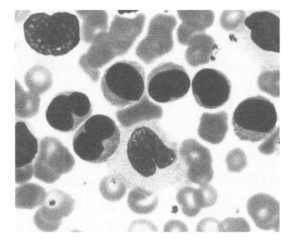

Figure 58.3 MGG, ×1000.

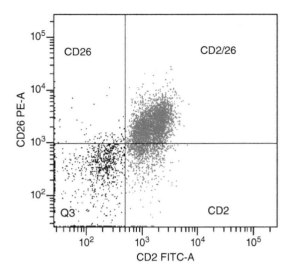

Figure 58.5 CD2/CD26.

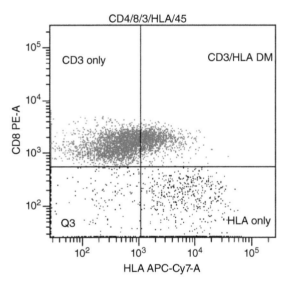

Figure 58.4 CD3/HLA-DR.

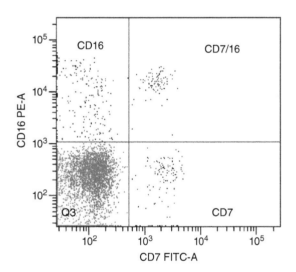

Figure 58.6 CD7/CD16.

co-expressing CD3, CD4 (Figures 58.10 and 58.11) and CD5 whilst CD7 and CD8 were both negative. There was a significant proportion of CD30⁺ cells, a small number of which had migrated into the epidermis. These appearances were in keeping with a T-cell lymphoma involving skin but with minimal epidermotropism.

Bone marrow trephine biopsy

The cellularity and composition of the marrow appeared essentially normal. However there were two small paratrabecular lymphoid infiltrates with associated eosinophils. The infiltrate had an identical phenotype to that described in the

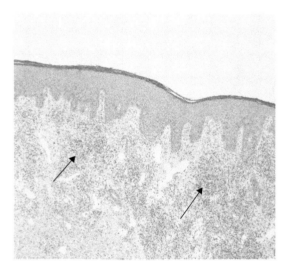

Figure 58.7 CD4/CD8.

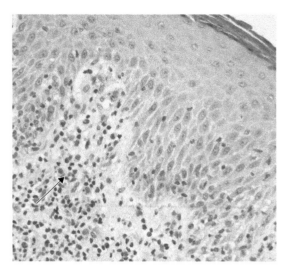

Figure 58.9 H&E, ×200.

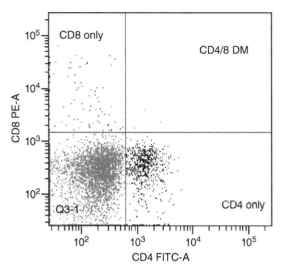

Figure 58.8 H&E, ×40.

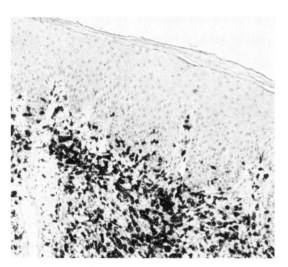

Figure 58.10 CD3, ×100.

blood (CD2⁺, CD5⁺, CD30⁺) but differed from that seen in skin in that CD4 was not expressed.

Discussion

Mycosis fungoides is a cutaneous T-cell lymphoma in which circulating lymphoma cells can sometimes be demonstrated at low levels using flow cytometry. These cells have a mature T-cell phenotype and usually express CD4, similarly to cells seen in Sézary syndrome. The abnormal circulating cells in this case showed pleomorphic morphology with prominent nuclear clefts/lobulation and the white cell count was significantly higher than that expected in chronic phase MF. The immunophenotype of these cells was also not in keeping with MF with loss of CD4 and gain of CD30. Cells with the same phenotype were seen to be involving the marrow

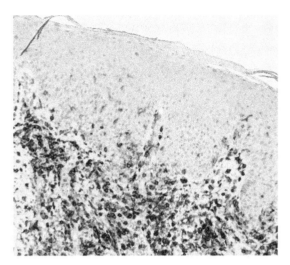

Figure 58.11 CD4, ×100.

in trephine biopsy sections but the skin biopsies merely showed features of residual MF. A distinct clinical deterioration had been noted in the patient with development of new lymphadenopathy and appearance in the peripheral blood of the lymphoid cells described above. This picture was in keeping with a progression/transformation of the pre-existing cutaneous T-cell lymphoma.

Final diagnosis

Progression of mycosis fungoides with nodal and peripheral blood involvement.

59

Case 59

A 10-year-old girl was assessed because of pallor and intermittent episodes of jaundice. On examination she appeared pale but well and the spleen tip was palpable.

Laboratory data

FBC: Hb 95 g/L, MCV 98 fl, WBC 8 × 10⁹/L and platelets 142 × 10⁹/L.

Reticulocytes 180 × 10⁹/L. Direct Coombs test was negative.

U&Es and bone profile normal.

Serum LDH 350 U/L.

LFTs: AST 70 U/L, ALT 40 U/L, ALP 180 U/L, albumin 38 g/L, bilirubin 35 μmol/L.

Blood film

This showed prominent spherocytes, occasional stomatocytes and mild polychromasia (Figures 59.1 and 59.2).

Flow cytometry (peripheral blood)

Red cell eosin-5-maleimide (EMA) binding studies were performed and showed a reduced value of 0.78 when expressed as a ratio to normal controls (NR >0.81).

Discussion

The clinical presentation, red cell morphology and EMA binding studies are all supportive of a diagnosis of hereditary spherocytosis (HS). This is a straightforward diagnosis in this

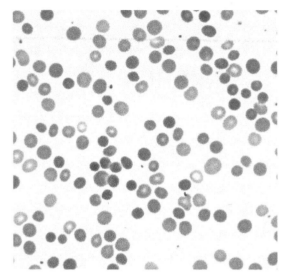

Figure 59.1 MGG, ×500.

case as the features were typical but the degree of anaemia and red cell morphology can be influenced by co-existent iron or folate deficiency. The latter is particularly common in patients before this diagnosis is established due to the demands on folate availability from marrow compensation and erythroid hyperplasia.

Another 30-year-old patient presented after a flu-like illness with severe anaemia (Hb 56 g/L), mild pancytopenia and reticulocytopenia (6 × 10⁹/L). She had been already transfused by the time a blood film was seen by a haematologist. We noted a previous history of cholecystectomy. There was a family history of hyperbilirubinaemia attributed to Gilbert's disease but a number of family members also had a history of splenectomy.

Practical Flow Cytometry in Haematology: 100 Worked Examples, First Edition. Mike Leach, Mark Drummond, Allyson Doig, Pam McKay, Bob Jackson and Barbara J. Bain.
© 2015 John Wiley & Sons, Ltd. Published 2015 by John Wiley & Sons, Ltd.

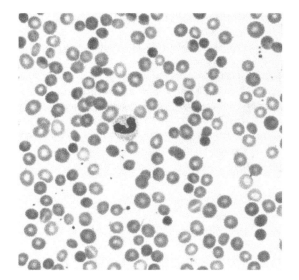

Figure 59.2 MGG, ×500.

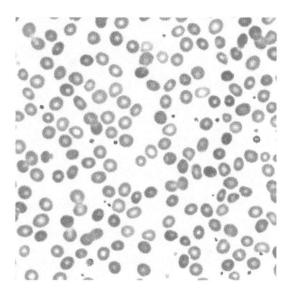

Figure 59.4 MGG, ×500.

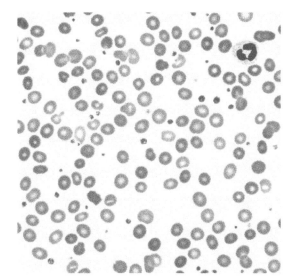

Figure 59.3 MGG, ×500.

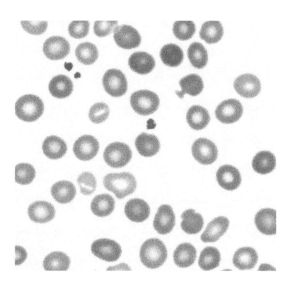

Figure 59.5 MGG, ×1000.

The film did not show many obvious spherocytes but a relatively small number of cells had a pinched, pincered or mushroom appearance depending on your preferred terminology (Figures 59.3–59.6). These cells are a particular morphological feature of band 3 deficiency hereditary spherocytosis and can be easily overlooked by those not familiar with this HS subtype.

The profound anaemia and reticulocytopenia in this second case were due to erythrovirus (parvovirus B19)

infection and after transfusion support she made an uneventful recovery thereafter. EMA studies performed on an EDTA-anticoagulated sample taken post-transfusion gave a binding ratio of 0.83, effectively a normal result but clearly shifted upward by the donor red cells. Repeat testing 2 months later, to allow clearance of donor cells and re-establishment of host erythropoiesis, gave a ratio of 0.68 fully in keeping with the working diagnosis.

Flow cytometry offers a rapid, reproducible diagnostic test which helps differentiate HS from other inherited haemolytic

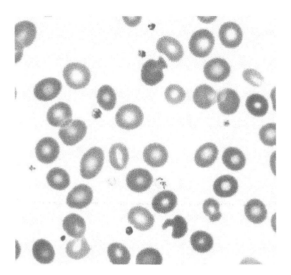

Figure 59.6 MGG, ×1000.

disorders; in particular the hereditary stomatocytoses. It has largely replaced osmotic fragility testing which is a poorly reproducible laboratory assay subject to various nuances of methodology that can be influenced by coexistent haematinic deficiency. Hereditary spherocytosis is a heterogeneous disorder that can result from a number of defects in the red cell membrane cytoskeleton including defects in actin, spectrin and band 3. The red cell morphology will vary to some degree depending on gene defect and the prominence of classic spherocytes varies accordingly. HS causes a chronic haemolytic anaemia with unconjugated hyperbilirubinaemia with a propensity to gall stone formation and splenomegaly. Aplastic crises can occur with erythrovirus infection and this can sometimes be the precipitant for a first thorough medical assessment and confirmation of this diagnosis (see also Case 16).

Final diagnosis

Hereditary spherocytosis.

60

Case 60

A 64-year-old woman attended her GP with a chest infection that was slow to settle. Clinical examination revealed infective signs at the right lung base but in addition there was widespread low volume lymphadenopathy.

Laboratory data

FBC: Hb 119 g/L, WBC 55 × 10^9/L (neutrophils 2.8 × 10^9/L, lymphocytes 47 × 10^9/L, monocytes, 5.5 × 10^9/L) and platelets 83 × 10^9/L.

U&Es, LFTs and bone profile were normal whilst CRP was 50 mg/L.

IgG 5 g/L, IgA 1 g/L, IgM 0.5 g/L; no paraprotein was detected.

Blood film

The film showed a prominent medium sized lymphoid population with condensed chromatin and minor nuclear irregularities (Figures 60.1 and 60.2). Nucleoli and nuclear clefts were not present, the neutrophils were unremarkable and the platelet count was accurate.

Flow cytometry

The abnormal lymphoid population were B cells (B cells 92%, T cells 8%) expressing CD19, CD20, CD22^{dim}, CD23 and HLA-DR. CD79b, CD5, CD10, FMC7 and surface

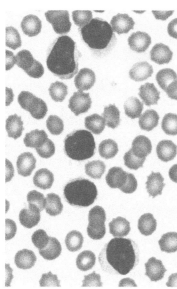

Figure 60.1 MGG, ×500.

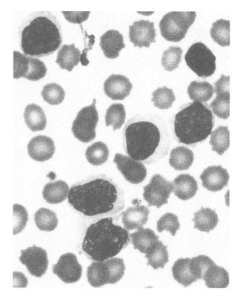

Figure 60.2 MGG, ×1000.

Practical Flow Cytometry in Haematology: 100 Worked Examples, First Edition. Mike Leach, Mark Drummond, Allyson Doig, Pam McKay, Bob Jackson and Barbara J. Bain.
© 2015 John Wiley & Sons, Ltd. Published 2015 by John Wiley & Sons, Ltd.

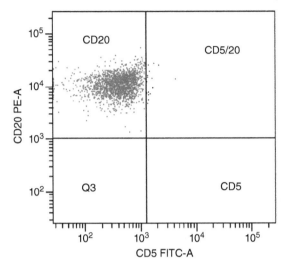

Figure 60.3 CD5/CD20.

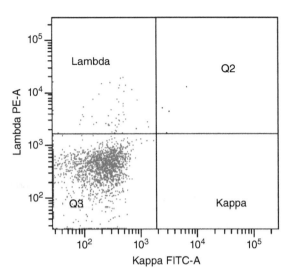

Figure 60.5 Kappa/lambda.

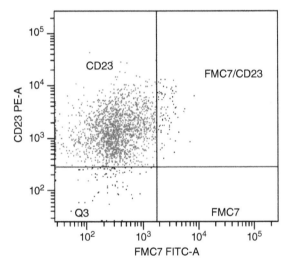

Figure 60.4 FMC7/CD23.

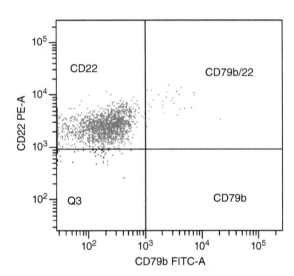

Figure 60.6 CD79b/CD22.

light chains were not expressed (Figures 60.3–60.6) but clonality was confirmed by demonstrating cytoplasmic lambda restriction (Figure 60.7).

The clonal B cells in this case show a number of significant characteristics. Unlike normal mature B cells, they show loss of FMC7 and CD79b and weak expression of CD22. This is typical of chronic lymphocytic leukaemia (CLL). Another typical feature of CLL is weak surface immunoglobulin/light chain expression and this case is an extreme example where surface expression has been lost altogether. What is also atypical in this case is the absence of CD5 expression but this

occurs in 10–15% of CLL cases and should not detract from this diagnosis as all the other features are typical, giving a CLL score of 4/5.

The aberrant phenotypic profile can be used to assess treatment response in CLL; in particular it allows the quantitation of minimal residual disease (MRD). The plots below, taken from a patient with 17p (*TP53*)-deleted CLL following alemtuzumab therapy, illustrate how a unique phenotype (in this case CD5$^+$, partial CD20^{dim} surface kappa^{dim}) allows the separation of disease cells (red events) from residual polyclonal B cells (blue events) in Figures 60.8 and 60.9.

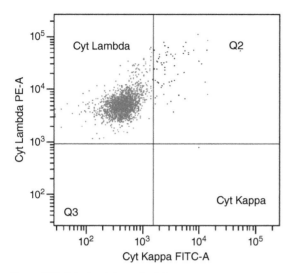

Figure 60.7 Cytoplasmic kappa/lambda.

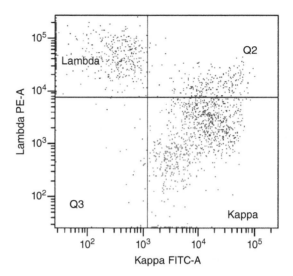

Figure 60.9 Kappa/lambda.

By using a sequential gating strategy with multiple antibodies, the residual CLL population can be quantified for MRD assessment. Such data is important in predicting progression-free survival and might inform management decisions. In this case the total B cells comprised just 2.7% of leucocytes with CLL cells constituting 16% of the total giving a 'CLL count' of 0.03×10^9/L (or 1 in 233 leucocytes).

Final diagnosis (main case)

CD5-negative chronic lymphocytic leukaemia.

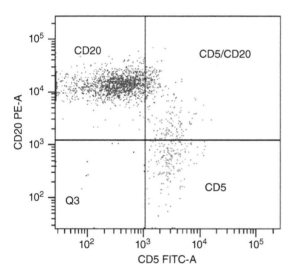

Figure 60.8 CD20/CD5.

Case 61

A 71-year-old man presented to his GP with a short history of fatigue and a purpuric rash. Prior medical history was unremarkable. An FBC sample was taken.

Laboratory data

FBC: Hb 92 g/L, WBC 22.2×10^9/L and platelets 8×10^9/L
Coagulation screen: normal.

Blood film

More than 90% of leucocytes were medium-sized blast cells.

Bone marrow aspirate

The bone marrow aspirate revealed that most cells (>85%) were blast cells of medium size (Figures 61.1 and 61.2), with agranular bluish grey cytoplasm and prominent nucleoli. No features indicative of myeloid differentiation could be seen.

Flow cytometry (bone marrow aspirate)

Flow cytometry was performed on a FSC/SSC blast gate, which comprised over 90% of all cells. They were noted to be CD45^{dim}, CD34$^+$, CD38$^+$, CD33^{dim} and weak HLA-DR with only 5–10% of cells expressing CD117 and CD15. MPO, CD13, CD14, CD64, CD11b, CD11c, TdT, CD56, CD1a, CD41, CD61, CD71 and all B- and T-Lineage markers were negative.

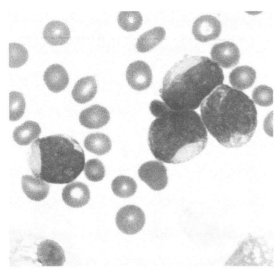

Figure 61.1 MGG, x1000.

Cytogenetic analysis (marrow aspirate)

No metaphase preparations were obtained.

Molecular analysis

PCR detected a *FLT3*-ITD mutation.

Discussion

The morphological assessment in this case failed to determine the likely blast cell lineage and diagnostic difficulty was compounded by a rare failure to obtain metaphases for

Practical Flow Cytometry in Haematology: 100 Worked Examples, First Edition. Mike Leach, Mark Drummond, Allyson Doig, Pam McKay, Bob Jackson and Barbara J. Bain.
© 2015 John Wiley & Sons, Ltd. Published 2015 by John Wiley & Sons, Ltd.

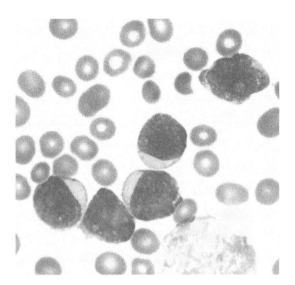

Figure 61.2 MGG, x1000.

G-banding analysis. In this circumstance an open mind is important and non-haemic or rare haematological tumours must be considered. There was no clumping of cells noted (a frequent observation in solid tumours) and the cells resembled haemic blasts. Flow cytometry confirmed a haemic origin (CD45^{dim}) of precursor cell stage (CD34$^+$) however it did not detect any lineage-specific antigens. The WHO has given criteria for assigning lineage in the context of suspected mixed phenotype acute leukaemia (MPAL) as follows (1):

1. Myeloid Lineage: MPO, or for monocytic lineage at least two of CD11c, CD14 or CD64.
2. T-Lineage: cytoplasmic or surface CD3.
3. B-Lineage: strong CD19, with at least one of CD79a, cCD22 or CD10. Weak CD19 with at least two of CD79a, cCD22 or CD10.

By these criteria leukaemic blasts may, in a small number of cases, be ascribed more than one lineage (because they express more than one lineage-specific marker) or no lineage (because they lack all criteria for lineage assignment). Such cases are termed acute leukaemia (AL) of ambiguous lineage, and these encompass MPAL and acute undifferentiated leukaemia (AUL). To recognise a lineage other than in the context of MPAL, the criteria are less stringent. For example, if CD13, CD33 and CD117 were expressed, the case would be recognised as myeloid. The reason for more stringent criteria for MPAL is that a distinction has to be made between genuine mixed phenotype AL and the not uncommon aberrant expression of a marker. For lineage assignment by flow cytometry, surface antigens are considered positive if at least 20% of cells are positive and for intracellular antigens (e.g., MPO and cCD3) if at least 10% of cells are positive. The only

suggestion of myeloid lineage in the immunophenotype of this patient is CD33^{dim} and expression of CD117 and CD15 in less than 10% of cells so classification as AUL might seem appropriate, and this would be the diagnosis assigned in the WHO classification. However, the situation is made more complex by the detection of *FLT3*-ITD (see below).

Before making a diagnosis of AUL, it is also important to exclude rare AML subtypes in which MPO is often negative. Pure erythroid leukaemia (glycophorin, CD235), acute megakaryoblastic leukaemia (CD41$^+$ and/or CD61$^+$) and acute basophilic leukaemia (CD13$^+$, CD33$^+$ and CD11b$^+$) all seemed unlikely from morphological examination and all were excluded by flow cytometry.

Failure of cytogenetic analysis in this situation demands a robust assessment of marrow cells by a panel of FISH probes and RT-PCR as appropriate. The ability to generate metaphase preparations on a cellular aspirate sample is influenced by multiple technical factors but it may also reflect the biology of the disease itself. Patients with unsuccessful cytogenetic analysis appear to have a poor prognosis, similar to that of patients with an unfavourable karyotype (2).

In this case the detection of a *FLT3*-ITD mutation, one of the commonest mutations in AML, indicated this might be the most likely diagnosis. Knowledge of the mutation profile of AUL is very limited due to the rarity of the disorder and it was felt that this case should be managed as a poorly differentiated AML. The patient was commenced on induction therapy with daunorubicin and cytarabine; unfortunately, his disease was refractory to induction and he died 2 months later.

Final diagnosis

Acute undifferentiated leukaemia, in view of *FLT3* ITD possibly actually acute myeloid leukaemia with minimal evidence of differentiation.

References

1 Borowitz, M.J., Béné, M.-C., Harris, N.L., Porwit, A., & Matutes, E. (2008) Acute leukaemia of ambiguous lineage. In: S.H. Swerdlow, E. Campo, N.L. Harris, E.S. Jaffe, S.A. Pileri, H. Stein, J. Thiele, & J.W. Vardiman (eds), *World Health Organization Classification of Tumours of Haematopoietic and Lymphoid Tissues*, pp. 150–155. IARC Press, Lyon.

2 Medeiros, B.C., Othus, M., Estey, E.H., Fang, M., Appelbaum, F.R. (2014) Unsuccessful diagnostic cytogenetic analysis is a poor prognostic feature in acute myeloid leukaemia. *British Journal of Haematology*, **164** (2), 245–250. PubMed PMID: 24383844.

Case 62

A 63-year-old man was referred for investigation of a persistent thrombocytosis, the platelet count having been above $600 \times 10^9/L$ for the previous year. This had come to light during investigation of a prostatic carcinoma that had been successfully surgically resected. There was no history of significant vascular disease, diabetes, hypertension or inflammatory disorders. Clinical examination was normal and the spleen was not palpable.

Laboratory data

FBC: Hb 140 g/L, WBC $9.7 \times 10^9/L$ and platelets $777 \times 10^9/L$.
  ESR: 8 mm/h.
  U&Es, LFTs, bone profile and CRP: all normal.

Blood film

This confirmed the thrombocytosis with significant anisothrombia and prominent larger forms. The red cell and leucocyte morphology were normal.

Bone marrow aspirate and trephine biopsy

The aspirate was particulate and cellular with a mildly expanded interstitium and prominent megakaryocytes. The trephine biopsy sections were mildly hypercellular for age with increased numbers of megakaryocytes with a tendency to clustering (Figures 62.1 and 62.2). The megakaryocytes tended to be large but otherwise had normal morphology (Figures 62.3 and 62.4). There was no abnormality of the

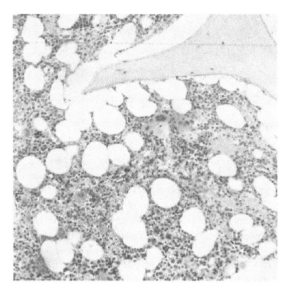

Figure 62.1 H&E, x100.

erythroid or myeloid series and reticulin staining was grade 0/1. These findings suggested a diagnosis of essential thrombocythaemia (ET) and at a later stage a *JAK2* V617F mutation was demonstrated, confirming the diagnosis.

Subsequent course

The patient was treated with hydroxycarbamide therapy with normalisation of the full blood count. The treatment was well tolerated until 4 years later when he developed anaemia and thrombocytopenia that did not respond to cessation of hydroxycarbamide therapy. The blood film did not initially show any specific features apart from hydroxycarbamide-related changes. Within the next 2 weeks, however, the film showed an evolving myeloblast

Practical Flow Cytometry in Haematology: 100 Worked Examples, First Edition. Mike Leach,
Mark Drummond, Allyson Doig, Pam McKay, Bob Jackson and Barbara J. Bain.
© 2015 John Wiley & Sons, Ltd. Published 2015 by John Wiley & Sons, Ltd.

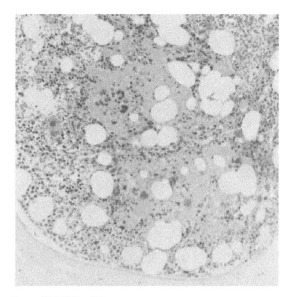

Figure 62.2 H&E, x100.

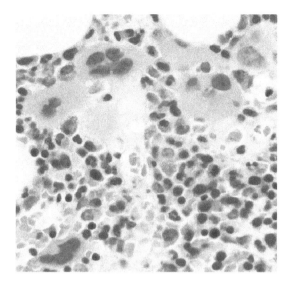

Figure 62.4 H&E, x400.

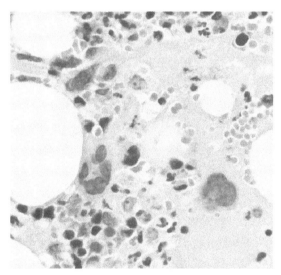

Figure 62.3 H&E, x400.

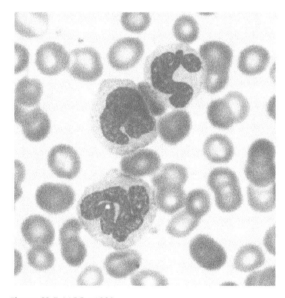

Figure 62.5 MGG, x1000.

population alongside abnormal cells of monocyte lineage (Figures 62.5–62.8).

Bone marrow aspirate

This confirmed a significant myeloblast infiltrate alongside monocytes, promonocytes and monoblasts indicating a diagnosis of secondary acute myelomonocytic leukaemia (Figures 62.9 and 62.10).

Flow cytometry

The morphological diagnosis was confirmed by flow studies as two populations of cells were identified using CD34/SSC (Figure 62.11) and FSC/SSC (Figure 62.12) analyses. The CD34+, low-SSC myeloblasts (red events) had a CD117+, CD33+, CD13+, HLA-DR+, CD15−, CD14−, CD64− phenotype, while the CD34−, moderate SSC monocytes and

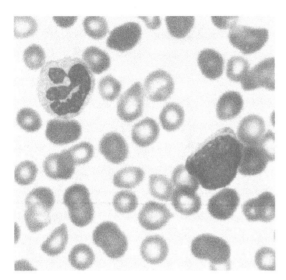

Figure 62.6 MGG, x1000.

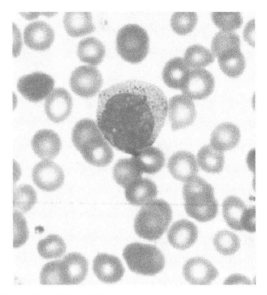

Figure 62.8 MGG, x1000.

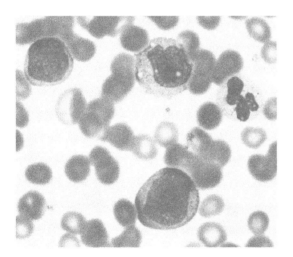

Figure 62.7 MGG, x1000.

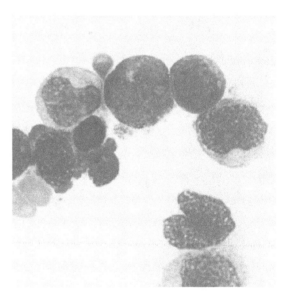

monoblasts (blue events) were CD117⁻, CD13ᵈⁱᵐ, CD33⁺, HLA-DR⁺, CD15⁺, CD14⁺ and CD64⁺.

Bone marrow trephine biopsy

The trephine biopsy sections were now markedly hypercellular with a diffuse blast cell infiltrate (Figures 62.13 and 62.14). Remarkably, small islands of residual megakaryocytes were still present (Figures 62.13, 62.15 and 62.16) reflecting the

Figure 62.9 MGG, x1000.

primary bone marrow pathology and these remained despite the secondary leukaemic progression.

Cytogenetic analysis

Metaphase preparations on the marrow aspirate cells showed 45,X,-Y in 14 cells and 46,XY in 6 cells of the 20 cells examined.

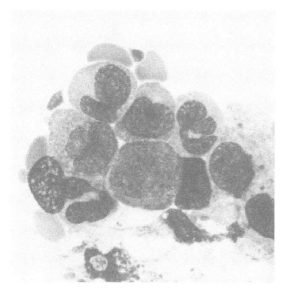

Figure 62.10 MGG, ×1000.

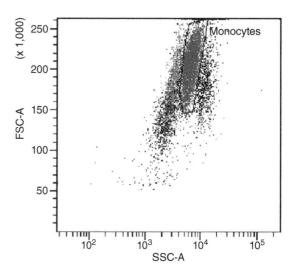

Figure 62.12 FSC/SSC.

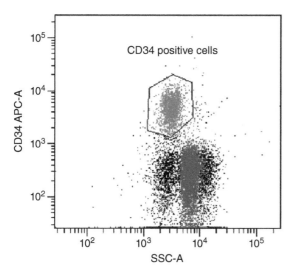

Figure 62.11 CD34/SSC.

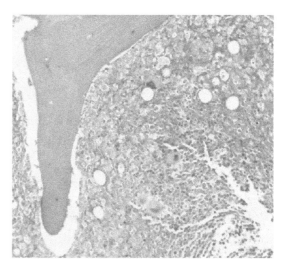

Figure 62.13 H&E, ×100.

Discussion

Essential thrombocythaemia is a chronic myeloproliferative neoplasm that involves primarily the megakaryocyte lineage. It produces an isolated thrombocytosis or, sometimes, thrombocytosis and mild leucocytosis, and is often an incidental finding. It predisposes to microvascular occlusion as well as major thromboses affecting both arteries and veins. It is an important condition to identify, particularly in older patients who have other cardiovascular risk factors, as normalisation of the platelet count and treatment with aspirin reduce these risks. The thrombocytosis generated has to be differentiated from the reactive thrombocytosis associated with neoplastic, infective and inflammatory disease. This differentiation has become substantially easier since the discovery of the *JAK2* V617F mutation (1) found in a large proportion of patients with myeloproliferative neoplasms and present in approximately 50% of patients with ET. This mutation, indicating a clonal disorder, generates

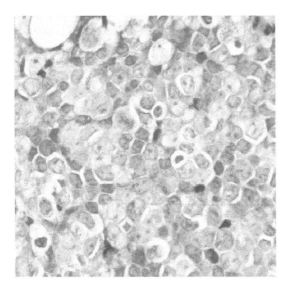

Figure 62.14 H&E, x500.

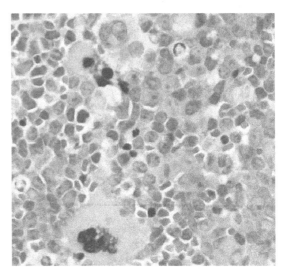

Figure 62.16 H&E, x500.

The prognosis in ET is normally excellent and in treated patients a normal life expectancy should be anticipated. Transformation to acute leukaemia is uncommon and occurs in less than 5% of patients. When it does occur it is sometimes related to the previous treatment and outdated therapies such as busulphan and radiophosphorus have particularly been implicated. There is no evidence that treatment with hydroxycarbamide increases the risk of this complication so evolution to an acute leukaemia in the case described is unusual. The outlook in such patients however is poor as these secondary leukaemias respond poorly to cytotoxic chemotherapy and these patients are often older than 60 years. The cytogenetic finding of acquired loss of chromosome Y in 14/20 cells is interesting. Loss of chromosome Y in a small proportion of cells can be seen in normal males and is increasingly found with ageing so it is not necessarily an indicator of a clonal disorder. When it occurs in the majority of metaphases examined (more than 75%) in patients with MDS and AML, it may be regarded as such (4, 5) and can be an indicator of clonal evolution, as in this case. This patient underwent an attempt at induction chemotherapy using fludarabine and cytarabine but the disease proved refractory and he died within two months of leukaemic transformation.

Final diagnosis

Transformation of essential thrombocythaemia to acute myeloid leukaemia.

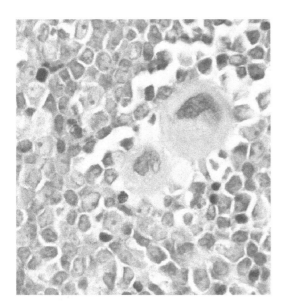

Figure 62.15 H&E, x100.

hypersensitivity to normal growth factors and is not found in patients with reactive thrombocytosis or leucocytosis or secondary polycythaemia (2). Furthermore, *JAK2*-negative ET can be further characterized by mutations in *MPL* rendering megakaryocytes hypersensitive to thrombopoietin and more recently by mutations in exon 9 of the calreticulin (*CALR*) gene (3).

References

1 Baxter, E.J., Scott, L.M., Campbell, P.J., East, C., Fourouclas, N., Swanton, S., *et al.* (2005) Acquired mutation of the tyrosine kinase JAK2 in human myeloproliferative disorders. *Lancet*, **365** (**9464**), 1054–1061. PubMed PMID: 15781101.

2 Tefferi, A., Thiele, J., Orazi, A., Kvasnicka, H.M., Barbui, T., Hanson, C.A., *et al.* (2007) Proposals and rationale for revision of the World Health Organization diagnostic criteria for polycythemia vera, essential thrombocythemia, and primary myelofibrosis: recommendations from an ad hoc international expert panel. *Blood*, **110** (4), 1092–1097. PubMed PMID: 17488875.

3 Klampfl, T., Gisslinger, H., Harutyunyan, A.S., Nivarthi, H., Rumi, E., Milosevic, J.D., *et al.* (2013) Somatic mutations of calreticulin in myeloproliferative neoplasms. *The New England Journal of Medicine*, **369** (**25**), 2379–2390. PubMed PMID: 24325356.

4 Wiktor, A., Rybicki, B.A., Piao, Z.S., Shurafa, M., Barthel, B., Maeda, K., *et al.* (2000) Clinical significance of Y chromosome loss in hematologic disease. *Genes, Chromosomes & Cancer*, **27** (**1**), 11–16. PubMed PMID: 10564581.

5 Wong, A.K., Fang, B., Zhang, L., Guo, X., Lee, S., Schreck, R. (2008) Loss of the Y chromosome: an age-related or clonal phenomenon in acute myelogenous leukemia/myelodysplastic syndrome? *Archives of Pathology & Laboratory Medicine*, **132** (**8**), 1329–1332. PubMed PMID: 18684036.

Case 63

A 32-year-old female presented to our institution at 10 weeks gestation in her first pregnancy. She had a lifelong history of epistaxis and spontaneous gingival bleeding. Dental extractions had precipitated bleeding for days and heavy menstrual bleeding had been troublesome from the menarche. She had received therapeutic platelet transfusions in childhood. She had no other past medical history of note and took no regular medications. There was no family history of a bleeding tendency. Physical examination was unremarkable.

Laboratory data

The FBC, coagulation screen, U&Es and LFTs were normal.

Blood film

The blood film (Figures 63.1 and 63.2) was normal. In particular the platelet count, size and morphology were normal. The peripheral blood leucocytes appeared normal; specifically no cytoplasmic inclusions were seen.

Platelet aggregation studies

Normal aggregation was seen as a response to ristocetin but was absent on exposure to epinephrine, collagen, ADP and arachidonic acid; shown schematically in Figure 63.3.

Flow cytometry studies

Flow cytometry analysis of surface glycoprotein (Gp) expression on fresh suspensions of patient citrated platelets showed

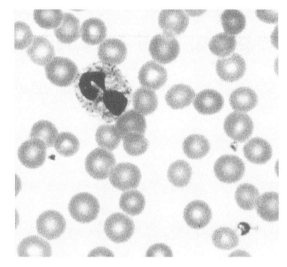

Figure 63.1 MGG, ×1000.

a marked reduction in expression of CD41 (GpIIb) and CD61 (GpIIIa) indicating defective expression of the platelet glycoprotein IIb/IIIa complex. Expression of CD42 (GpIb) was normal.

Discussion

The clinical presentation with a history of mucosal type bleeding from an early age is in keeping with the diagnosis of an inherited platelet disorder. The platelet count was consistently normal and the patient's platelets were of normal size and morphology excluding the macro-thrombocytopenic disorders and grey platelet syndrome. The absence of a relevant family history of bleeding suggests an autosomal

Practical Flow Cytometry in Haematology: 100 Worked Examples, First Edition. Mike Leach, Mark Drummond, Allyson Doig, Pam McKay, Bob Jackson and Barbara J. Bain.

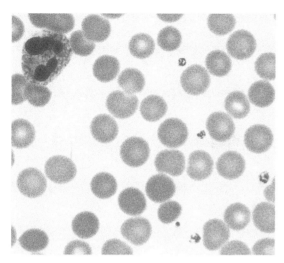

Figure 63.2 MGG, ×1000.

recessive condition and the platelet aggregation and flow cytometry studies indicate a diagnosis of Glanzmann thrombasthenia, which was subsequently confirmed on genetic testing.

Glanzmann thrombasthenia is a rare autosomal recessive disorder due to deficiency or abnormality of the platelet glycoprotein IIb/IIIa integrin complex. Normal platelet activation induces a conformational change in the complex that allows binding of fibrinogen, von Willebrand factor and fibronectin. The binding of fibrinogen allows it to bridge platelets and to initiate primary and secondary phases of aggregation. The absence of the normal complex explains the absence of platelet aggregation to ADP, collagen, epinephrine and arachidonic acid: all these factors are dependent on fibrinogen binding in order to promote aggregation in vitro. Aggregation (sometimes designated agglutination) with ristocetin is preserved as this is dependent on an intact Gp Ib/IX complex but is independent of Gp IIb/IIIa.

The severity of this disorder is variable between patients and is influenced to some degree by the nature of the genetic defect on chromosome 17q21-23. Heterozygous carriers are asymptomatic as they show near normal platelet Gp IIb/IIIa levels. Affected individuals can suffer repeat episodes of severe mucosal bleeding that may require treatment with platelet transfusion. Surgical procedures and pregnancy generate a substantial bleeding challenge that requires prophylactic platelet transfusion cover but this generates risk of HLA and/or platelet alloimmunisation. There is a particular risk that patients may develop anti-Gp IIb/IIa antibodies that will render them refractory to subsequent platelet therapy. Similarly, exposure to fetal platelets during pregnancy can result in neonatal alloimmune thrombocy-

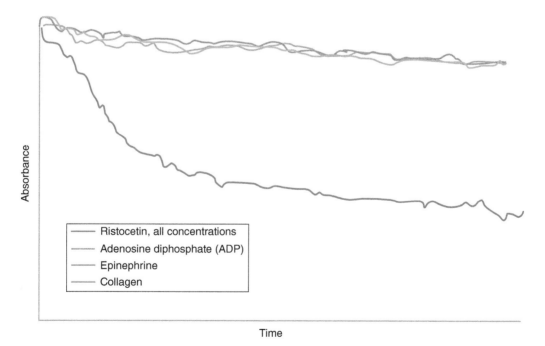

Figure 63.3 Platelet aggregation studies

topenia. Once identified, these patients need to be managed by specialist haemostasis units who have experience of managing this disorder. Pregnancy poses a particular challenge that requires careful planning by the haematology and obstetric teams with a management algorithm to cover all eventualities that may arise.

The patient was treated with weekly infusions of intravenous immunoglobulin from 24 to 38 weeks gestation to reduce the risk of alloimmunisation against the normal fetal platelet Gp IIb/IIIa antigen complex inherited from the father. She underwent an elective Caesarean section with general anaesthetic at 38 weeks with two pools of platelets preoperatively and a further pool at the time of skin incision. She was given intravenous tranexamic acid pre-operatively then oral tranexamic acid for seven days post-delivery. She was delivered of a healthy baby with a normal platelet count. There was no excess blood loss, intra- or post-operatively and the puerperium was uneventful.

Final diagnosis

Glanzmann thrombasthenia.

Case 64

A 44-year-old woman with a history of mild chronic obstructive pulmonary disease was admitted acutely via her GP with severe pancytopenia. A blood film showed infrequent myeloblasts. A bone marrow aspirate and trephine biopsy were performed.

Laboratory data

FBC: Hb 79 g/L, WBC 3.1×10^9/L and platelets 26×10^9/L. U&Es, LFTs, bone profile and LDH: normal.

Bone marrow aspirate at diagnosis

A marrow aspirate demonstrated over 80% of cells to be myeloblasts, many of which exhibited maturation, with granular cytoplasm and frequent Auer rods (Figures 64.1–64.3). Flow cytometry confirmed >80% of cells to be CD34+, CD117dim, CD13+, CD33+ and MPO+ blast cells. In addition, significant numbers of smaller cells were noted with intensely basophilic and granular cytoplasm (arrow, Figure 64.3), characteristics typical of mast cells, were noted in bone marrow films.

Histopathology at diagnosis

Bone marrow trephine biopsy sections confirmed maximal cellularity due to extensive infiltration by a partially differentiated blast population (Figures 64.4 and 64.5). A more intensely staining paratrabecular population of cells with more condensed nuclei was noted in some areas (arrows, Figures 64.4 and 64.5). CD117 IHC demonstrated differential staining suggesting two populations (Figures 64.6–64.8):

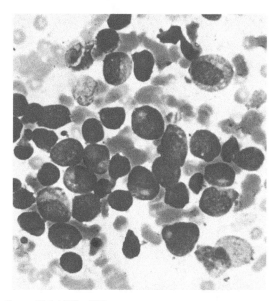

Figure 64.1 MGG, ×500.

the CD117dim myeloblasts and the CD117bright mast cells, the latter being seen particularly in the paratrabecular and perivascular areas. The mast cells were noted to be positive for CD25 and tryptase, but were CD2 negative (not shown).

Bone marrow aspirate following induction chemotherapy

AML induction therapy in the form of daunorubicin and cytarabine successfully achieved remission. A post-induction

Practical Flow Cytometry in Haematology: 100 Worked Examples, First Edition. Mike Leach, Mark Drummond, Allyson Doig, Pam McKay, Bob Jackson and Barbara J. Bain.
© 2015 John Wiley & Sons, Ltd. Published 2015 by John Wiley & Sons, Ltd.

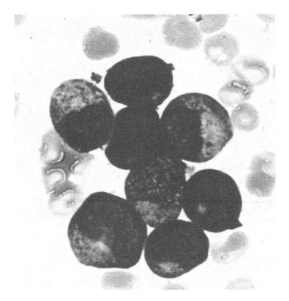

Figure 64.2 MGG, ×1000.

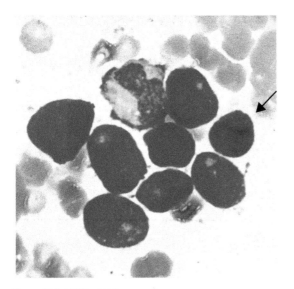

Figure 64.3 MGG, ×1000.

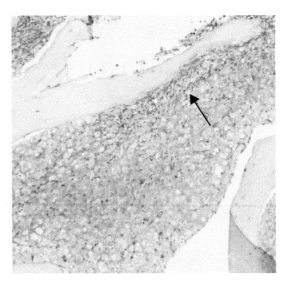

Figure 64.4 H&E, ×100.

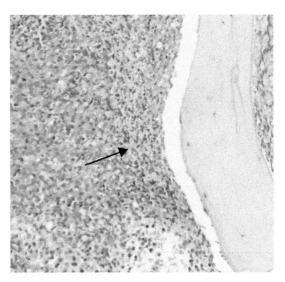

Figure 64.5 H&E, ×200.

Flow cytometry at remission

Flow cytometric analysis of the remission marrow sample confirmed a $CD117^+$, $CD2^-$, $CD25^+$ population of abnormal mast cells (Figures 64.13–64.15). Cell numbers using this methodology are notoriously low due to the fragility of the target population and their close association with marrow particles and trabecular areas making analysis of free cells in suspension problematical.

marrow aspirate showed infrequent myeloblasts (<2%) and a more readily appreciated mast cell infiltrate (Figures 64.9 and 64.10), particularly in and around the marrow particles. Tryptase IHC on a post-remission trephine biopsy specimen confirmed the paratrabecular and perivascular clustering of mast cells (Figures 64.11 and 64.12).

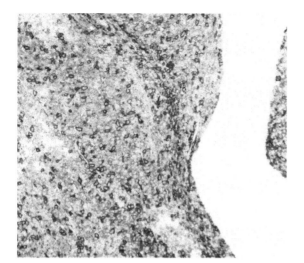

Figure 64.6 CD117, ×100.

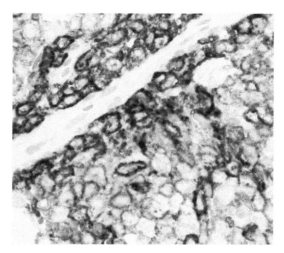

Figure 64.8 CD117 perivascular, ×500.

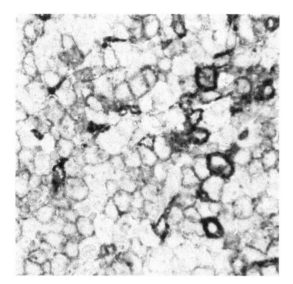

Figure 64.7 CD117, ×500.

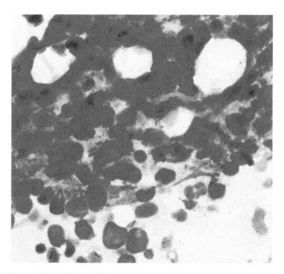

Figure 64.9 MGG, ×500.

Cytogenetic analysis

t(8;21)(q22;q22) was identified in 20/20 cells of the marrow aspirate at diagnosis.

Molecular studies

PCR on marrow confirmed the presence of an activating point mutation in codon 816 of *KIT* (the D816V mutation).

Discussion

This case initially appeared to be a straightforward 'good-risk' AML, with t(8;21)(q22;q22). However careful morphological assessment identified a second abnormal population, confirmed by IHC and flow cytometry as being a clonal mast cell infiltrate. Aberrant CD25 expression was detected on the mast cells by IHC and flow cytometry, although in this case the mast cells were negative for CD2, which is another commonly expressed aberrant antigen in systemic mastocytosis (SM). These characteristics fulfilled the

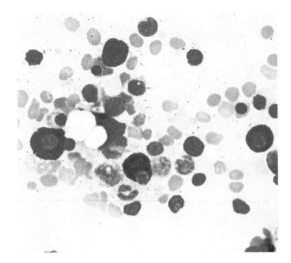

Figure 64.10 MGG, ×500.

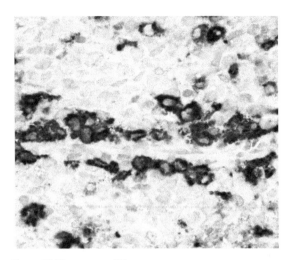

Figure 64.12 tryptase, ×400.

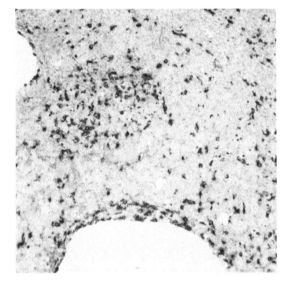

Figure 64.11 tryptase, ×100.

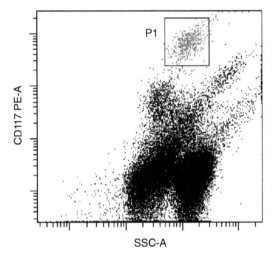

Figure 64.13 CD117/SSC.

criteria for SM, which when found in conjunction with another haematological malignancy is termed SM with associated clonal haematological non-mast cell lineage disease (SM-AHNMD). This strange condition is not fully understood, in particular the relationship between the two malignancies at the molecular genetic level. Attempts to perform cell sorting on this sample (followed by targeted FISH) to determine whether the mast cell compartment carried t(8;21) were technically unsuccessful. There is, however, known to be a specific association between SM and AML with t(8;21).

In our case there was no prior clinical history to suggest SM; specifically no history of rash, flushing, diarrhoea, allergies or anaphylaxis. At baseline, serum tryptase was significantly elevated at 119 ng/ml (NR <13 ng/L). CT imaging demonstrated no evidence of organ infiltration. Dual-energy X-ray absorptiometry (DEXA) scanning did demonstrate significant ostopenia however, and the patient was commenced on prophylactic therapy.

The patient underwent four cycles of AML chemotherapy in total, incorporating high-dose cytarabine. Post-chemotherapy she was commenced on dasatinib 100 mg daily, in an attempt to reduce mast cell burden and reduce the

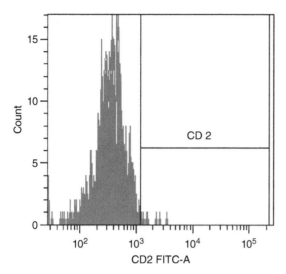

Figure 64.14 CD2/CD117 histogram.

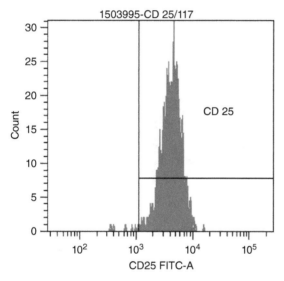

Figure 64.15 CD25/CD117 histogram.

risk of AML relapse. There is now, however, little evidence for use of this drug in SM, and treatment was stopped after 2 years. Molecular monitoring of marrow disease, RQ-PCR for *RUNX1-RUNX1T1*, resulting from t(8;21), demonstrated a slow but steady fall in transcript levels. Indeed after 5 years of follow up post-chemotherapy, low-level transcripts are still detectable although at a level associated with a low risk of relapse. Tryptase remains elevated at around 60–80 ng/ml, and the patient remains symptom free.

Typically AML arising on a background of a chronic myeloproliferative neoplasm (e.g. PV, primary myelofibrosis) is generally associated with a dismal prognosis, with allogeneic stem cell transplantation offering the only hope of long-term survival. AML in this case however is not necessarily 'secondary' disease, and good outcomes reported in the literature and in our case would support an approach akin to that for *de novo* AML.

Final diagnosis

Acute myeloid leukaemia with t(8;21) as a systemic mastocytosis-associated clonal haematological non-mast cell lineage disease (SM-AHNMD).

Case 65

A 50-year-old man presented with dyspnoea, ankle swelling and two episodes of collapse. On examination, he had pitting oedema to his thighs, bilateral pleural effusions and ascites. His tongue was enlarged and showed depressions along the lateral margins due to pressure from his teeth. He was in atrial fibrillation, had a raised jugular venous pressure and had symptomatic postural hypotension on standing.

Laboratory data

FBC: Hb 105 g/L, WBC 6×10^9/L (neutrophils 3.0×10^9/L, lymphocytes 1.8×10^9/L, monocytes 0.8×10^9/L) and platelets 112×10^9/L.

U&Es: Na 134 mmol/l, K 4.1 mmol/L, urea 6.4 mmol/L, creatinine 61 µmol/L.

Bone profile: calcium 2.51 mmol/L, phosphate 1.52 mmol/L.

LFTs: AST 46 U/L, ALP 483 U/L, albumin 9 g/L, total protein 12 g/L.

Immunoglobulins: IgG 2 g/L, IgA 0.3 g/L, IgM 0.2 g/L.

Serum electrophoresis: no intact paraprotein identified, but lambda free light chains present in excess (kappa 6.1 mg/L, lambda 979 mg/L).

Urine total protein: 11.7 g/L. Urine protein/creatinine ratio: 12,247 mg/mmol.

Blood film

This showed a normocytic anaemia but there were no specific findings.

Imaging

A CXR showed bilateral pleural effusion to the mid zones. A skeletal survey showed no bone abnormality whilst a CT confirmed pleural effusions and showed ascites. There was no mediastinal lymphadenopathy or pleural abnormality. Both kidneys appeared uniformly enlarged suggesting a renal infiltrative process (Figure 65.1).

Bone marrow aspirate

This showed a number of important features. On low magnification an amorphous purple staining material (MGG stain)

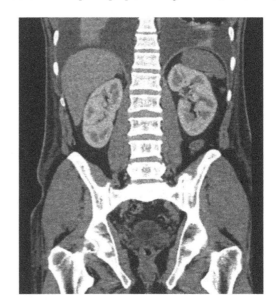

Figure 65.1 CT.

Practical Flow Cytometry in Haematology: 100 Worked Examples, First Edition. Mike Leach, Mark Drummond, Allyson Doig, Pam McKay, Bob Jackson and Barbara J. Bain.
© 2015 John Wiley & Sons, Ltd. Published 2015 by John Wiley & Sons, Ltd.

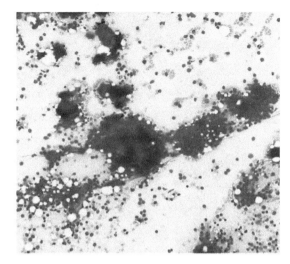

Figure 65.2 MGG, ×100.

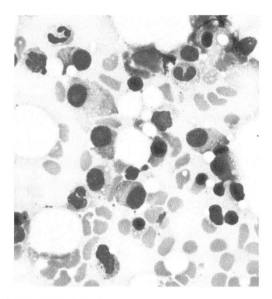

Figure 65.4 MGG, ×500.

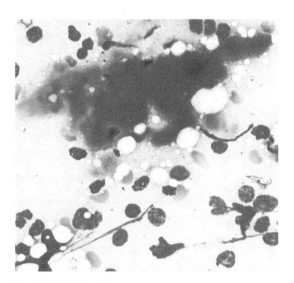

Figure 65.3 MGG, ×500.

Flow cytometry (bone marrow aspirate)

Plasma cells were quantified at 3.1% of events by flow cytometry. These had a neoplastic phenotype as follows: CD138$^+$, CD38$^+$, CD19$^-$, CD45$^-$ and weak CD56$^+$.

Bone marrow trephine biopsy

This trephine biopsy sections were remarkable in that they demonstrated perivascular foci of amorphous pink material interspersed between the cellular areas (Figure 65.5, H&E); this stained positively with Sirius red (Figure 65.6), for amyloid P (Figure 65.7) and weakly for lambda light chains (Figure 65.8). This amorphous material corresponded to that seen in the aspirate, which was thus identified as amyloid. Immunostaining for AA protein was negative.

On higher power examination the plasma cells were apparent (Figure 65.9) and in some parts of the sections showed a focal nodular distribution, highlighted using CD138 (Figure 65.10).

Discussion

This patient presented with nephrotic syndrome, autonomic neuropathy and cardiac failure at an early age. Bone marrow

was dispersed throughout the marrow particles (Figures 65.2 and 65.3). There was also a plasma cell population present; as an absolute percentage these constituted less than 5% of cells (Figure 65.4) but they were more prominent in some parts of the aspirate than others. The normal marrow elements were largely preserved.

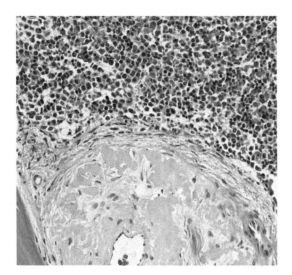

Figure 65.5 H&E, ×100.

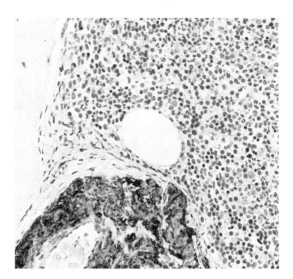

Figure 65.7 Amyloid P, ×100.

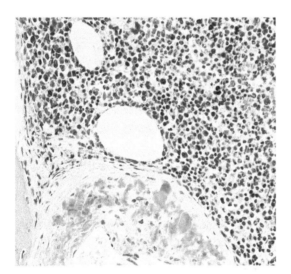

Figure 65.6 Sirius red, ×100.

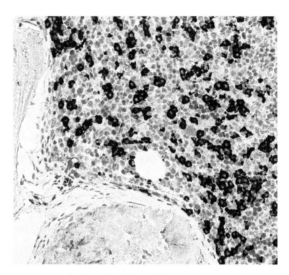

Figure 65.8 Lambda light chains, ×100.

examination identified a small but significant clone of neo-plastic plasma cells alongside perivascular accumulations of amyloid. He did not have bone pain, hypercalcaemia or radi-ological evidence of bone destruction. These findings are all in keeping with a diagnosis of primary AL amyloidosis.

The amyloidoses are a group of conditions charac-terised by tissue deposition of fibrillar proteins with a beta pleated sheet structure. Amyloid is resistant to digestion or phagocytosis and accumulates in tissue causing a progressive loss of function. The four main types of amyloid are as follows:

1. AL amyloid (immunoglobulin light chain derived) seen in plasma cell neoplasms.

2. AA amyloid (serum amyloid A protein derived, an acute phase reactant) seen in chronic inflammatory disease and with chronic infection.

3. Beta 2 microglobulin type, seen in renal dialysis patients.

4. ATTR amyloid derived from transthyretin, the amyloido-sis of ageing.

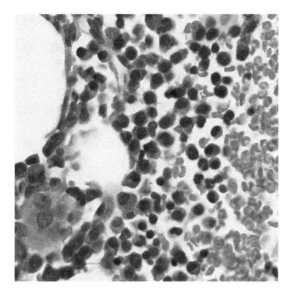

Figure 65.9 H&E, ×400.

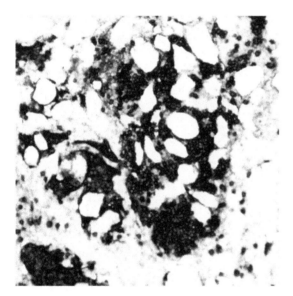

Figure 65.10 CD138, ×100.

AL amyloid is most often seen in patients with multiple myeloma and tends to accumulate throughout the duration of the illness and cause symptoms late in the disease. It is more frequently seen in patients with lambda free light chains or lambda paraproteins but the differing propensity to the formation of amyloid between patients is poorly understood. Primary AL amyloidosis is a rare plasma cell neoplasm where a relatively small neoplastic plasma cell clone produces a paraprotein (or free light chain) with a particular ability to generate amyloid deposition in tissues. Patients do not normally suffer the consequences of direct bone damage and pain as seen in myeloma but typically present with symptoms relating to advanced tissue damage due to amyloid deposition: the kidneys, heart, liver and peripheral nervous system are particularly affected; indentations of the tongue are also typical and suggestive of the diagnosis. Patients presenting with established heart failure have a poor prognosis but it important that therapy is not denied as a sub-group of chemotherapy-responsive patients show a significant improvement in outcome (1). This patient, however, succumbed to a fatal arrhythmia within a few weeks of diagnosis.

Final diagnosis

Primary AL amyloidosis

Reference

1 Wechalekar, A.D., Schonland, S.O., Kastritis, E. *et al.* (2013) A European collaborative study of treatment outcomes in 346 patients with cardiac stage III AL amyloidosis. *Blood*, **121**(17), 3420–3427. PubMed PMID: 23479568.

Case 66

A 58-year-old woman was diagnosed with mycosis fungoides (MF), the most commonly encountered cutaneous T-cell lymphoma (CTCL). She responded to treatment with phototherapy. Nine years later she presented with erythroderma. She failed to respond to weekly methotrexate and was commenced on interferon alpha and extracorporeal photopheresis.

Laboratory investigations

FBC: Hb 126 g/L, WBC 32.9×10^9/L, platelets 409×10^9/L

WBC differential: neutrophils 15.2×10^9/L, lymphocytes 5.4×10^9/L, 'monocytes' 4.2×10^9/L, eosinophils 10.3×10^9/L.

The blood film showed a reactive picture. There was a neutrophilia, marked eosinophilia and, in addition, a population of atypical lymphoid cells with cerebriform nuclei was noted (Figures 66.1 – 66.4). These accounted for 65% of all lymphocytes.

Imaging

A CT scan showed small volume lymphadenopathy in the axillae and groins, but no organomegaly.

Flow cytometry

An abnormal CD4+ lymphoid population with loss of CD7 and CD26 was identified (Figures 66.5 – 66.7). Note some residual normal T cells remain (CD7/CD16 positive). The CD4:CD8 ratio was in excess of 10:1.

Histopathology

Skin biopsy

At low power there was an atypical lymphoid infiltrate within the papillary dermis with focal epidermotropism (Figures 66.8 and 66.9). Note the linear arrangement of the haloed T cells at the dermal/epidermal junction with encroachment into the basal layer of the epidermis (seen best in Figure 66.9 (arrow). Some eosinophils were noted within the dermis. At high power the lymphoid cells were of intermediate size and co-expressed CD2, CD3, CD4 and CD5 with loss of CD7. The location of the neoplastic cells is highlighted using CD4 and CD3 in Figures 66.10 and 66.11, respectively.

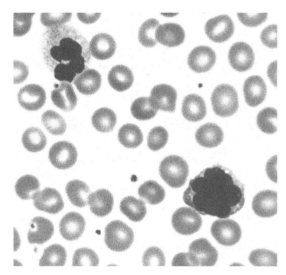

Figure 66.1 MGG, ×1000

Practical Flow Cytometry in Haematology: 100 Worked Examples, First Edition. Mike Leach, Mark Drummond, Allyson Doig, Pam McKay, Bob Jackson and Barbara J. Bain.
© 2015 John Wiley & Sons, Ltd. Published 2015 by John Wiley & Sons, Ltd.

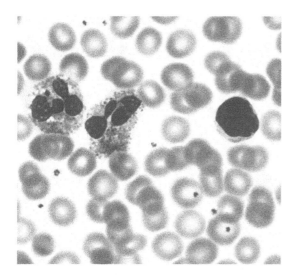

Figure 66.2 MGG, ×1000

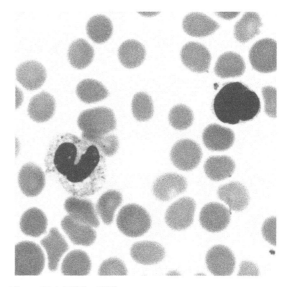

Figure 66.4 MGG, ×1000

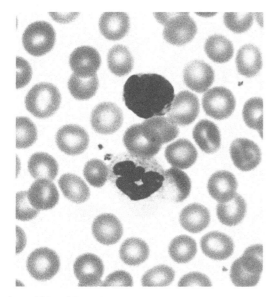

Figure 66.3 MGG, ×1000

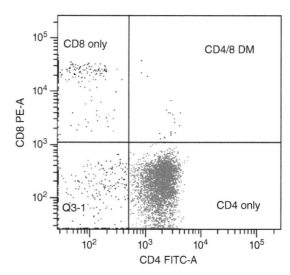

Figure 66.5 CD4/CD8

Lymph node biopsy

There were florid dermatopathic changes. However, a proportion of the cells had lost CD7 raising the possibility of early nodal involvement by T-cell lymphoma.

Molecular studies

PCR for T-cell receptor gene (TCR) rearrangement on peripheral blood identified a single peak using primers for TCR gamma, in keeping with the presence of a monoclonal T-cell proliferation. PCR studies on the skin and lymph node biopsies showed an identical clone to that demonstrated in peripheral blood.

Discussion

The skin biopsies confirmed a diagnosis of CTCL. There also appeared to be early peripheral nodal involvement. A

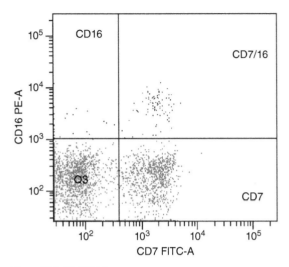

Figure 66.6 CD7/CD16

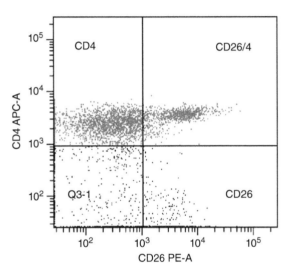

Figure 66.7 CD4/CD26

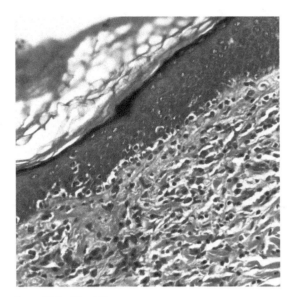

Figure 66.8 H&E, ×200

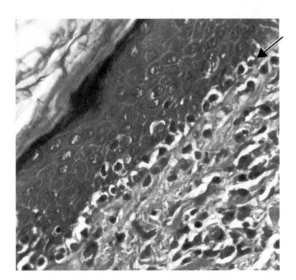

Figure 66.9 H&E, ×400

neoplastic population of T cells was detected in the peripheral blood by a combination of morphology, flow cytometry and PCR. Significant blood involvement (>1000 Sézary cells/mm³ or >20% Sézary cells) is an adverse independent prognostic feature in CTCL (1). Loss of expression of CD7 and CD26 is typical of Sézary cells but it must be remembered that CD7 loss or weak expression may also be seen in peripheral blood T cells from patients with benign dermatoses. Loss of CD26 expression may be a more robust marker of neoplasia (2). Detection of a T-cell clone in the peripheral blood by PCR may also be found in

benign inflammatory conditions. The clinical significance of such a result is however enhanced if an identical clone is detected in both skin and blood. Distinguishing mycosis fungoides with nodal involvement and erythroderma from Sézary syndrome is difficult on purely pathological grounds. Clinicopathological correlation is required. Given the long history of patch/plaque disease in this patient with recent development of erythroderma and circulating atypical lymphoid cells, a diagnosis of erythrodermic MF is preferred.

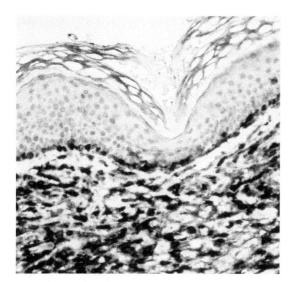

Figure 66.10 CD4, ×200

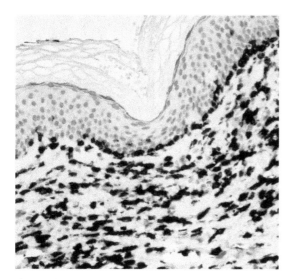

Figure 66.11 CD3, ×200

Determining prognosis in MF/Sézary syndrome depends on accurate clinical staging. A recent proposal for staging has been published by the ISCL and EORTC and this has been validated in a large clinical series (3, 4). The described patient with erythroderma and lymph node and significant peripheral blood involvement would be expected to run a relatively aggressive course.

Final diagnosis

Erythrodermic mycosis fungoides.

References

1 Kim, Y.H., Liu, H,L., Mraz-Gernhard, S.*et al.* (2003) Long-term outcome of 525 patients with mycosis fungoides and Sezary syndrome: clinical prognostic factors and risk for disease progression. *Archives of Dermatology*, **139** (7), 857–866. PubMed PMID: 12873880.

2 Jones, D., Dang, N.H., Duvic, M. *et al.* (2001) Absence of CD26 expression is a useful marker for diagnosis of T-cell lymphoma in peripheral blood. *American Journal of Clinical Pathology*, **115** (6), 885–892. PubMed PMID: 11392886.

3 Olsen, E., Vonderheid, E., Pimpinelli, N. *et al.* (2007) Revisions to the staging and classification of mycosis fungoides and Sezary syndrome: a proposal of the International Society for Cutaneous Lymphomas (ISCL) and the cutaneous lymphoma task force of the European Organization of Research and Treatment of Cancer (EORTC). *Blood*, **110** (6), 1713–1722. PubMed PMID: 17540844.

4 Agar, N.S., Wedgeworth, E., Crichton, S. *et al.* (2010) Survival outcomes and prognostic factors in mycosis fungoides/Sezary syndrome: validation of the revised International Society for Cutaneous Lymphomas/European Organisation for Research and Treatment of Cancer staging proposal. *Journal of Clinical Oncology: Official Journal of the American Society of Clinical Oncology*, **28** (31), 4730–4739. PubMed PMID: 20855822.

Case 67

A 78-year-old woman presented to her GP with fatigue and easy bruising. She had a history of diffuse large B-cell lymphoma 4 years previously, treated successfully with eight cycles of R-CHOP chemotherapy.

Laboratory data

FBC: Hb 104 g/L, WBC 3.1×10^9/L, (neutrophils 0.6×10^9/L, monocytes 0.4×10^9/L) and platelets 43×10^9/L.

U&Es, LFTs, bone profile and LDH were all normal.

Blood film

This confirmed the cytopenias; many neutrophils showed abnormalities of nuclear segmentation and reduced granulation (not shown).

Bone marrow aspirate

The aspirate demonstrated relative myeloid hyperplasia with a left shift. Myeloblasts and monoblasts were frequent, together comprising 15% of cells (Figures 67.1 and 67.2). Hypolobated dysplastic neutrophils were prominent as were monocytes, which likewise exhibited dysplastic changes (Figures 67.3 and 67.4). Overall the monocytic lineage comprised 17% of all cells. The erythroid series exhibited less obvious dysplastic change, although nuclear irregularity and poor haemoglobinisation were evident (Figure 67.3). Mitotic figures were frequent (Figure 67.5). In this patient monoblasts were more prominent than myeloblasts (Figure 67.6). Note the neutrophil nucleus in Figure 67.7.

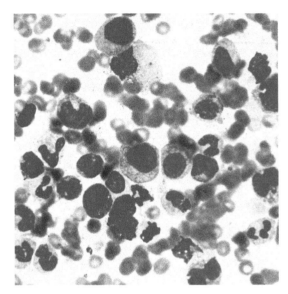

Figure 67.1 MGG, ×500.

Flow cytometry (marrow aspirate)

Gating was carried out using CD45/SSC: lymphocytes (green), monocytes (blue) and granulocytes (red) and this is shown in Figure 67.8. Monocytes were not present in excess in the peripheral blood, but, like the bone marrow cells (Figure 67.9) they did demonstrate aberrant CD56 expression. Notably a significant CD45^{dim} monocyte population was not apparent in peripheral blood, although it was present in the bone marrow.

Cytogenetic analysis

Metaphase studies showed 46,XX in 20 cells examined.

Practical Flow Cytometry in Haematology: 100 Worked Examples, First Edition. Mike Leach, Mark Drummond, Allyson Doig, Pam McKay, Bob Jackson and Barbara J. Bain.

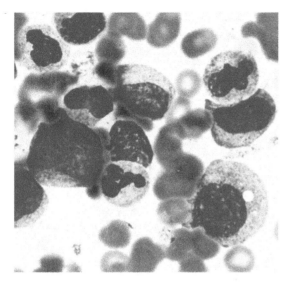

Figure 67.2 MGG, ×1000.

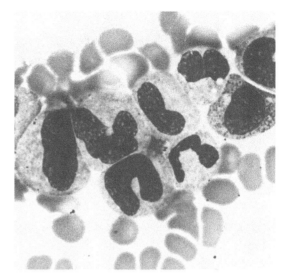

Figure 67.4 MGG, ×1000.

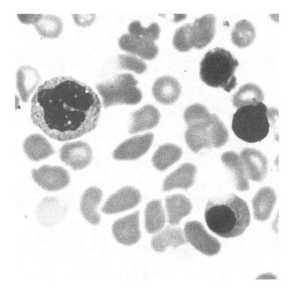

Figure 67.3 MGG, ×1000.

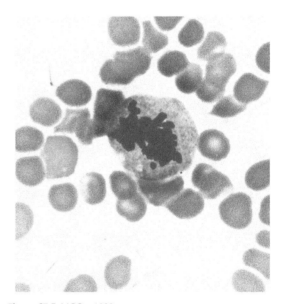

Figure 67.5 MGG, ×1000.

Discussion

Myelodysplastic syndromes (MDS) can arise *de novo* or be secondary to anti-cancer therapy (therapy-related MDS, t-MDS). Approximately 10% of all MDS cases are t-MDS, which is generally characterised by a poor outcome not least due to its association with a high frequency of complex karyotypes. It is worth noting that the most widely used MDS prognostic score (the IPSS) did not incorporate cases of 'secondary' MDS, although it is commonly applied in this setting. The IPSS in this patient would be intermediate 1, which appears reassuringly low and does not reflect the anticipated poor prognosis indicated by our experience of

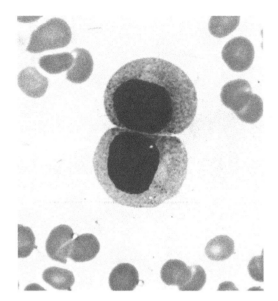

Figure 67.6 MGG, ×1000.

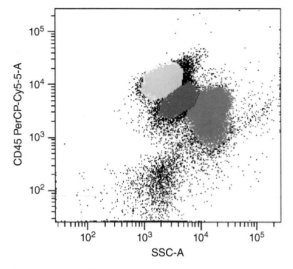

Figure 67.8 CD45/SSC.

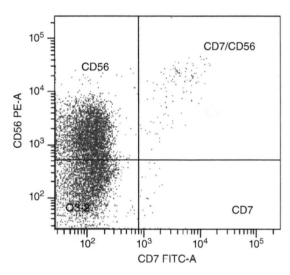

Figure 67.9 Monocyte CD7/CD56.

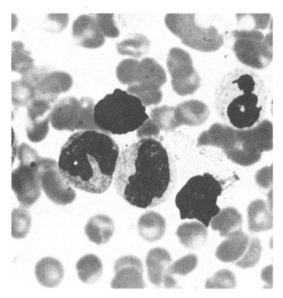

Figure 67.7 MGG, ×1000.

t-MDS with multi-lineage cytopenias. In fact, the prognosis of t-MDS is so poor that the WHO groups such cases with t-AML. The normal cytogenetic profile can also be falsely reassuring as the very clones of interest might be less able to generate metaphases for analysis whilst the normal residual cells generate mitoses in culture.

Both morphology and flow cytometry confirmed a high frequency of abnormal monocytes and their precursors in this case. Immaturity was indicated by CD64^{bright}/CD14$^-$ or CD64$^+$/CD14^{dim} patterns of expression (data not shown), most likely correlating with the monoblastic and promonocytic/dysplastic monocyte morphology, respectively. Aberrant expression of CD56 was also seen on the monocytic population, providing an objective marker for dysplastic maturation at least of this sub-population.

An overview of CD56 expression has been given elsewhere in this book (see Case 29). Flow cytometric analysis in MDS is technically challenging, not least because of the requirement to analyse multiple populations in a very heterogeneous cell background that varies markedly from case to case. A general theme in MDS flow cytometric studies is that abnormalities are most marked in the most advanced and dysplastic cases, precisely the group where the diagnosis is usually most obvious morphologically.

Final diagnosis

Therapy-related myelodysplastic syndrome (t-MDS).

Case 68

A 46-year-old male presented with a short history of night sweats, fatigue and increasing dyspnoea. He had a dry cough but no sputum production. He had a history of uveitis of unknown aetiology but otherwise had no past medical history of note. He was taking prednisolone 20 mg daily at the time of admission. On examination, he appeared unwell and febrile at 38.5°C but there was no palpable lymphadenopathy or organomegaly. He had fine bibasal crepitations and oxygen saturations on air were 90%. His CXR showed fine interstitial shadowing throughout both lung fields.

Laboratory investigations

FBC: Hb 71 g/L, WBC 1.35×10^9/L, neutrophils 0.14×10^9/L, lymphocytes 1.03×10^9/L, monocytes 0.18×10^9/L, platelets 38×10^9/L. Ferritin >20,000 µg/L.

Coagulation screen: PT 16 s, APTT 40 s, TT 24 s, fibrinogen 0.79 g/L and D-dimer 4112 ng/ml.

U&Es: Na 127 mmol/L, K 4.0 mmol/L, urea 7.2 mmol/L, creatinine 87 µmol/L.

LFTs: AST 359 U/L, ALT 262 U/L, ALP 222 U/L, bilirubin 29 µmol/L, albumin 14 g/L.

LDH 1486 U/L, calcium 2.1 mmol/L, phosphate 1.35 mmol/L, CRP 63 mg/L.

Blood cultures: no growth.

PCR studies on viral gargle for a spectrum of viral pathogens: negative.

Sputum culture: light growth of *Candida albicans*.

HIV, hepatitis B, hepatitis C serology: all negative.

EBV serology: IgG antibodies present, IgM absent.

CMV serology: IgM antibodies absent.

Blood EBV PCR log 5.66, CMV PCR log 3.79

The blood film showed no circulating blasts and there were no informative features. His clinical condition continued to deteriorate despite broad-spectrum antibiotic therapy with progressive pulmonary shadowing and worsening hypoxia. Computed tomography imaging confirmed a pneumonitis but did not identify lymphadenopathy or enlargement of the liver or spleen. A bone marrow aspirate and trephine biopsy were obtained. The most notable feature of the aspirate was a significant increase in macrophages with profound haemophagocytosis, some cells having ingested multiple nucleated marrow cells (Figures 68.1 and 68.2). In addition there was a population of large blastoid cells with prominent pink granules, which accounted for 5–10% of all cells (Figures 68.3 and 68.4) (arrows). A differential count was particularly difficult in view of the number of cells ingested by macrophages and the amount of cell debris evident.

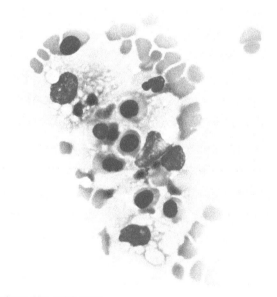

Figure 68.1 MGG, ×500.

Practical Flow Cytometry in Haematology: 100 Worked Examples, First Edition. Mike Leach, Mark Drummond, Allyson Doig, Pam McKay, Bob Jackson and Barbara J. Bain.
© 2015 John Wiley & Sons, Ltd. Published 2015 by John Wiley & Sons, Ltd.

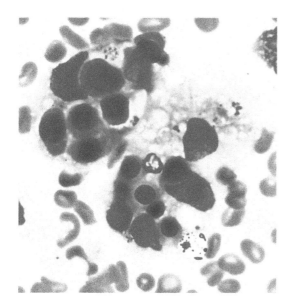

Figure 68.2 MGG, ×500.

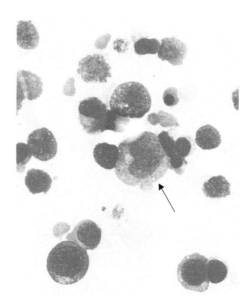

Figure 68.4 MGG, ×500.

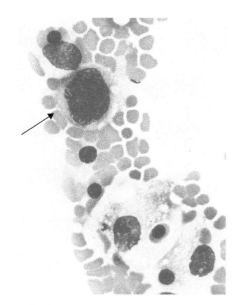

Figure 68.3 MGG, ×500.

Flow cytometry

Flow cytometry studies on the bone marrow aspirate were inconclusive. There was no precursor neoplasm apparent. In view of the clinical presentation we were keen to exclude a natural killer (NK)- or T-cell leukaemia or lymphoma but using a blast or CD2 gating strategy neither could be confirmed. We were aware that the analyses and scatter plots were showing a lot of debris and free cell nuclei that could not be accurately categorised. A second aspirate was taken but was hypocellular and diluted by blood.

The working diagnosis was of overwhelming EBV infection with a secondary haemophagocytic syndrome and DIC. The patient continued to deteriorate clinically despite intravenous ganciclovir with persistent fever, worsening hypoxia and cytopenias. The coagulopathy was resistant to replacement therapy with fresh frozen plasma, cryoprecipitate and platelets and the patient developed bleeding from multiple sites.

Bone marrow trephine biopsy

This was processed rapidly in view of the clinical urgency. The cellularity was increased at 70% overall; there was a diffuse interstitial infiltrate of highly pleomorphic large cells with vesicular nuclei that had one or more nucleoli (Figure 68.5) (arrows). These were expressing CD2, CD56 (Figure 68.6) and granzyme B (Figure 68.7) but were negative for CD3, CD5, CD7, CD4, CD8 and TdT. *In situ* hybridisation for EBV EBER revealed strong nuclear positivity in all tumour cells (Figure 68.8). These findings are in keeping with a diagnosis of aggressive NK-cell leukaemia.

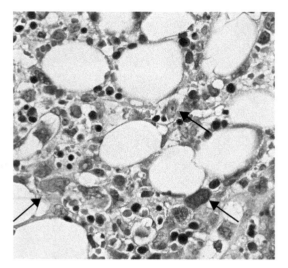

Figure 68.5 H&E, ×400.

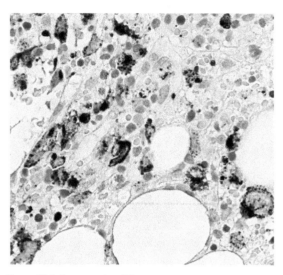

Figure 68.7 Granzyme B, ×400.

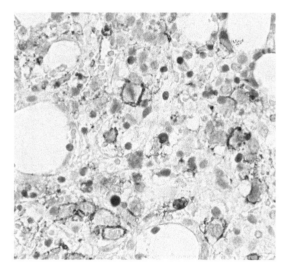

Figure 68.6 CD56, ×400.

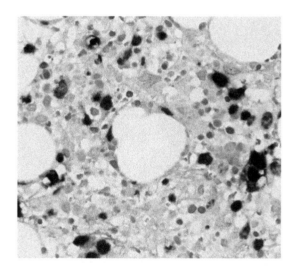

Figure 68.8 EBV EBER, ×400.

Cytogenetic analysis

Bone marrow aspirate metaphase preparations identified a complex karyotype with near tetraploidy (Figure 68.9).

The patient was treated with high dose methylprednisolone followed by ESHAP with asparaginase. Complete remission was achieved with recovery of blood counts and resolution of the haemophagocytosis and coagulopathy. The viraemias resolved and the abnormal karyotype was no longer evident. Treatment was consolidated using 4 cycles of

the SMILE regimen and a sibling donor allogeneic transplant was undertaken.

At 90 days post-transplant the patient again became unwell with fatigue, fever, pancytopenia, EBV viraemia and DIC. A bone marrow aspirate showed haemophagocytosis and re-appearance of large granular lymphoid cells with vacuolated pale blue cytoplasm indicative of relapsed disease (Figures 68.10 and 68.11) (arrows).

Flow cytometry on this occasion clearly identified these cells using a CD56 versus SSC gating approach (P1, Figure 68.12) now showing a CD2+, CD16+, CD56+, CD45+

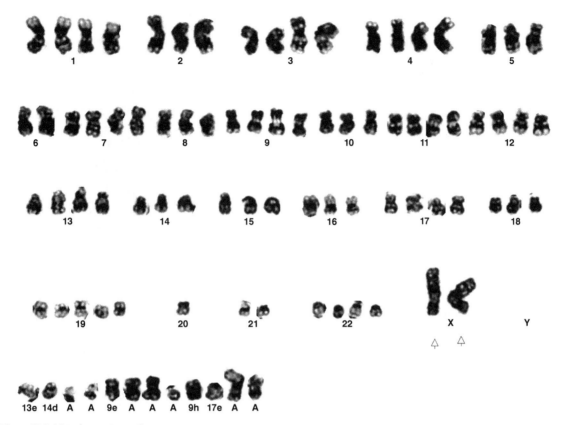

Figure 68.9 Metaphase cytogenetics.

phenotype. The variable size and granularity of these cells is reflected by their appearance in multiple zones of the FSC/SSC plot (Figure 68.13).

Despite the re-introduction of high dose steroids the patient deteriorated rapidly and died within a few days.

Discussion

This case illustrates some of the difficulties in confirming a diagnosis of this rare disorder even when it is clinically suspected. The clinical presentation with a short history of fever, sweats and pneumonitis together with the laboratory findings of pancytopenia, DIC, extreme hyperferritinaemia and striking haemophagocytosis in the bone marrow generated a relatively narrow differential diagnosis. This presentation may be the result of a profound reaction to a viral infection (sometimes in the context of an inherited immunodeficiency) or as a cytokine-driven response to a T- or NK-cell leukaemia or lymphoma. The EBV viraemia

was misleading as it was assumed initially that this was the primary pathogen being one of the viruses most cited as causing a haemophagocytic syndrome. However, the bone marrow aspirate did show suspicious cells with morphology in keeping with NK-cell leukaemia/lymphoma. Despite early attempts to identify these cells using flow cytometry studies, they proved elusive possibly due to their size and fragility and relative under-representation in the aspirate sample. The specimens were relatively hypocellular and the quality of the aspirate was clearly compromised by the disturbed bone marrow environment. A more accurate representation of marrow cellularity was achieved with the trephine biopsy specimen and this enabled a diagnosis to be made. At relapse the marrow aspirate was more cellular and neoplastic NK cells could be easily demonstrated both morphologically and using flow cytometry.

The EBV viraemia is a regular finding in NK-cell leukaemia; the virus is implicated in the proliferation of the NK cells. The pneumonitis may well have been caused by reactivation of CMV in the context of the gross immune

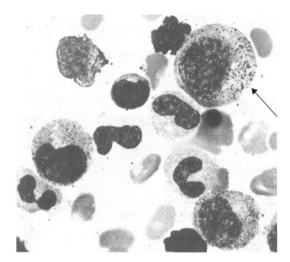

Figure 68.10 MGG, ×1000.

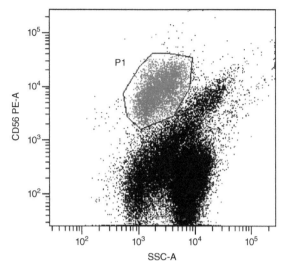

Figure 68.12 CD56/SSC.

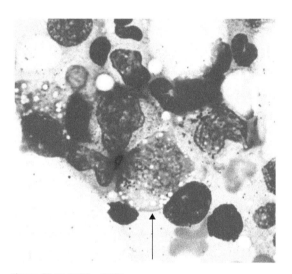

Figure 68.11 MGG, ×1000.

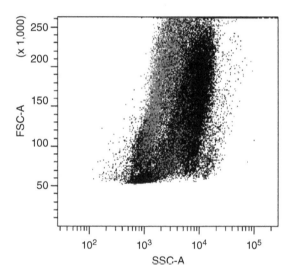

Figure 68.13 FSC/SSC.

dysregulation that is seen in T and NK neoplasms. This case also demonstrates the difficulties in managing this condition. Despite the initial response to therapy and achievement of a complete remission we elected to proceed to allogeneic transplant. Despite this 'maximal therapy' approach the disease relapsed early and the patient could not be rescued a second time.

Final diagnosis

Aggressive NK-cell leukaemia with secondary haemophago-cytic syndrome.

Case 69

A 79-year-old man presented with increasing back pain, anorexia and nausea. He had a history of diet-controlled diabetes but had otherwise been previously well. Physical examination showed kyphosis. He had no palpable lymphadenopathy or organomegaly.

Laboratory data

FBC: Hb 105 g/L, WBC 5×10^9/L, platelets 190×10^9/L.
 U&Es; creatinine 200 μmol/L with eGFR 20 ml/min.
 LFTs: normal except albumin 28 g/L. Glucose 28 mmol/L.
 Serum electrophoresis: IgM kappa paraprotein 39 g/L, with immune paresis.
 Serum free kappa light chains were 2977 mg/L.
 Plasma viscosity was 3.21 mPAS.
 A skeletal survey confirmed kyphosis and osteoporosis with a wedge fracture of the T11 vertebra but no focal lytic lesions.
 The differential diagnosis here was between a low-grade lymphoma and multiple myeloma. As the former seemed most likely, flow cytometry studies were not performed on the first bone marrow aspirate. A lymphoplasmacytic lymphoma (Waldenström macroglobulinaemia) appeared to be the likely diagnosis.

Histopathology

The bone marrow trephine biopsy showed interstitial involvement by a population of small lymphocytes and plasma cells with prominent Dutcher bodies (arrows, Figure 69.1); the plasma cells expressed CD138 (Figure 69.2), CD20 (Figure 69.3), cyclin D1 (Figure 69.4) and kappa light

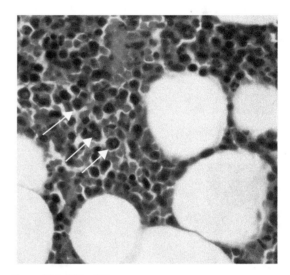

Figure 69.1 H&E, ×400.

chains (Figure 69.5). A diagnosis of a cyclin D1$^+$, CD20$^+$ IgM myeloma was now favoured so a repeat bone marrow aspirate was taken and submitted for flow studies.

Bone marrow aspirate

The aspirate was rather hypocellular. The cells that were present had lymphoplasmacytic morphology: there was a spectrum of cells some resembling mature lymphoid cells whilst others, though small, had plasma cell morphology and yet others had intermediate characteristics (Figures 69.6–69.8). On morphological assessment these cells accounted for approximately 20% of cells in the aspirate.

Practical Flow Cytometry in Haematology: 100 Worked Examples, First Edition. Mike Leach, Mark Drummond, Allyson Doig, Pam McKay, Bob Jackson and Barbara J. Bain.
© 2015 John Wiley & Sons, Ltd. Published 2015 by John Wiley & Sons, Ltd.

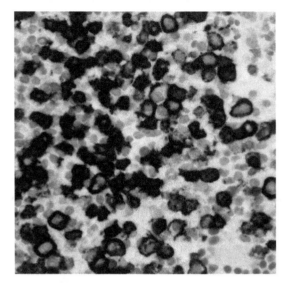

Figure 69.2 CD138, ×400.

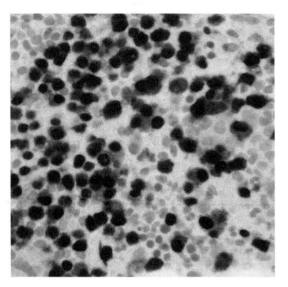

Figure 69.4 Cyclin D1, ×400.

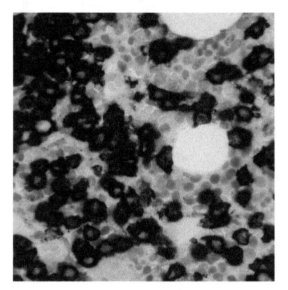

Figure 69.3 CD20, ×400.

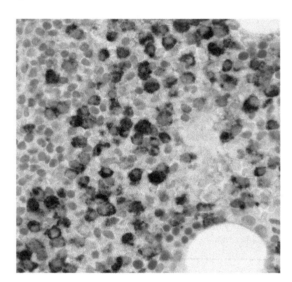

Figure 69.5 Kappa, ×400.

Flow cytometry

Two different strategies were used to assess this case. Firstly, a mature lymphoid panel gating on the CD19$^+$ cell population was performed. This showed that CD19$^+$ cells accounted for just 1.1% of events. These had a mature B-cell phenotype with no aberrant antigen expression and were polyclonal in terms of surface immunoglobulin expression: kappa 43%,

lambda 50%. Secondly, we used a myeloma panel gating on CD138$^+$ cells (versus side scatter) and these cells accounted for 11% of all events. They had the phenotype CD45$^-$, CD19$^-$ (Figure 69.9), CD20$^+$, CD38$^+$ and CD56$^+$ (Figure 69.10).

Discussion

The neoplastic plasma cells of multiple myeloma typically have a CD138$^+$, CD38$^+$, CD45$^-$, CD19$^-$, CD56$^+$ phenotype,

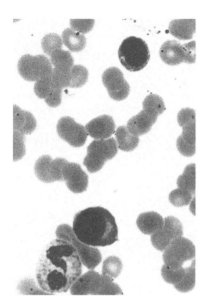

Figure 69.6 MGG, ×1000.

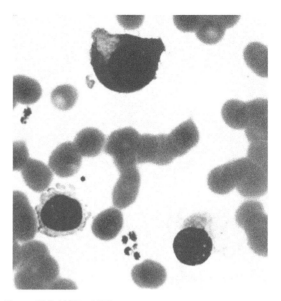

Figure 69.8 MGG, ×1000.

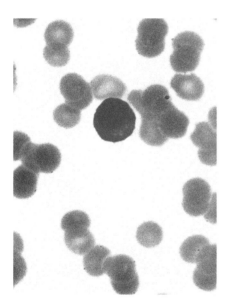

Figure 69.7 MGG, ×1000.

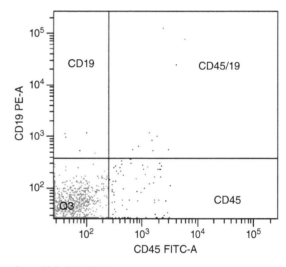

Figure 69.9 CD45/CD19.

easily differentiating them from normal plasma cells that are CD138+, CD38+, CD45dim, CD19+, CD56−; the latter show a mixed polyclonal expression of cytoplasmic kappa and lambda. Assessment of cytoplasmic light chain expression is not normally required as the myeloma cell phenotype is easily identified.

This case is unusual in two respects. Firstly, this neoplasm is producing an IgM paraprotein and although IgM myeloma is well recognised it is extremely rare. An IgM paraprotein is much more frequently associated with low-grade lymphomas, namely lymphoplasmacytic lymphoma, marginal zone lymphoma or small lymphocytic lymphoma/CLL. Secondly, this neoplasm is expressing CD20 and cyclin D1, though importantly CD19 and other pan-B markers were not expressed. This curiosity, cyclin D1+ CD20+ myeloma

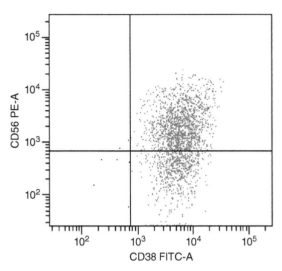

Figure 69.10 CD56/CD38.

to recognise and to differentiate from lymphoplasmacytic lymphoma (1), as the treatment of these conditions is different. Misinterpretation as CD5⁻ mantle cell lymphoma is also possible due to the strong cyclin D1 positivity; the morphology and expression of plasmacytic markers (CD138) should help to exclude this entity. In view of the strong expression of CD20, the utility of rituximab is already being explored as an adjunct to established therapies in the treatment of this variant of multiple myeloma.

Final diagnosis

IgM multiple myeloma with t(11;14)(q13;q32) and CD20 positivity.

Reference

1 Schuster, S.R., Rajkumar, S.V., Dispenzieri, A. et al. IgM multiple myeloma: disease definition, prognosis, and differentiation from Waldenstrom's macroglobulinemia. *American Journal of Hematology*, 2010, **85** (**11**), 853–855. PubMed PMID: 20842638.

accounts for approximately 20% of myeloma cases and the cyclin D1 over expression is the result of a t(11;14)(q13;q32) translocation. It is often associated with a small plasma cell or lymphoplasmacytoid morphology. It does not appear to carry an adverse prognosis but is an important condition

Case 70

A 17-year-old male with a history of treated T lymphoblastic lymphoma presented with facial weakness, skin nodules and breathlessness. Clinical examination showed features of lower motor neurone facial and oculomotor nerve palsies. His primary presentation had been with superior vena cava obstruction secondary to a large mediastinal mass due to cortical-T lymphoblastic lymphoma. He had achieved remission with ALL-type induction and consolidation therapy and had been proceeding through maintenance chemotherapy when new signs and symptoms developed. Brain CT and MRI studies were normal, showing no mass lesion or meningeal enhancement so a lumbar puncture was performed and a CSF specimen was acquired.

Laboratory data

FBC: Hb 120 g/L, WBC 4.9 × 10⁹/L (neutrophils 3.5 × 10⁹/L), platelets 540 × 10⁹/L.

U&Es, LFTs, bone profile and LDH were all normal.

CSF: WBC 0.086 × 10⁹/L, protein 0.7 g/L and glucose 1.8 mmol/L.

CSF cytospin morphology

The CSF was cellular with a markedly increased cell count (normal less than 0.001 × 10⁹/L). Morphological assessment showed a pleomorphic population of large lymphoid cells with cytoplasmic protrusions and fronds, partly exacerbated by the cytospin process (Figures 70.1–70.4). Occasional apoptotic forms were present (Figure 70.3).

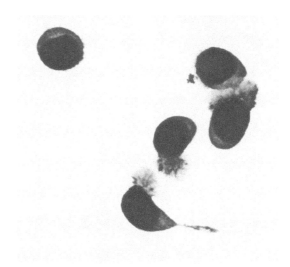

Figure 70.1 MGG, ×1000.

Flow cytometry

Flow studies on CSF identified the same population of large lymphoid cells expressing CD2, CD3, CD5, CD7ᵈⁱᵐ, CD8 and CD1a. This is not in keeping with a reactive T-cell population in view of the CD8 restriction and CD1a expression. This phenotype is identical to that of the cortical-T lymphoblastic lymphoma seen at the primary diagnosis and as such this indicates a meningeal relapse of this disease.

Bone marrow aspirate

The bone marrow aspirate showed normal morphology with no excess of blasts or abnormal infiltrate.

Practical Flow Cytometry in Haematology: 100 Worked Examples, First Edition. Mike Leach, Mark Drummond, Allyson Doig, Pam McKay, Bob Jackson and Barbara J. Bain.
© 2015 John Wiley & Sons, Ltd. Published 2015 by John Wiley & Sons, Ltd.

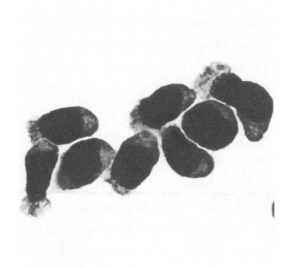

Figure 70.2 MGG, ×1000.

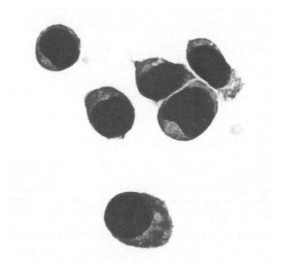

Figure 70.4 MGG, ×1000.

Cytogenetic analysis

47,XY,del(2)(q?34q?36),del(6)(q?15q?16),add(9)(q34),
+mar[5] on a lymph node preparation.

Discussion

This case illustrates the ability of flow cytometry to clearly define the nature and phenotype of abnormal lymphoid cells involving the CSF at relatively low levels and to correlate this with the characteristics of the initial tumour diagnosis. This clonal restricted CD8+, CD1a+ phenotype clearly differentiates these malignant cells from a reactive T-cell infiltrate where a mixture of CD4+ and CD8+ cells would be anticipated without expression of CD1a. Skin biopsies confirmed involvement by lymphoid cells with an identical phenotype. Reinduction chemotherapy, with intensive CNS-directed therapy, was commenced with full resolution of cranial nerve symptomatology and normalisation of CSF parameters and flow studies. Unfortunately a further disease relapse occurred and the disease proved refractory to subsequent therapy.

A number of cytogenetic abnormalities carry prognostic significance in B lymphoblastic leukaemia/lymphoma. Patients with a t(9;22)(q33;q13), t(4;11)(q21;q23), t(8;14) (q24.1;q32), complex karyotypes or low hypodiploidy/near triploidy all have inferior outcomes whilst those with high

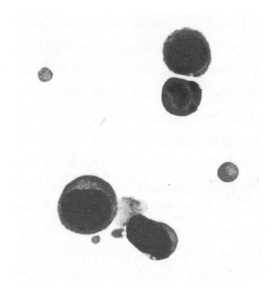

Figure 70.3 MGG, ×1000.

Skin lesions

Biopsy of the newly developed skin nodules identified malignant cells with an immunophenotype identical to that described above.

hyperdiploidy, t(12;21)(p13;q22) or a del(9p) appear to have a significantly improved outcome (1). These cytogenetic abnormalities, however, relate specifically to B-cell lineage disease, which constitutes the majority of cases in the reported series. Up to 50% of patients with T lymphoblastic leukaemia/lymphoma actually have a normal karyotype. In the remaining patients complex karyotypes are common and detailed analysis is required in order to identify which findings are prognostically important. A high proportion of cryptic abnormalities, particularly those involving breakpoints near the telomere, can be identified using targeted FISH studies. Mutations involving T-cell receptor (*TCR*) genes (*TCRA* and *TCRD* at 14q11, *TCRG* at 7p14 and *TCRB* at 7q32), *TAL1* at 1p32, *HOX11 (TLX1)* at 10q24, *HOX11L2 (TLX3)* at 5q35 and *NOTCH1* (a gene encoding one of a family of proteins regulating cell fate and differentiation) located at 9q34 appear important amongst a myriad of others (2, 3). The add(9)(q34) reported in this case may have involved the *NOTCH1* locus but the other abnormalities do not appear to have carried any definite specificity (though del(6q) may involve a tumour suppressor gene) and thus impact on prognosis at the outset. Clearly relapse of disease during maintenance therapy, particularly as the CNS was involved, was a devastating development for this patient.

Final diagnosis

Meningeal and cutaneous relapse of cortical-T lymphoblastic lymphoma.

References

1 Moorman, A.V., Harrison, C.J., Buck, G.A. *et al.* (2007) Karyotype is an independent prognostic factor in adult acute lymphoblastic leukemia (ALL): analysis of cytogenetic data from patients treated on the Medical Research Council (MRC) UKALLXII/Eastern Cooperative Oncology Group (ECOG) 2993 trial. *Blood*, **109** (8), 3189–3197. PubMed PMID: 17170120.

2 Graux, C., Cools, J., Michaux, L., Vandenberghe, P. & Hagemeijer, A. (2006) Cytogenetics and molecular genetics of T-cell acute lymphoblastic leukemia: from thymocyte to lymphoblast. *Leukemia: Official Journal of the Leukemia Society of America, Leukemia Research Fund, UK*, **20** (9), 1496–1510. PubMed PMID: 16826225.

3 Cave, H., Suciu, S., Preudhomme, C. *et al.* (2004) Clinical significance of HOX11L2 expression linked to t(5;14)(q35;q32), of HOX11 expression, and of SIL-TAL fusion in childhood T-cell malignancies: results of EORTC studies 58881 and 58951. *Blood*, **103** (2), 442–450. PubMed PMID: 14504110.

Case 71

A 19-year-old female, who had previously been a blood donor presented with progressive fatigue of a few months' duration. She gave no history of bleeding apart from menstruation that was not heavy. She took no regular medication and had no past medical history of note. There were no other specific symptoms but on examination her skin had a lemon yellow tinge.

Laboratory data

FBC: Hb 70 g/L, MCV 102 fl, WBC 4×10^9/L (neutrophils 2×10^9/L, lymphocytes 1.5×10^9/L, monocytes 0.38×10^9/L) and platelets 87×10^9/L.

Serum ferritin 8 ng/ml, serum folate 4 ng/ml and serum vitamin B_{12} 300 pg/ml.

Reticulocytes 120×10^9/L. Direct Coombs test was negative.

U&Es and bone profile: normal.

LFTs: normal except AST 85 U/L, bilirubin 50 μmol/L. Serum LDH 630 U/L.

Blood film

This showed polychromasia, moderate anisopoikilocytosis, with macrocytes, teardrop poikilocytes and pencil cells but without spherocytes (Figures 71.1 and 71.2). The small number of cells that lack central pallor are the result of the blood film being thinly spread, in turn due to the significant anaemia; a similar false impression of spherocytosis can result from examining the tail of the film. The features seen are relatively non-specific but the polychromasia and confirmed reticulocytosis indicate an attempt at bone marrow

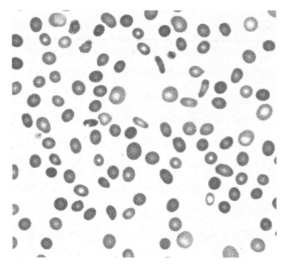

Figure 71.1 MGG, ×500.

compensation for the anaemia. The serum ferritin indicated iron deficiency but clearly this is not the sole diagnosis. There are a number of features here to suggest a haemolytic disorder. The poor reticulocyte response for anaemia of this severity is likely to be the result of absent bone marrow iron.

Bone marrow aspirate and trephine biopsy

The aspirate showed erythroid hyperplasia with a minor degree of dysplasia such as is often seen in a stressed bone marrow (Figures 71.3 and 71.4). There was no abnormal infiltrate and the myeloid and megakaryocyte series were normal. Stainable iron was absent.

Practical Flow Cytometry in Haematology: 100 Worked Examples, First Edition. Mike Leach, Mark Drummond, Allyson Doig, Pam McKay, Bob Jackson and Barbara J. Bain.
© 2015 John Wiley & Sons, Ltd. Published 2015 by John Wiley & Sons, Ltd.

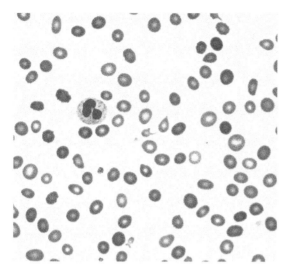

Figure 71.2 MGG, ×500.

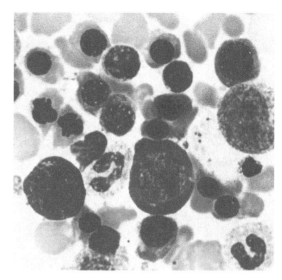

Figure 71.4 MGG, ×500.

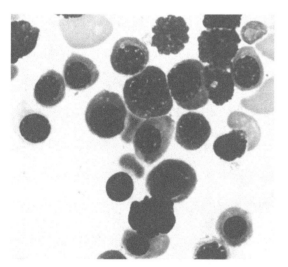

Figure 71.3 MGG, ×500.

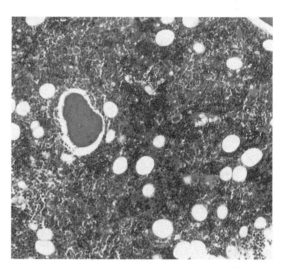

Figure 71.5 H&E, ×100.

Similarly, the trephine biopsy sections were hypercellular due to gross expansion of the erythroid lineage (Figures 71.5 and 71.6). Note the prominent haloes which, although they are a shrinkage artefact, help to distinguish erythroblasts from lymphocytes (Figure 71.6).

The findings were therefore of an acquired non-immune haemolytic anaemia with incomplete compensation due to coexistent iron deficiency. A diagnosis of paroxysmal nocturnal haemoglobinuria (PNH) was considered.

Flow cytometry (peripheral blood)

Peripheral blood granulocytes were examined using fluorochrome-linked antibodies to CD24 and CD66 together with FLAER (fluorochrome-linked aerolysin). CD24 and CD66 are antigens bound to the glycosylphosphatidylinositol (GPI) anchor in the cell membrane whilst FLAER binds directly to the GPI anchor itself. This patient's neutrophils

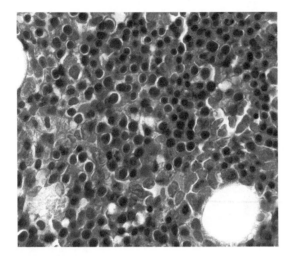

Figure 71.6 H&E, ×400.

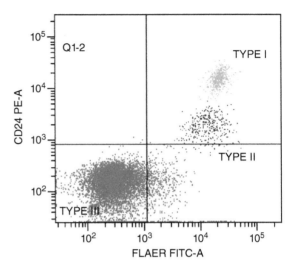

Figure 71.8 CD24/FLAER.

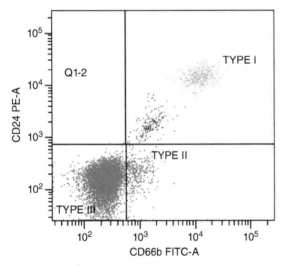

Figure 71.7 CD24/CD66b.

Figure 71.9 Perls stain, ×500.

showed a type III PNH clone (red events) affecting over 90% of cells whilst a small type II population was also seen (blue events) (Figures 71.7 and 71.8). The residual normal (type I) cells are shown in green. These findings, with a very large type III PNH clone, are in keeping with the haemolytic presentation.

Urine haemosiderin

The sediment from a fresh urine specimen was stained for iron using Perls stain (Figure 71.9). This shows a marked excess of urinary iron (bright blue); this iron has been partially reabsorbed by the urothelial cells (nuclei counterstained red) in the presence of recurrent episodes of haemoglobinuria, and has been converted by them to haemosiderin, which then appears in the urine when cells are shed. This test is useful in the investigation of chronic haemolytic disorders, and will remain abnormal for some time after an acute episode of intravascular haemolysis.

Discussion

Paroxysmal nocturnal haemoglobinuria is a rare acquired stem cell disorder producing the triad of haemolytic anaemia, thrombosis and bone marrow hypoplasia. It is characterised by loss of the GPI anchor from the cell membrane: the degree of loss, partial or complete, can be assessed using flow cytometry studies quantifying antigens bound to GPI. Some of these antigens such as CD55 (decay accelerating factor, DAF) and CD59 (membrane inhibitor of reactive lysis, MIRL) have known functions in protecting red cells from inappropriate activation of complement and their loss results in an intravascular haemolysis. The function of other linked antigens is less clear but must contribute in some way to the clinical manifestations of PNH. Patients with large PNH clones typically present with haemolytic anaemia but are also at high risk of venous thrombosis; the latter can carry a high mortality as the thrombosis can be serious, affecting splanchnic vessels and cerebral venous sinuses.

This patient was planned to commence eculizumab therapy but whilst this was being formalised and despite heparin anticoagulation she represented with a progressive headache. An MRI study showed a right sigmoid sinus and early posterior sagittal sinus thrombosis. This was treated promptly using heparin, warfarin and eculizumab and serious sequelae were prevented. Treatment with systemic anticoagulation and eculizumab will need to continue indefinitely.

Final diagnoses

1. Paroxysmal nocturnal haemoglobinuria due to a large type III clone.
2. Iron deficiency resulting from urinary iron loss.

Case 72

A previously fit 32-year-old man developed left shoulder and chest discomfort. On examination he had signs of a small right pleural effusion and small volume neck lymphadenopathy.

Laboratory data

FBC: Hb 168 g/L, WBC 12×10^9/L (neutrophils 3.15×10^9/L, 'lymphocytes' 5.25×10^9/L, 'monocytes' 3.56×10^9/L) and platelets 365×10^9/L.

U&Es, LFTs and bone profile: normal. Serum LDH: 350 U/L.

Blood film

A population of large nucleolated blast cells was evident, some showing cytoplasmic granules in keeping with a myeloid lineage (Figures 72.1–72.3). Neutrophils were preserved and did not show significant dysplastic morphology (Figures 72.3 and 72.4).

Imaging

A CXR showed mediastinal widening and blunting of the right costophrenic angle. More detailed assessment using CT showed the unexpected finding of a mediastinal mass (arrows, Figures 72.5–72.7), together with a right pleural effusion and neck lymphadenopathy. The mass was of heterogeneous density with possible necrosis. There was no involvement of the pericardium or compromise of the great vessels. From a radiological perspective, a high-grade

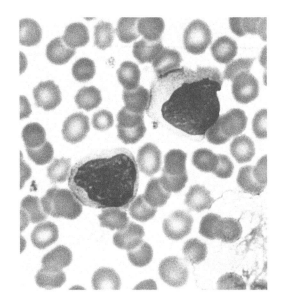

Figure 72.1 MGG, ×1000.

lymphoma was felt to be the most likely diagnosis so a percutaneous supraclavicular lymph node core biopsy was undertaken.

Bone marrow aspirate

The aspirate was heavily involved by blast cells similar to those in the peripheral blood (66% of cells). These again showed prominent nucleoli, cytoplasmic granules (Figures 72.8 and 72.9) and, in addition, some had Auer rods (arrow, Figure 72.9)

Practical Flow Cytometry in Haematology: 100 Worked Examples, First Edition. Mike Leach, Mark Drummond, Allyson Doig, Pam McKay, Bob Jackson and Barbara J. Bain.
© 2015 John Wiley & Sons, Ltd. Published 2015 by John Wiley & Sons, Ltd.

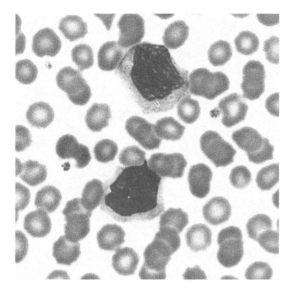

Figure 72.2 MGG, ×1000.

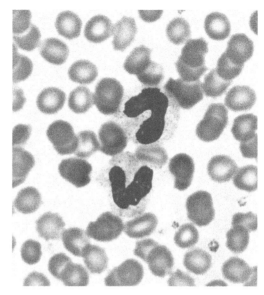

Figure 72.4 MGG, ×1000.

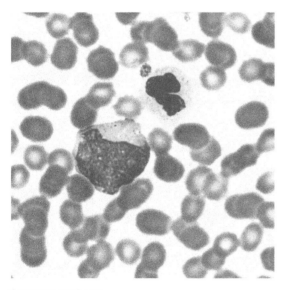

Figure 72.3 MGG, ×10.

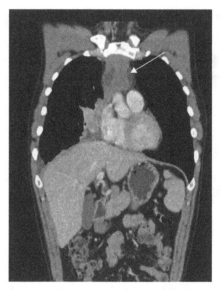

Figure 72.5 CT.

Flow cytometry (peripheral blood and bone marrow)

We now had a diagnostic dilemma in that there was a morphological diagnosis of acute myeloid leukaemia whilst CT had identified a mediastinal mass and lymphadenopathy, suggestive of lymphoma. Auer rods are only seen in myeloid neoplasms.

Flow cytometry showed the blasts to have a CD34+, CD38+, CD117+, CD15dim, CD33+, CD7+, CD13+, HLA-DR+, MPO+ and CD19+ phenotype. Surface CD14, CD64, CD20, CD10, cCD3, cCD79a and nuclear TdT were not expressed. This was therefore acute myeloid leukaemia (AML) with aberrant CD7 and CD19 expression. It is not a mixed phenotype acute leukaemia (MPAL), B/myeloid

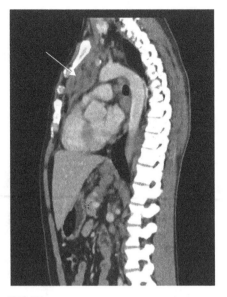

Figure 72.6 CT.

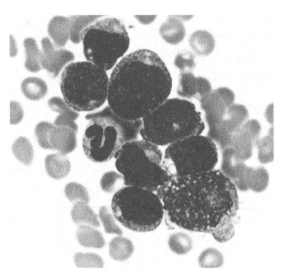

Figure 72.8 MGG, ×1000.

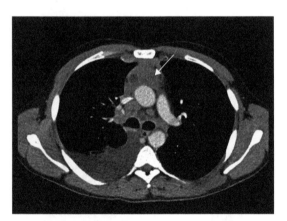

Figure 72.7 CT.

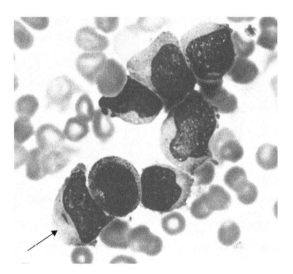

Figure 72.9 MGG, ×1000.

or T/myeloid, as cytoplasmic CD3 was not detected and expression of CD19 is not in itself sufficient to satisfy the WHO criteria for MPAL; there must be expression of CD79a (a cytoplasmic epitope is detected), cCD22 or CD10 or, if CD19 expression is weak, coexpression of at least two of these antigens. The lymph node biopsy and cytogenetic studies were critical for a unifying diagnosis. We did consider a t(8;21)(q22;q22) AML with a mediastinal myeloid sarcoma, particularly as we had documented aberrant CD19 positivity on the myeloid blasts (this being a relatively common finding in this type of AML). The aberrant CD7 expression would, however, have been atypical, in our experience, for t(8;21)

AML. Another consideration was of the 8p11 syndrome. This is a rare stem cell leukemia/lymphoma syndrome, an aggressive neoplasm associated with chromosomal translocations involving the fibroblast growth factor receptor 1 (*FGFR1*) tyrosine kinase gene at 8p11.23-11.22. These patients can present with a simultaneous myeloproliferative neoplasm or AML together with lymphoblastic leukaemia/lymphoma. Multiple partner genes of *FGFR1* have been described.

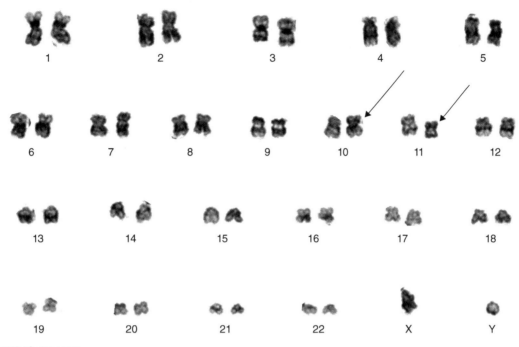

Figure 72.10 Karyogram.

Histopathology

The lymph node cores showed effacement by a blast cell population with irregular nuclei and eosinophilic cytoplasm. The tumour cells were positive for CD45 (weak), CD43, CD34 and CD117 and negative for CD3, CD5, CD10, CD8, CD79a and CD20. This was in keeping with nodal involvement by acute myeloid leukaemia and presumably this was also responsible for the mediastinal mass.

Cytogenetic analysis

Cytogenetic studies identified neither a t(8;21) nor a translocation involving 8p11. They did identify a t(10;11)(p13;q21) translocation (arrows, Figure 72.10).

Discussion

Acute myeloid leukaemia with t(10;11)(p13;q21) is a rare entity. The translocation generates a *PICALM-MLL10* fusion gene and cases are characterised by an AML with aberrant T-cell and B-cell antigen expression, young age at presentation and the presence of a mediastinal mass (1). All of these features were present in the patient described. Central nervous system involvement has also been described in a series of cases.

This leukaemia often proves refractory to therapy with either difficulty in achieving remission or early relapse (2). A selected bone marrow blast flow cytometric profile at diagnosis is shown in Figure 72.11a. There was only partial clearance of blasts following induction chemotherapy (17% of marrow cells (CD34+) following induction course 1, Figure 72.11b) and the mediastinal mass was slow to resolve. Morphological remission was achieved following a second course of chemotherapy (1.5% of marrow cells CD34+ following induction course 2, Figure 72.11c) but a small abnormal blast population could still be identified by following the CD34+, CD19+, CD7+ subset, which enabled us to distinguish neoplastic cells from normal recovering marrow myeloblasts (CD34+, CD19−, CD7−) and haematogones (purple events, H in Figure 72.11c).

Although the number of published cases is small, the current evidence indicates that this leukaemia carries a poor prognosis. In addition, the slow response of bone marrow and mediastinal disease to therapy and the persistence of

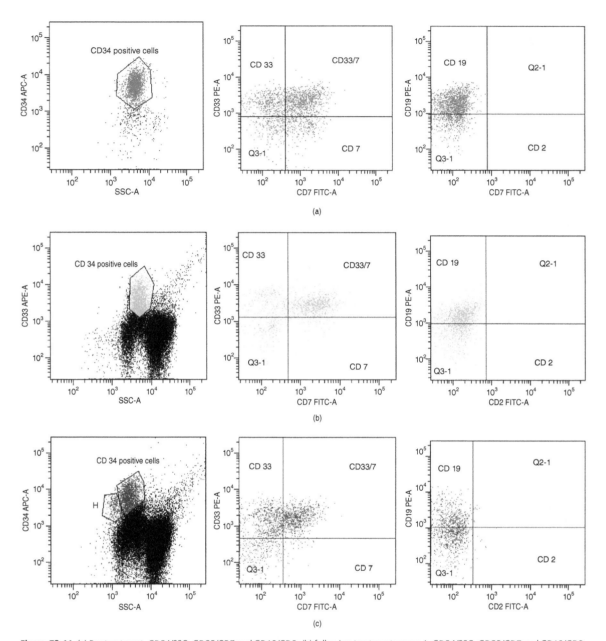

Figure 72.11 (a) Pre-treatment, CD34/SSC, CD33/CD7 and CD19/CD2; (b) following treatment course 1, CD34/SSC, CD33/CD7 and CD19/CD2; (c) following treatment course 2, CD34/SSC, CD33/CD7 and CD19/CD2.

disease at low levels (defined by flow cytometry) suggested a high risk of relapse. A sibling donor has been identified and a cyclophosphamide/TBI-conditioned transplant is scheduled for the patient.

Final diagnosis

Acute myeloid leukaemia with t(10;11)(p13;q21) showing aberrant CD19 and CD7 expression with associated lymphadenopathy and a mediastinal mass.

References

1 Savage, N.M., Kota, V., Manaloor, E.J. *et al.* (2010) Acute leukemia with PICALM-MLLT10 fusion gene: diagnostic and treatment struggle. *Cancer Genetics and Cytogenetics*, **202** (**2**), 129–132. PubMed PMID: 20875875.

2 Borel, C., Dastugue, N., Cances-Lauwers, V. *et al.* (2012) PICALM-MLLT10 acute myeloid leukemia: a French cohort of 18 patients. *Leukemia Research*, **36** (**11**), 1365–1369. PubMed PMID: 22871473.

Case 73

An 82-year-old woman with known multiple myeloma on cyclophosphamide/thalidomide/dexamethasone (CTD) therapy was admitted for investigation of increasing breathlessness. Clinical examination identified a left pleural effusion and this was confirmed on CXR.

Laboratory data

FBC: Hb 106 g/L, MCV 106 fl, WBC 11.6 × 10⁹/L (neutrophils 8.9 × 10⁹/L, lymphocytes 1.8 × 10⁹/L, monocytes 0.8 × 10⁹/L, eosinophils 0.1 ×10⁹/L) and platelets 118 × 10⁹/L.

U&Es: Na 150 mmol/l, K 4.2 mmol/L, urea 14.1 mmol/L, creatinine 128 μmol/L.

Bone profile: normal. LFTs: normal except albumin 28 g/L.

Blood film

There were no specific features to report.

Flow cytometry (pleural fluid)

A diagnostic pleural aspiration was undertaken showing a fluid with cell count of 0.42 × 10⁹/L, total protein of 42 g/L and LDH of 5,800 U/L.

Morphological assessment of a cytospin preparation showed a significant population of pleomorphic apparently undifferentiated cells with convoluted nuclei and basophilic cytoplasm. No significant plasma cell population was seen, nor was there a significant reactive lymphocyte response (Figures 73.1–73.4).

Flow cytometry showed a large CD45⁻ cell population on CD45/SSC analysis (Figure 73.5) suggesting a

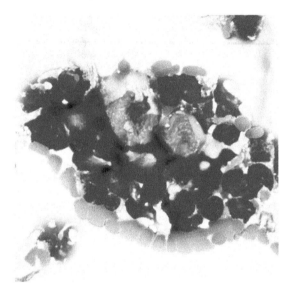

Figure 73.1 MGG, ×500.

non-haemopoietic neoplasm but on further assessment these cells gave negative results with the EpCAM (epithelial cell adhesion molecule) antibody (Figure 73.6). The cells did not express CD138, CD38 or CD56 thus excluding a plasma cell population.

Cytology

Cytomorphology identified a population of large atypical undifferentiated cells, some with blast like characteristics alongside a population of inflammatory cells. There were no specific features to define the origin of the tumour and insufficient material was available for immunocytochemistry.

Practical Flow Cytometry in Haematology: 100 Worked Examples, First Edition. Mike Leach, Mark Drummond, Allyson Doig, Pam McKay, Bob Jackson and Barbara J. Bain.
© 2015 John Wiley & Sons, Ltd. Published 2015 by John Wiley & Sons, Ltd.

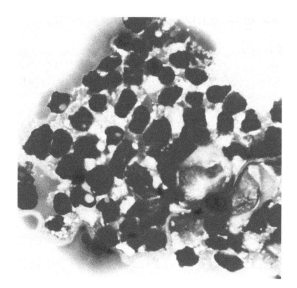

Figure 73.2 MGG, ×500.

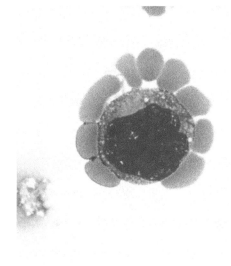

Figure 73.4 MGG, ×1000.

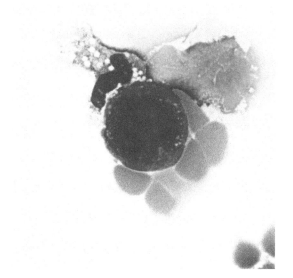

Figure 73.3 MGG, ×1000.

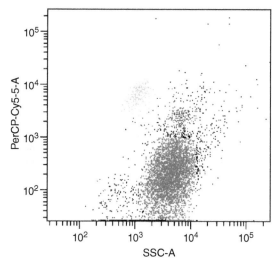

Figure 73.5 CD45/SSC.

Clinical course

The patient was already rather frail as a result of the myeloma and her condition continued to decline such that more detailed imaging using CT was not undertaken. In view of the combined cytological and flow immunocytometric findings and the remote likelihood of any meaningful therapy being available for a non-haemopoietic tumour affecting the pleura, a plan of supportive care was felt to be most appropriate. The exact primary origin of the neoplasm was never clarified but a squamous carcinoma of lung was considered most likely.

Discussion

Histopathological examination of tissue with an extensive immunohistochemistry panel is the accepted gold standard

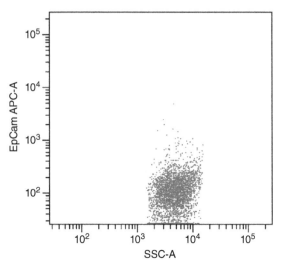

Figure 73.6 EpCAM/SSC.

for the diagnosis of solid tumours. Flow cytometry has played a relatively minor role in the accurate identification of non-haemopoietic tumours largely because such cells are not often available in suspension and an array of appropriate fluorochrome-linked antibodies has not been commercially available. It does, however, have a role to play alongside cytology and the findings from the two methodologies can compliment each other. Flow cytometry does actually offer some advantages. Immunophenotyping can provide a rapid analysis of cells in suspension so is very suitable for analysing cells in pleural fluid, ascitic fluid or CSF and for analysing suspensions of cells from fine needle lymph node aspirates. The results can be available in a few hours and can guide subsequent investigations. It is suitable for examining paucicellular specimens and for defining small populations of neoplastic cells admixed with reactive cells, for example a minor population of carcinoma cells together with large numbers of reactive T cells. It is perhaps better at defining intensity of antigen expression than immunohistochemistry and it can confirm co-expression of antigens on a single cell.

EpCAM is capable of binding to cells of a number of tumours of epithelial origin, particularly those originating in breast, lung, colon and prostate. It normally gives negative reactions with squamous carcinomas, however, so this remained a possible diagnosis in this patient. By considering the clinical presentation and past oncological history of a patient and using of a panel of antibodies (such as anti-CD99, anti-myogenin and anti-CD56) in addition to EpCAM in CD45 tumours, the likely derivation can often de determined (1).

Final diagnosis

Pleural metastasis of a non-haemopoietic tumour in a patient with multiple myeloma.

Reference

1 Chang, A., Benda, P.M., Wood, B.L. & Kussick, S.J. (2003) Lineage-specific identification of nonhematopoietic neoplasms by flow cytometry. *American Journal of Clinical Pathology*, **119** (5), 643–655.. PubMed PMID: 12760282.

Case 74

A 34-year-old male presented to the ENT department with the recent onset of right sided otalgia, hearing difficulty and facial weakness. He was found to have a partial right facial nerve palsy and a right sensorineural hearing loss was apparent. Examination of the nasal space, pharynx and larynx was unremarkable. A provisional diagnosis of mastoiditis was considered although the typical mastoid erythema and tenderness with associated fever were not seen.

Laboratory data

FBC: Hb 89 g/L, WBC 2.6×10^9/L (neutrophils 0.69×10^9/L, lymphocytes 1.6×10^9/L, monocytes 0.34×10^9/L) and platelets 237×10^9/L.

Coagulation profile: normal.

U&Es, LFTs and bone profile: normal. Serum LDH was 220 U/L and CRP 15 mg/L.

Blood film

This confirmed neutropenia but showed neither specific features nor leucoerythroblastosis.

Imaging

A mass was seen on CT involving the right parapharyngeal and right carotid space, surrounding the carotid artery with compression of the internal jugular vein (Figure 74.1, arrow) with opacification of the mastoid air cells (Figure 74.2, arrow). The mass could be seen to extend up to the base of the skull (Figure 74.3, arrow) The cause of this appearance was not clear but a neoplastic process was considered likely.

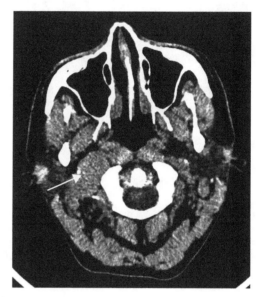

Figure 74.1 CT.

In view of the uncertainty regarding a diagnosis, the mass was explored surgically and multiple biopsies were taken. A frozen section on biopsied lymph nodes was reported as showing reactive features only.

A bone marrow aspirate was performed on account of the unexplained anaemia and neutropenia.

Bone marrow aspirate

An infiltrate of myeloid blasts with granular cytoplasm and prominent nucleoli was seen. There was limited granulocytic differentiation and minor dysplasia of the erythroid lineage (Figures 74.4–74.6). Megakaryocytes were preserved.

Practical Flow Cytometry in Haematology: 100 Worked Examples, First Edition. Mike Leach, Mark Drummond, Allyson Doig, Pam McKay, Bob Jackson and Barbara J. Bain.
© 2015 John Wiley & Sons, Ltd. Published 2015 by John Wiley & Sons, Ltd.

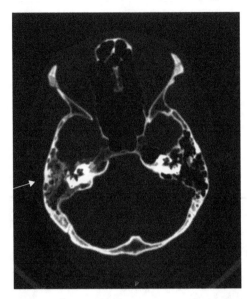

Figure 74.2 CT (bone windows).

Flow cytometry

Bone marrow aspirate examination confirmed a large blast cell population (43% of events) expressing CD34, CD117/CD15, partial CD13, partial CD33, HLA-DR, MPO and partial CD19 (Figures 74.7–74.10). Cytoplasmic CD79a and CD3 were not expressed.

This indicates a diagnosis of acute myeloid leukaemia with aberrant CD19 expression. Note the asynchronous co-expression of CD117 and CD15 on the blast cells; in our experience this is a frequent characteristic of FAB M2 AML with dysplastic myeloid maturation (which can be used for monitoring minimal residual disease). The absence of cytoplasmic CD3 and CD79a, CD22 and CD10 excludes the possibility of a T/myeloid or B/myeloid mixed phenotype leukaemia, respectively.

Histopathology

Examination of paraffin-embedded material from the paracarotid mass revealed several reactive lymph nodes in keeping with the initial frozen section assessment. Within the perinodal fat, however, there was a diffuse infiltrate of immature nucleolated blast cells and granular myeloid cells showing some loss of detail due to incipient necrosis (Figure 74.11). Immunohistochemistry showed positivity for CD34 (weak), CD117 (Figure 74.12), MPO and CD15

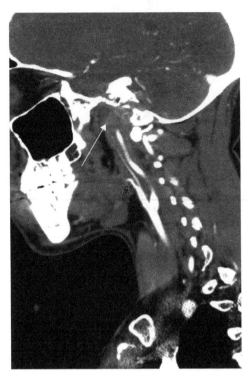

Figure 74.3 CT.

(Figure 74.13) whilst CD79a, CD20, CD3, CD43, CD68 and TdT were not expressed. The proliferation fraction was 40%. These features were in keeping with a myeloid neoplasm and the clinical presentation was in keeping with a diagnosis of myeloid sarcoma.

Cytogenetic analysis (marrow aspirate)

t(8;21)(q22;q22) was identified in 18 of 20 cells examined.

Discussion

Myeloid sarcoma, also known as granulocytic sarcoma and chloroma, is defined by the WHO classification as a tumour mass consisting of myeloid blasts, with or without maturation, occurring at an anatomical site other than bone marrow. In addition, the presentation should be with tumour masses in which the tissue architecture is effaced. It can occur *de novo*, simultaneously to, or preceding, acute

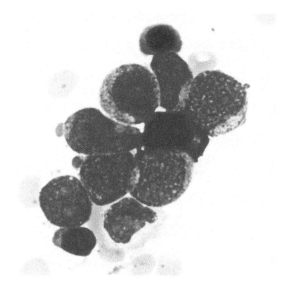

Figure 74.4 MGG, ×1000.

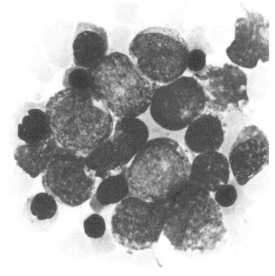

Figure 74.6 MGG, ×1000.

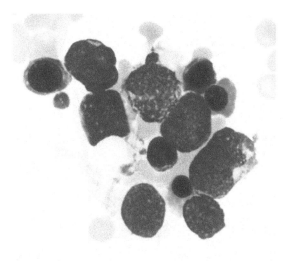

Figure 74.5 MGG, ×1000.

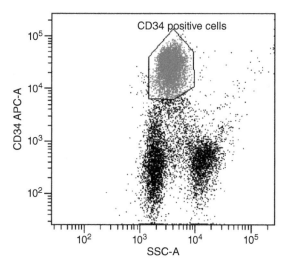

Figure 74.7 CD34/SSC.

myeloid leukaemia (AML), or can occur as an acute blastic transformation of a myelodysplastic or myeloproliferative neoplasm. It can also be an isolated manifestation of relapse in patients with a history of treated AML. Virtually any tissue can be involved and depending on the site can cause significant diagnostic difficulty. Patients with involvement of the brain, dura and cauda equina have all been described.

A variety of cytogenetic abnormalities similar to those seen in acute myeloid leukaemia and other myeloid neoplasms have been identified in myeloid sarcoma. In our, and others (1) experience, t(8;21)(q22;q22) has often been implicated. It should be noted that aberrant CD19 expression is a recognised feature of this molecular subtype of AML.

Myeloid sarcoma does not necessarily carry an adverse prognosis as long as the condition is promptly identified.

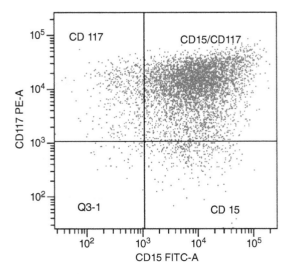

Figure 74.8 CD15/CD117.

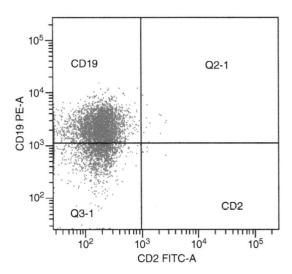

Figure 74.10 CD2/CD19.

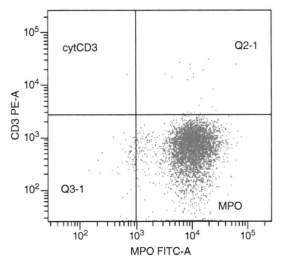

Figure 74.9 cCD3/MPO.

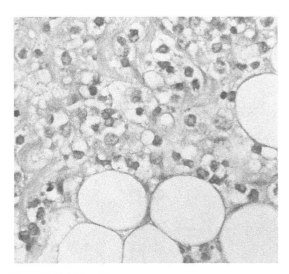

Figure 74.11 H&E, ×400.

The outcome is influenced by the associated cytogenetic abnormality and by whether it represents transformation of a preceding haematological disease. Patients with t(8;21) myeloid sarcoma/AML frequently show a good response to therapy and have durable remissions. Patients presenting with isolated myeloid sarcoma require AML type therapy (2). Any attempt at local treatment with excision or radiotherapy is likely to result in failure as the subsequent development of AML is inevitable.

The patient described was treated with four cycles of AML therapy and achieved marrow remission following the first course. The neck mass resolved rapidly and he is well 4 years later with no residual cranial nerve deficit.

Final diagnosis

Myeloid sarcoma at presentation of acute myeloid leukaemia associated with t(8;21)(q22;q22).

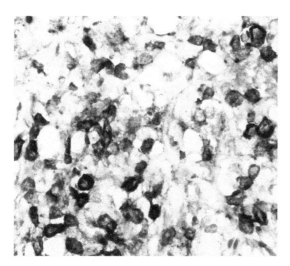

Figure 74.12 CD117, ×400.

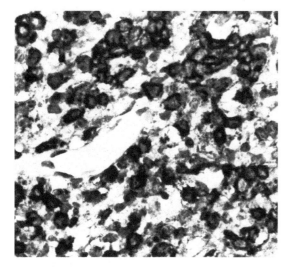

Figure 74.13 CD15, ×400.

References

1 Tallman, M.S., Hakimian, D., Shaw, J.M., Lissner, G.S., Russell, E.J. & Variakojis, D. (1993) Granulocytic sarcoma is associated with the 8;21 translocation in acute myeloid leukemia. *Journal of Clinical Oncology*, **11** (**4**), 690–697. PubMed PMID: 8478662.

2 Bakst, R.L., Tallman, M.S., Douer, D. & Yahalom, J. (2011) How I treat extramedullary acute myeloid leukemia. *Blood*, **118** (**14**), 3785–3793. PubMed PMID: 21795742.

Case 75

A 50-year-old Afro-Caribbean woman presented with a history of itchy skin lesions, fatigue, nausea and constipation. On examination she had a number of raised erythematous skin papules, low volume lymphadenopathy and a palpable spleen.

Laboratory data

FBC: Hb 103 g/L, WBC 13.3 × 10^9/L (neutrophils 2.5 × 10^9/L, lymphocytes 9.9 × 10^9/L, monocytes 0.5 × 10^9/L) and platelets 173 × 10^9/L.

U&Es: Na 136 mmol/l, K 4.0 mmol/L, urea 8 mmol/L, creatinine 120 µmol/L.

Bone profile: calcium 2.9 mmol/L, phosphate 1.5 mmol/L, ALP 350 U/L.

LFTS: normal except albumin 30 g/L.

Serum LDH 650 U/L.

Blood film

This showed a number of small to medium sized abnormal lymphoid cells with multiple prominent nuclear clefts. Flower-shaped nuclei were seen in the majority of cells examined (Figures 75.1–75.3). In addition there was a degree of red cell crenation and fragmentation but minimal polychromasia.

Flow cytometry (peripheral blood)

The abnormal cells were captured using the lymphoid gate on FSC versus SSC. They were shown to be CD4$^+$ T cells

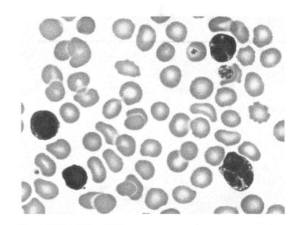

Figure 75.1 MGG, ×1000.

(CD4:CD8 ratio was 15:1) expressing CD2, CD3^{dim}, CD5 and CD25. CD7, CD26 and CD56 were not expressed. The findings are therefore indicative of a clonal CD4$^+$ proliferation showing loss of CD7 but gain of CD25. The loss of CD26 also indicates likely clonality.

Discussion

The presentation here is of a clonal mature CD4$^+$ T-cell disorder showing leukaemic and lymphomatous components. A number of mature CD4$^+$ T-cell disorders are known to involve skin and blood including T-prolymphocytic leukaemia (T-PLL), Sézary syndrome (SS), mycosis fungoides (MF) and HTLV-1-related adult T-cell leukaemia/lymphoma (ATLL). All of these entities can show cells with polylobated nuclei. These conditions can partly be distinguished by the pattern of skin involvement typically

Practical Flow Cytometry in Haematology: 100 Worked Examples, First Edition. Mike Leach, Mark Drummond, Allyson Doig, Pam McKay, Bob Jackson and Barbara J. Bain.
© 2015 John Wiley & Sons, Ltd. Published 2015 by John Wiley & Sons, Ltd.

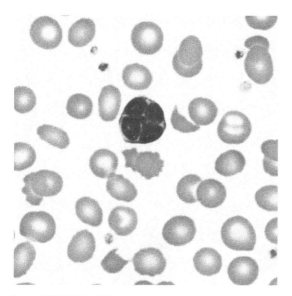

Figure 75.2 MGG, ×1000.

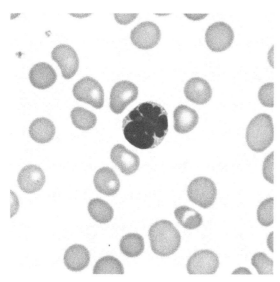

Figure 75.3 MGG, ×1000.

with diffuse erythroderma in SS, plaques and nodules in MF and a mixed pattern in T-PLL and ATLL. It should be noted that ATLL, as well as SS, can show epidermotropism.

These entities can often be separated by immunophenotyping studies in that T-PLL typically shows no antigen loss and expresses uniform CD26; SS and MF frequently show loss of CD7 and CD26 but absence of CD25; ATLL shows loss of CD7 and loss of CD26 but is consistently CD25+. The clinical presentation, morphology and immunophenotype in this case were strongly suggestive of a diagnosis of ATLL and human T-cell lymphotropic virus 1 (HTLV-1) serology proved positive. Another regular characteristic of this condition at presentation is the presence of hypercalcaemia.

Adult T-cell leukaemia/lymphoma is a rare T-cell lymphoproliferative disorder caused by HTLV-1 infection. This is a virus that can be acquired through exposure to blood, semen or breast milk but most cases are probably acquired vertically from the mother *in utero* or at birth. The majority of cases are seen in regions where the virus is endemic, and in individuals originating from these regions, notably the Caribbean basin, south-eastern United States, South America, parts of central Africa, Iran, central Asia and south-western Japan. Host susceptibility, or possibly random genetic events, are important in the pathogenesis of ATLL as only a proportion of those latently infected develop the neoplasm. The tumour possibly arises from CD4+ CD25+ FOXP3+ regulatory T cells that are normally important in controlling the tendency to autoimmunity. There is currently no effective therapy for this condition, although interferon plus zidovudine has some efficacy, and the outlook is poor in most cases. In addition to the effects of this disease, HTLV-1 infected patients are also at high risk of immunodeficiency-related opportunistic infections and HTLV-1-related myelopathy.

Final diagnosis

HTLV-1 associated adult T-cell leukaemia/lymphoma.

76

Case 76

A 61-year-old man, previously well, presented via his GP with a 4-week history of malaise, weight loss, fever and bone pain. An FBC was taken.

Laboratory data

FBC: Hb 127 g/L, WBC 4.5×10^9/L (neutrophils 2.2×10^9/L) and platelets 26×10^9/L

Coagulation screen: PT 12 s, APTT 25 s, fibrinogen 1.41 g/L and D-dimers 32,764 ng/ml.

U&Es, bone profile, LFTs normal except albumin 29 g/L. Serum LDH was 453 U/L.

Blood film

Initial blood film examination identified occasional blast cells (<10% of all cells); these showed prominent nucleoli, cytoplasmic granules and irregular nuclear margins (Figure 76.1). Auer rods were not seen. There were frequent nucleated red cells and myelocytes (not shown) comprising a leucoerythroblastic picture.

Bone marrow aspirate

This showed extensive marrow infiltration by large hypergranular blasts, including occasional bilobed and vacuolated forms (not shown).

Flow cytometry on blood and bone marrow aspirate

Flow cytometry on blood and bone marrow (not shown) identified a significant blast population with the follow-

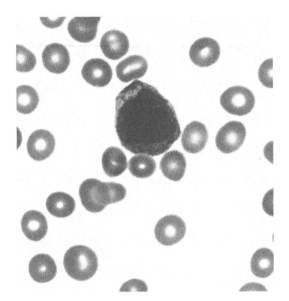

Figure 76.1 MGG, ×1000.

ing phenotype: CD34⁻, CD117⁻, HLA-DR^{dim}, CD13^{dim}, CD33⁺, MPO⁺, CD64⁺, CD56^{bright}.

Cytogenetic analysis

Chromosome analysis of cultured bone marrow cells revealed a complex abnormal karyotype with loss of Y and multiple structural abnormalities in 8 out of 10 cells examined.

45,X,-Y,inv(2)(p?13q?23),t(6;22)(p?12.2;p?11.2),del(11)(p?11.2p?13)del(13)(q?14q?21)[8]/46XY[2].

This complex karyotype gave no specific diagnostic information but t(15;17) was not detected by cytogenetic or FISH analyses and *PML-RARA* was absent by RT-PCR.

Practical Flow Cytometry in Haematology: 100 Worked Examples, First Edition. Mike Leach, Mark Drummond, Allyson Doig, Pam McKay, Bob Jackson and Barbara J. Bain.
© 2015 John Wiley & Sons, Ltd. Published 2015 by John Wiley & Sons, Ltd.

Immediate clinical course

The morphological review of blast morphology, plus evidence of DIC, prompted initial administration of ATRA. Cell markers were not typical of APL however (HLA-DR^{dim}, CD56^{bright}) and there was no evidence of a translocation involving chromosome 17 by FISH. Intensive AML-type induction chemotherapy was started and the patient underwent a total of 4 cycles in total, with CR after cycle 1. Severe systemic upset persisted through cycle 1, however, with severe hypoalbuminaemia, ascites, DIC and fever. Aggressive supportive care was required through initial chemotherapy.

Four months from completion of chemotherapy, having remained well and out of hospital, the patient re-presented with persistent headaches. CT and MRI imaging was normal (not shown). A lumbar puncture was performed.

CSF cytospin

The CSF leucocyte count was grossly elevated (0.81×10^9/L). The majority of cells present were hypergranular blasts, with morphology identical to that of the blast population at initial presentation (Figures 76.2–76.4).

Flow cytometry (CSF)

This demonstrated cells with an identical immunophenotype to that at diagnosis. The cells had blast morphology and

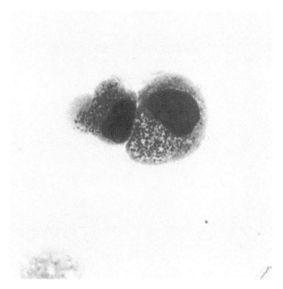

Figure 76.3 MGG, ×1000.

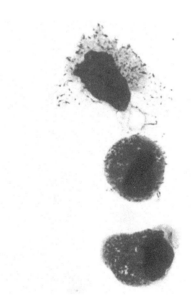

Figure 76.4 MGG, ×1000.

FSC/SSC characteristics (Figure 76.5). Heterogeneous CD13 and HLA-DR expression was again seen (Figure 76.6) and the cells were CD34$^-$ (histogram analysis shown, Figure 76.7). CD14 was negative but heterogeneous CD64 expression was noted (Figure 76.8). CD56 was strongly expressed (Figure 76.9).

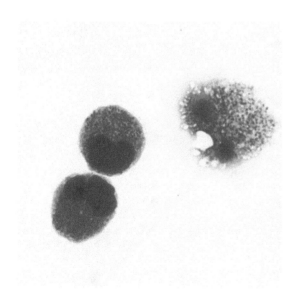

Figure 76.2 MGG, ×1000.

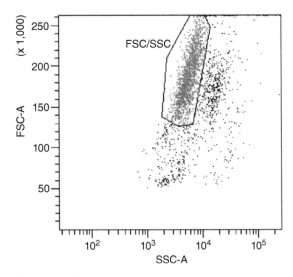

Figure 76.5 FSC/SSC.

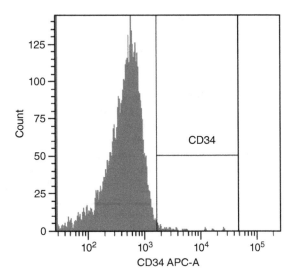

Figure 76.7 CD34 histogram.

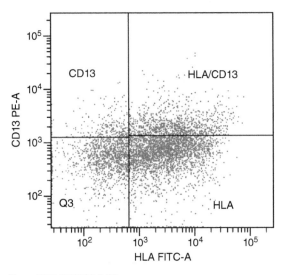

Figure 76.6 CD13/HLA-DR.

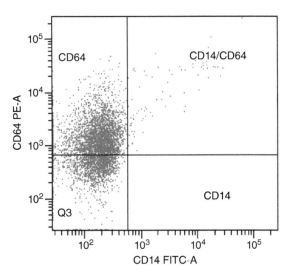

Figure 76.8 CD14/CD64.

Bone marrow aspirate (at CNS relapse)

Bone marrow examination confirmed florid disease relapse with a large population of hypergranular blast cells again being present (Figures 76.10 and 76.11).

Discussion

This case presented a number of diagnostic issues, not least the 'APL-like' morphology in conjunction with DIC, leading to early introduction of ATRA pending definitive investigation. Extensive genetic investigation excluded the presence of t(15;17) or alternative translocation involving *RARA*. The patient was extremely unwell initially, with a marked wasting illness and florid DIC. This is an unusual clinical scenario in AML, yet no infective cause was identified.

CD56 expression was unusually strong in this case, raising the possibility of an NK/myeloid phenotype acute leukaemia. This is a rare leukaemia thought to be derived from a common NK/myeloid precursor. The literature is confusing in that two different NK/myeloid entities have

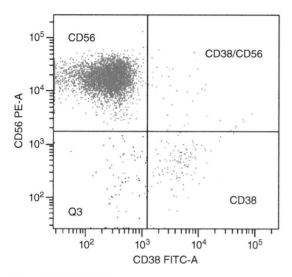

Figure 76.9 CD56/CD38.

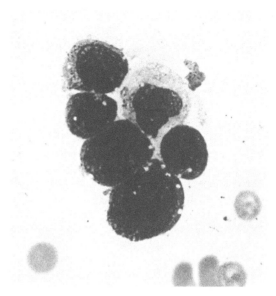

Figure 76.11 MGG, ×1000.

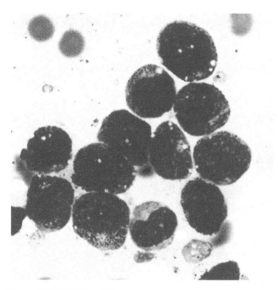

Figure 76.10 MGG, ×1000.

described here closely resembles the former type with 'APL-like' morphology, immunophenotype and associated DIC. Furthermore, this case showed CD64 positivity, another usual feature of APL. The authors have encountered a series of similar cases with this morphology and phenotype; in particular the universal CD34 negativity with heterogeneous expression of CD13 and HLA-DR together with expression of CD56, CD64, CD33 and MPO. In addition to the original description and our unpublished series this leukaemia has also been described by others (4, 5).

Meningeal relapse of acute leukaemia can only be reliably diagnosed by CSF examination using cytomorphology and flow cytometry. Note the insensitivity of MRI in picking up the CNS disease, which is well recognised (see case 47 for a more comprehensive discussion on this topic). The development of meningeal and bone marrow relapse just 4 months from the completion of chemotherapy presented serious challenges for subsequent management. The patient reported early symptomatic improvement from the first dose of intrathecal cytarabine but on day 2 developed a rapid decline in conscious level. CT imaging identified a massive intra-cerebral haemorrhage from which he could not be rescued.

It should be noted that, pending the results of definitive investigation, it is important that patients with APL-like AML receive treatment with ATRA in order that patients who do have APL are not left untreated. There is still a high early death rate in APL and pre-emptive treatment should therefore be given while awaiting results of specialised tests.

been described. This term was first used to describe an acute leukaemia resembling APL variant which had a CD34^{dim}, HLA-DR$^-$, CD56$^+$, CD33$^+$, CD13^{dim}, CD15$^+$, CD16$^-$, MPO$^+$ phenotype (1). The second was a 'M0' type acute leukaemia having a CD34$^+$, HLA-DR$^+$, CD56$^+$, CD7$^+$, CD33$^+$, CD16$^-$, MPO$^-$ phenotype (2, 3). Although neither entity has a recurring cytogenetic or molecular aberration these two leukaemias are clearly different; they are not currently recognised in the WHO classification. The case

Final diagnosis

Acute myeloid leukaemia with maturation (NK/myeloid type).

(See also Case 47 for discussion)

References

1 Scott, A.A., Head, D.R., Kopecky, K.J. *et al.* (1994) HLA-DR-, CD33+, CD56+, CD16- myeloid/natural killer cell acute leukemia: a previously unrecognized form of acute leukemia potentially misdiagnosed as French-American-British acute myeloid leukemia-M3. *Blood*, **84** (**1**), 244–255. PubMed PMID: 7517211.

2 Suzuki, R. & Nakamura, S. (1999) Malignancies of natural killer (NK) cell precursor: myeloid/NK cell precursor acute leukemia and blastic NK cell lymphoma/leukemia. *Leukemia Research*, **23** (7), 615–624. PubMed PMID: 10400182.

3 Inaba, T., Shimazaki, C., Sumikuma, T. *et al.* (2001) Clinico-pathological features of myeloid/natural killer (NK) cell precursor acute leukemia. *Leukemia Research*, **25** (2), 109–113. PubMed PMID: 11166825.

4 Chen, B., Xu, X., Ji, M. & Lin, G. (2009) Myeloid/NK cell acute leukemia. *International Journal of Hematology*, **89** (**3**), 365–367. PubMed PMID: 19326059.

5 Tang, G., Truong, F., Fadare, O., Woda, B. & Wang, S.A. (2008) Diagnostic challenges related to myeloid/natural killer cells, a variant of myeloblasts. *International Journal of Clinical and Experimental Pathology*, **1** (6), 544–549. PubMed PMID: 18787634.

77

Case 77

A 70-year-old man with a history of chronic lymphocytic leukaemia (CLL) treated with fludarabine and cyclophosphamide 4 years earlier, presented with a rapidly enlarging lymph node mass in the right supraclavicular fossa and the recent onset of night sweats.

Laboratory results

FBC: Hb 109 g/L, WBC 4.5 × 10^9/L (lymphocytes 0.9 × 10^9/L) and platelets 220 × 10^9/L.

U&Es and bone profile: normal. Liver function mildly deranged (AST 77 U/L). LDH was raised at 656 U/L.

Imaging

CT scan showed widespread lymphadenopathy throughout the neck, thorax, abdomen and pelvis with the largest (symptomatic) nodal mass in the right supraclavicular fossa. In addition there was collapse of the lower lobe of the right lung associated with a moderately large pleural effusion.

Pleural fluid aspirate

The fluid was straw coloured. Total protein content was 48 g/L with albumin 22 g/L (serum albumin 28). Glucose was 1.3 mmol/L and LDH 1838 U/L. Microscopy showed pleomorphic medium to large vacuolated lymphoid cells with occasional macrophages and neutrophils. A low glucose level and high LDH are in keeping with malignant effusions but these parameters are not entirely specific. The morphological appearances, however, were suggestive of a malignant lymphoid effusion (Figures 77.1–77.3).

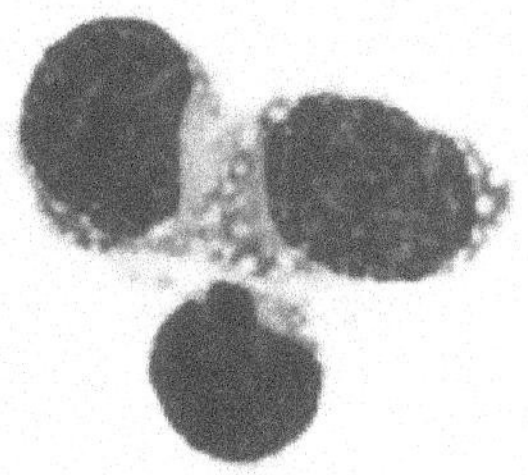

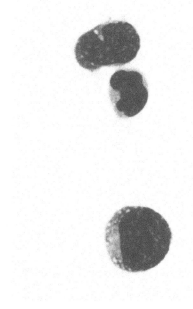

Figure 77.1 MGG, ×1000.

Figure 77.2 MGG, ×1000.

Practical Flow Cytometry in Haematology: 100 Worked Examples, First Edition. Mike Leach, Mark Drummond, Allyson Doig, Pam McKay, Bob Jackson and Barbara J. Bain.
© 2015 John Wiley & Sons, Ltd. Published 2015 by John Wiley & Sons, Ltd.

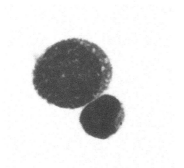

Figure 77.3 MGG, ×1000.

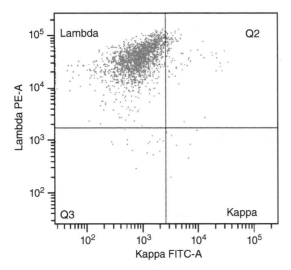

Figure 77.4 Kappa/lambda.

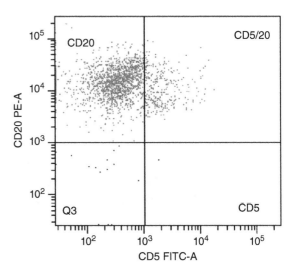

Figure 77.5 CD20/CD5.

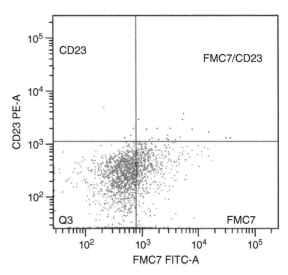

Figure 77.6 CD23/FMC7.

Flow cytometry (pleural fluid)

The pleural fluid leucocyte count was 13.9×10^9/L. There was an equal mix of T cells and B cells, indicating a significant B-cell excess. Gating on the B cells demonstrated a lambda^{bright}, CD20$^+$, CD10$^+$, partial FMC7^{dim}, CD38$^+$, partial CD5^{dim}, CD23$^-$ B-cell disorder (Figures 77.4–77.6). The accompanying T cells were reactive in nature.

Histopathology

Core biopsy from the right supraclavicular fossa lymph node mass showed a diffuse infiltrate of medium sized lymphoid cells with numerous apoptoses. Immunohistologically, these cells were positive for CD20, BCL2, BCL6, CD10 and MUM1 and negative for CD5, CD23, cyclin D1, TdT and EBV LMP. The proliferation index was high at 95%.

The morphology and immunophenotyping were in keeping with diffuse large B-cell lymphoma (DLBCL), germinal centre subtype.

Discussion

The flow cytometry and core biopsy findings identified a high-grade mature B-cell neoplasm with a germinal centre phenotype. It is important to consider a diagnosis of DLBCL in any CLL patient who shows a rapid onset of a localised lymphoid or extranodal mass, B symptoms or rapid clinical decline. The site of transformation is obvious in some but PET/CT imaging is useful in showing the differing intensity of isotopic uptake of transformed disease compared to native CLL. Such imaging can help direct biopsies (1).

There are three main types of DLBCL seen in CLL. The first is a direct transformation of the CLL clone (Richter transformation) and shows aggressive behaviour with rapid clinical decline, very high serum LDH and refractoriness to therapy. Some cases have a phenotype that relates to the CLL cell of origin and the transformation may relate to secondary acquired *CDKN2A* loss, *TP53* disruption, *MYC* activation or *NOTCH1* mutations (2). The second is an immunosuppression-related DLBCL which may be EBV driven and can follow previous therapy with T-cell depleting agents such as fludarabine and alemtuzumab. The third is a *de novo* DLBCL, which may show a germinal centre phenotype (GCB), as in this case, rather than the activated B-cell phenotype (ABC) commonly seen in the first two situations. This third group may be unrelated to the CLL. This subgroup tends to show a better response to therapy so determining the possible origin of the tumour may help decide on the intensity and intent of treatment in any given case (3).

Final diagnosis

Diffuse large B-cell lymphoma occurring in a patient with a history of treated chronic lymphocytic leukaemia. The two diseases were probably unrelated.

References

1 Papajik, T., Myslivecek, M., Urbanova, R. *et al.* (2014) 2-[18F]fluoro-2-deoxy-D-glucose positron emission tomography/computed tomography examination in patients with chronic lymphocytic leukemia may reveal Richter transformation. *Leukemia & Lymphoma*, **55** (**2**), 314–319. PubMed PMID: 23656196.

2 Chigrinova, E., Rinaldi, A., Kwee, I. *et al.* (2013) Two main genetic pathways lead to the transformation of chronic lymphocytic leukemia to Richter syndrome. *Blood*, **122** (**15**), 2673–2682. PubMed PMID: 24004666.

3 Parikh, S.A., Kay, N.E. & Shanafelt, T.D. (2014) How we treat Richter syndrome. *Blood*, **123** (**11**), 1647–1657. PubMed PMID: 24421328.

78

Case 78

A 74-year-old man of Chinese origin was admitted to hospital with a short history of dizziness and fatigue. No organomegaly was present on examination. His past medical history included hypertension, diabetes mellitus, chronic renal impairment and alpha thalassaemia trait.

Laboratory data

FBC: Hb 79 g/L (MCV 78 fl, MCH 24.7 pg), WBC 14.1 × 10^9/L (neutrophils 7.2 × 10^9/L) and platelets 267 × 10^9/L

U&Es: Na 135 mmol/L, K 4.3 mmol/L, urea 13.1 mmol/L and creatinine 181 mmol/L. Bone profile: normal. LFTs: normal except albumin 29 g/L.

Blood film

The film demonstrated marked dysplastic changes in the neutrophil series, with abnormal nuclear segmentation, hypogranularity and pseudo-Pelger forms easily seen together with a small population of blast cells (11% of all cells) (Figures 78.1–78.5). There were occasional macropolycytes, that shown in Figure 78.6 being binucleated. Red cells were microcytic and occasionally hypochromic, in keeping with known alpha thalassaemia trait. There were no tear drop forms present and the frequent echinocytes were thought to reflect underlying the renal dysfunction.

Bone marrow aspirate

This was essentially a dry tap with few cells available for comment. Blasts were 21% of cells present and dysplastic changes in the myeloid and erythroid lineages were notable.

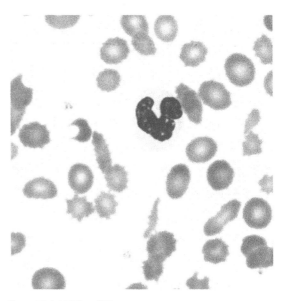

Figure 78.1 MGG, ×1000.

Flow cytometry (bone marrow)

Flow studies highlighted a population of CD34+ cells comprising 18% of all events; these were co-expressing HLA-DR, CD13, CD56 and CD7.

Histopathology

The trephine biopsy sections showed cellularity to be grossly increased at 99% (Figures 78.7 and 78.8). The most striking abnormality was a marked increase in megakaryocytes displaying clustering (Figures 78.8 and 78.9) and abnormal

---

Practical Flow Cytometry in Haematology: 100 Worked Examples, First Edition. Mike Leach, Mark Drummond, Allyson Doig, Pam McKay, Bob Jackson and Barbara J. Bain.
© 2015 John Wiley & Sons, Ltd. Published 2015 by John Wiley & Sons, Ltd.

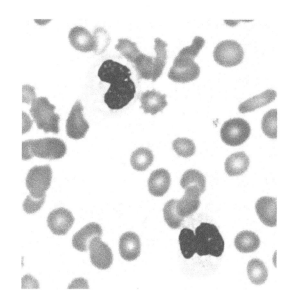

Figure 78.2 MGG, ×1000.

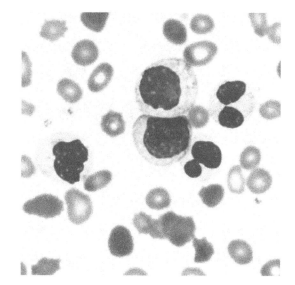

Figure 78.4 MGG, ×1000.

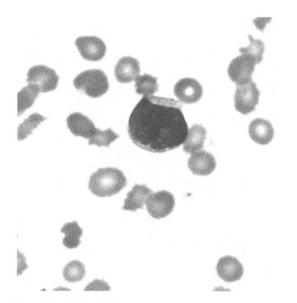

Figure 78.3 MGG, ×1000.

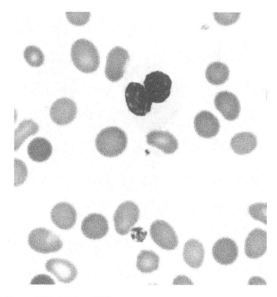

Figure 78.5 MGG, ×1000.

localisation. A patchy increase in myeloid precursors was evident (Figure 78.10), with greatly thickened paratrabecular myeloid seams (Figure 78.7). Reticulin was increased at grade 2, with focal areas of grade 3 (Figure 78.11). CD34 IHC highlighted areas of focal blast clustering (20 to 30% of cells, Figure 78.12) and marked increase in vascularity (endothelial staining, Figure 78.13). Numerous atypical megakaryocytes (including micromegakaryocytes) were highlighted by CD42b (Figure 78.14, note staining of small mononuclear cells and individual platelets also). Glycophorin IHC (not shown) highlighted clusters of erythroid precursors including larger less mature forms.

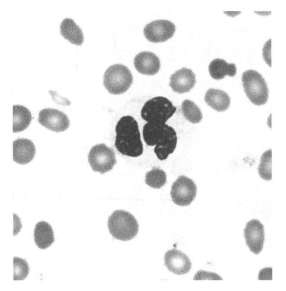

Figure 78.6 MGG, ×1000.

Figure 78.8 H&E, ×200.

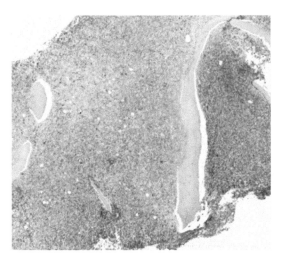

Figure 78.7 H&E, ×100.

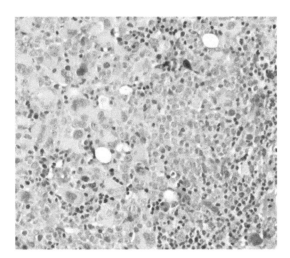

Figure 78.9 H&E, ×300.

Cytogenetic analysis

Metaphase cytogenetics revealed a complex karyotype in 10/10 cells examined: 45,XY,del(2)(q32q33),del(3)(q21q26), del(5)(q23q31),-7,-12,-20,-22,+mar1,+mar2,+mar3.

Discussion

This case presents a complex pathological and cytogenetic picture. The differential diagnosis includes a transforming myelofibrosis or MDS/MPN, acute panmyelosis with myelofibrosis (a sub-type of AML), high grade MDS or AML with MDS-related changes. A transforming myelofibrosis may be discounted given the lack of splenomegaly, teardrop forms and leucoerythroblastosis and a recent unremarkable pre-morbid FBC. The latter also goes against a pre-existing MDS/MPN. Morphology alone might favour acute panmyelosis, which is characterised by an increase in all marrow myeloid cells including erythroid, granulocyte and megakaryocytic elements, dysplastic myeloid series, 20–25% myeloblasts and reticulin fibrosis. It is however the

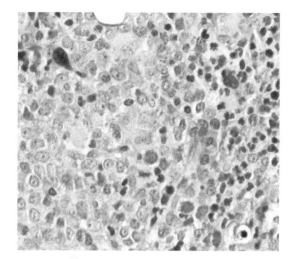

Figure 78.10 H&E, ×400.

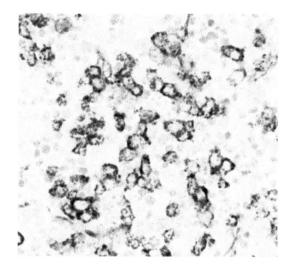

Figure 78.12 CD34, ×400.

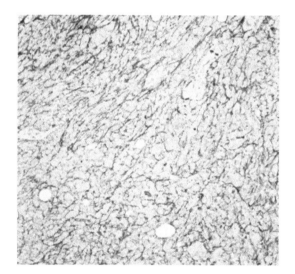

Figure 78.11 reticulin, ×100.

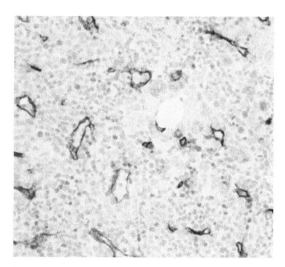

Figure 78.13 CD34, ×100.

complex MDS-related cytogenetic picture in this case that must be considered in determining classification, together with the marrow blast percentage: the case is best classified as AML with MDS-related changes. Note the monosomy 7 and del(5q) abnormalities, which are the most common abnormalities defined in MDS. Within the cytogenetic profile the prefix 'mar' refers to marker chromosome, indicating the presence of a structurally abnormal chromosome in which no part can be identified. It should be noted that it is the morphological blast count (in this patient 21% in the bone marrow) that must be considered in judging

if the criteria for AML, rather than high grade MDS, are met, not the percentage of CD34-positive cells (in this patient's bone marrow 18%). In addition, comparison with the trephine biopsy sections suggests that the reticulin fibrosis may have led to blast cells being under-represented in the aspirate. It is also of interest that CD13 was the only myeloid marker detected on flow cytometry and yet the severe granulocytic dysplasia, the dysplastic megakaryocytes on trephine biopsy and the specific cytogenetic abnormalities demonstrated leave no doubt that the blast cells were myeloid.

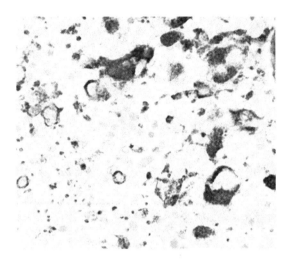

Figure 78.14 CD42b, ×400.

There are a number of ways to 'arrive' at the definition of AML with MDS-related changes: prior MDS, morphological features of MDS or MDS-related cytogenetic abnormalities (any or all of these features). Given this, the WHO recommend that it be indicated under what criteria the diagnosis is reached (1). Unsurprisingly, CR rates are low and outcomes poor.

The reticulin fibrosis in this case was striking. Not infrequently this leads the inexperienced to make a hasty diagnosis of primary myelofibrosis, however the differential diagnosis remains wide (including MPNs, MDS/MPN, acute panmyelosis, MDS with secondary fibrosis, acute megakaryoblastic leukaemia, systemic mastocytosis, hairy cell leukaemia and Hodgkin lymphoma). Marrow spread of non-haemic tumours, HIV infection and autoimmune disorders (e.g. SLE) may also be associated with fibrotic changes. It is therefore of great importance to consider all of these potential causes in the diagnostic work up.

After being counselled with regards the extremely poor prognosis associated with this cytogenetic profile, the patient elected to receive no active therapy and succumbed to his disease only 6 weeks later.

Final diagnosis

AML with MDS-related changes (MDS-associated cytogenetic abnormalities and multilineage dysplasia).

Reference

1 Arber, D.A., Brunning, R.D., Orazi, A. *et al.* (2008) Acute myeloid leukaemia with myelodysplasia-related changes. In: Swerdlow, S.H., Campo, E., Harris, N.L., Jaffe, E.S., Pileri, S.A., Stein, H., Thiele, J. & Vardiman, J.W. (eds), *World Health Organization Classification of Tumours of Haematopoietic and Lymphoid Tissues*. IARC Press, Lyon, pp. 124–126.

Case 79

A 70-year-old man presented with visual difficulty and diplopia. On examination he had bilateral partial palsies of the sixth cranial nerve.

He had initially presented 9 months earlier with pancytopenia, small volume lymphadenopathy and extensive bone marrow infiltration by mantle cell lymphoma (MCL). The immunohistochemistry at that time had been typical of MCL (CD20+, CD79a+, BCL2+, CD5+ and cyclin D1+). In addition the tumour expressed CD10 and had pleomorphic morphology with a high proliferating fraction (60%) in keeping with the blastoid variant. He achieved complete remission following 4 cycles of rituximab with high dose cytarabine.

Laboratory results

FBC normal.

U&Es, LFTs, bone profile and LDH were all normal.

Imaging

MRI scan of brain showed multiple non specific white matter changes of uncertain significance. There was no space-occupying lesion and the meninges appeared normal.

CSF analysis

CSF protein was raised at 1.6 g/L and glucose reduced at 1.2 mmol/L. The cell count was 0.046×10^9/L. Morphological assessment of a cytospin preparation revealed two populations of lymphoid cells. The first were small with little cytoplasm and were in keeping with reactive T cells whilst the second were much larger with moderate amounts of cytoplasm, nuclear clefts and lobes and prominent nucleoli (Figures 79.1 and 79.2).

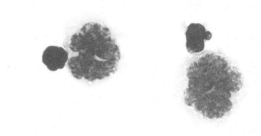

Figure 79.1 MGG, ×1000.

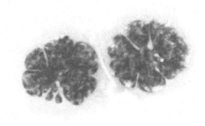

Figure 79.2 MGG, ×1000.

Practical Flow Cytometry in Haematology: 100 Worked Examples, First Edition. Mike Leach,
Mark Drummond, Allyson Doig, Pam McKay, Bob Jackson and Barbara J. Bain.
© 2015 John Wiley & Sons, Ltd. Published 2015 by John Wiley & Sons, Ltd.

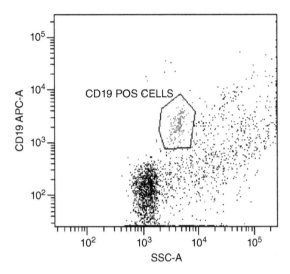

Figure 79.3 CD19/SSC.

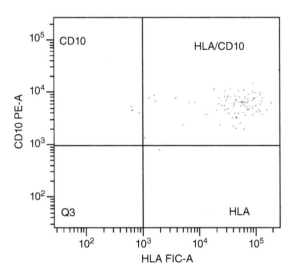

Figure 79.5 CD10/HLA-DR.

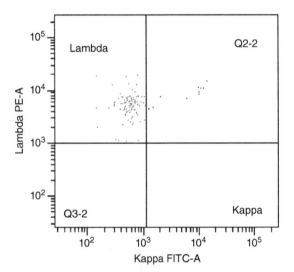

Figure 79.4 kappa/lambda.

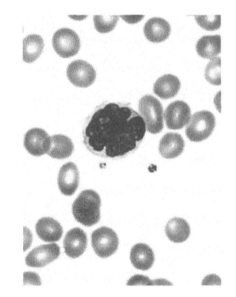

Figure 79.6 MGG, ×1000.

Flow cytometry (cerebrospinal fluid)

A CD19⁺ population was identified accounting for just 5% of all leucocytes, the remainder being reactive T lymphocytes (Figure 79.3) and cell debris. These cells were lambda light chain-restricted (Figure 79.4) and co-expressed CD5, CD20, HLA-DR, CD10 (Figure 79.5), CD79b and CD22.

His presentation blood film from 9 months earlier, taken at the time of initial immunophenotyping, was reviewed. This showed large pleomorphic mantle cells identical to those now present in CSF (Figures 79.6 and 79.7).

Discussion

Blastoid variant mantle cell lymphoma is an aggressive clinical entity associated with advanced stage disease, extranodal

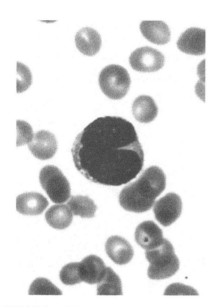

Figure 79.7 MGG, ×1000.

involvement and B symptoms. In the laboratory it carries all the typical hallmarks of MCL with a pan-B phenotype with aberrant cyclin D1 expression due to t(11;14)(q32;q11). In addition, CD5 is expressed, the proliferation fraction is often high, CD10 may be expressed and additional cytogenetic abnormalities, sometimes complex and involving *MYC* at 8q24, are seen.

Central nervous system involvement by blastoid MCL is rare but well documented and carries a poor prognosis. Flow cytometry on CSF was able to characterise the disease cells in this case when MRI imaging was inconclusive. Always consider CSF analysis by flow cytometry in any patient presenting with cranial nerve palsies where a lymphomatous meningitis is a possibility. Do not discount this diagnosis because of a normal brain MRI.

Final diagnosis

Meningeal relapse of blastoid mantle cell lymphoma.

A 55-year-old man, previously well, attended his GP with a 3-month history of fatigue and malaise. In addition, over the previous 4 weeks, there had been a history of significant night sweats and weight loss (5 kg). On clinical examination the spleen was palpated 3 cm below the left costal margin. An FBC was taken.

Laboratory data

FBC: Hb 54 g/L, WBC 18.3×10^9/L (neutrophils 13.5×10^9/L, basophils 0.4×10^9/L) and platelets 245×10^9/L.

U&Es, LFTs, bone profile: normal. Serum LDH was 350 U/L.

Blood film

The blood film showed a left shifted myeloid series, neutrophilia (Figure 80.1) and the presence of occasional agranular medium sized blast cells (Figures 80.2 and 80.3). The basophilia was confirmed. Platelet numbers were preserved and occasional large forms were noted (Figure 80.4).

Bone marrow aspirate

This was difficult to acquire but a small aparticulate sample was available for flow analysis. A trephine biopsy roll showed the presence of medium sized to large agranular blast cells (not shown).

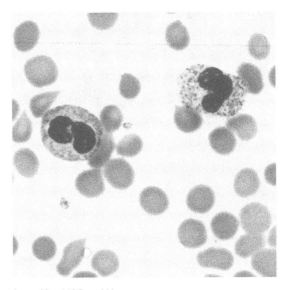

Figure 80.1 MGG, ×1000.

Flow cytometry (marrow aspirate)

Using CD34$^+$ gating (Figure 80.5), a lymphoblast population comprising 35% of all events was easily identified with the immunophenotype being CD34$^+$, CD79a$^+$, CD20$^+$ (heterogeneous), CD10$^+$ and TdT$^+$ (Figures 80.6 and 80.7).

Bone marrow trephine biopsy

A good quality 1.5 cm core demonstrated >90% cellularity (Figures 80.8 and 80.9), with a monotonous infiltrate

Practical Flow Cytometry in Haematology: 100 Worked Examples, First Edition. Mike Leach, Mark Drummond, Allyson Doig, Pam McKay, Bob Jackson and Barbara J. Bain.
© 2015 John Wiley & Sons, Ltd. Published 2015 by John Wiley & Sons, Ltd.

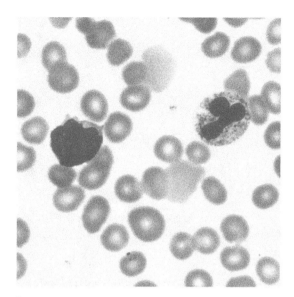

Figure 80.2 MGG, ×1000.

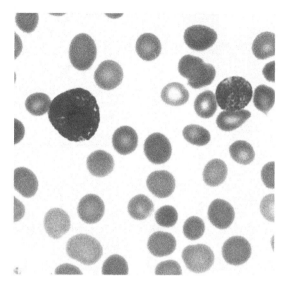

Figure 80.4 MGG, ×1000.

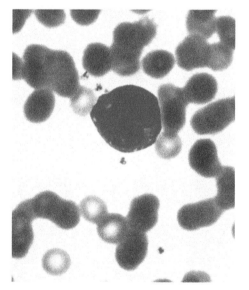

Figure 80.3 MGG, ×1000.

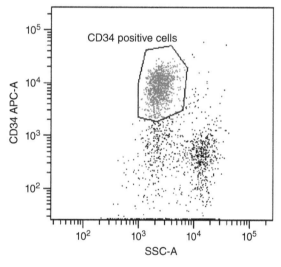

Figure 80.5 CD34/SSC.

of small lymphoblasts noted. All other lineages were present and myeloid maturation to neutrophils was readily seen. Reticulin was increased to grade 2 (Figure 80.10). The immunophenotype of the blast cells was shown by IHC to be identical to that obtained by flow cytometry (Figures 80.11–80.14).

Cytogenetic analysis

46,XY,inv(3)(p?24q?23), t(9;22)(q34;q11)[7]/45,idem,dic(7;9)(p11–13;p11), del(11)(q23)[2]/46,XY[1].

These findings indicated a male karyotype with the presence of two related abnormal cell lines. The presence

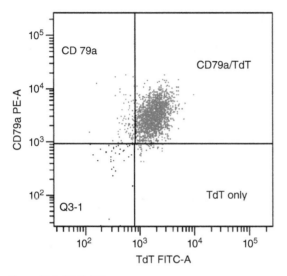

Figure 80.6 CD79a/TdT.

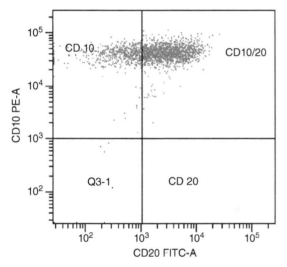

Figure 80.7 CD10/CD20.

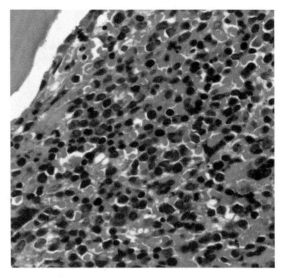

Figure 80.8 H&E, ×400.

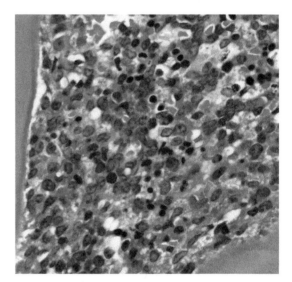

Figure 80.9 H&E, ×400.

of t(9;22) together with inv(3), a recognised abnormality associated with transformation of chronic myeloid leukaemia (CML) was in keeping with clonal evolution of CML; there was an additional more minor clone showing further cytogenetic evolution. FISH analysis confirmed loss of 11q including the *MLL* gene at 11q23.3 (4/7 metaphases) and a *BCR-ABL1* rearrangement involved the M-BCR (major breakpoint cluster region) which is more commonly seen in chronic myeloid leukaemia. It is of interest that although inv(3) is associated with myeloid leukaemias, dic(7;9)(p11-13;p11) is associated with acute lymphoblastic leukaemia and has been recognised in association with t(9;22) (with p190 *BCR-ABL1* transcripts) in four previous patients (1).

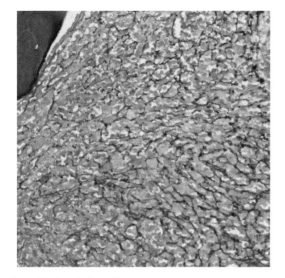

Figure 80.10 Reticulin, ×200.

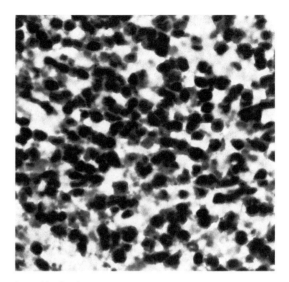

Figure 80.12 TdT, ×400.

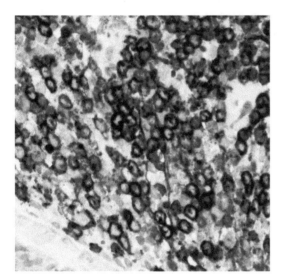

Figure 80.11 CD34, ×400.

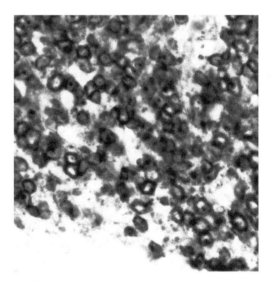

Figure 80.13 CD10, ×400.

Molecular studies

RT-PCR demonstrated *BCR-ABL1*, p210 type.

Additional investigations

CT neck/chest/abdomen/thorax showed splenomegaly (16 cm in long axis) but no other significant abnormality and in particular no lymphadenopathy.

Discussion

This case illustrates a well recognised diagnostic dilemma in haematological malignancy, namely how to differentiate at first presentation between *de novo* Philadelphia⁺ (Ph⁺) ALL and lymphoid blast phase (BP) of undiagnosed CML. Although ultimately management strategies converge (optimally allogeneic transplant for suitable candidates) initial management with chemotherapy may differ, as may

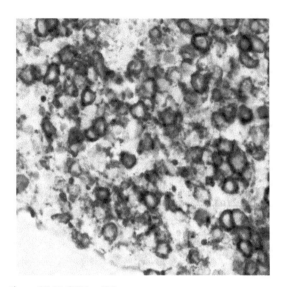

Figure 80.14 CD20, ×400.

eligibility for particular clinical trials. A number of features supported this case being classified as likely BP-CML, namely:

1. A clinical history of symptoms measured in months rather than weeks, in keeping with symptoms of a chronic rather than acute process.
2. Presence of significant splenomegaly at diagnosis.
3. Left shifted myeloid blood film with neutrophilia and preserved platelet count.
4. Peripheral blood basophilia.
5. A background of myeloid proliferation in the marrow, in addition to large numbers of lymphoblasts.

6. Evidence of cytogenetic clonal evolution with two related abnormal cell lines.
7. The presence of p210 *BCR-ABL1* transcripts rather than p190 (the latter more typically associated with Ph[+] ALL).

Note that none of these features is definitive for BP-CML. The cytogenetic abnormalities are suggestive of secondary progression of a pre-existent chronic phase CML, with additional abnormalities becoming apparent in the context of lymphoblastic progression.

The patient was commenced on dasatinib 140 mg daily, along with pulsed vincristine and prednisone. Prior to allogeneic SCT, the response was consolidated with a single course of FLAG chemotherapy. A reduced intensity sibling allograft was performed, and 8 months later the patient was well and in complete molecular remission (RQ-PCR for *BCR-ABL1* in marrow).

Final diagnosis

Lymphoid blast phase as presentation of chronic myeloid leukaemia.

Reference

1 Pan, J., Xue, Y., Wu, Y., Wang, Y. & Shen, J. (2006) Dicentric (7;9)(p11;p11) is a rare but recurrent abnormality in acute lymphoblastic leukemia: a study of 7 cases. *Cancer Genetics and Cytogenetics*, **169**, 159–163.

Case 81

A 55-year-old man with a history of recently treated stage IVB diffuse large B-cell lymphoma presented some 8 months after completion of R-CHOP chemotherapy. His initial presentation had included bone marrow involvement and extranodal disease, both known risk factors for CNS relapse. The best approach to prevention of CNS relapse of occult CNS disease at presentation remains a topic of intense debate. His new complaint was of progressive weakness in his lower limbs with difficulty walking. There was no significant bladder or bowel disturbance.

On examination he appeared well and was without palpable lymphadenopathy or organomegaly. The most notable feature was of a lower limb paresis and sensory disturbance without a clear sensory level. His leg muscle groups were wasted and lower limb power was impaired. As he had been treated with vinca alkaloid therapy he was generally hyporeflexic rendering this modality of assessment less reliable. He reported no significant lower limb pain.

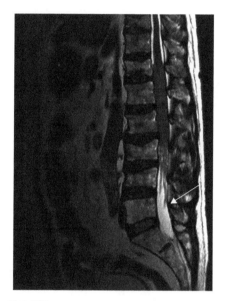

Figure 81.1 MRI.

Laboratory investigations

The FBC and blood film were unremarkable.

U&Es, LFTs, bone profile, LDH and CRP were all normal.

A bone marrow aspirate (being a site of disease at presentation) showed no abnormal lymphoid population, or other significant abnormality.

Imaging

Lower spinal cord pathology was suspected. MRI imaging showed a lesion affecting the lower cord and conus medullaris

(arrow, Figure 81.1); this would explain the clinical presentation, although the sparing of bladder and bowel function was somewhat unusual. CT imaging of the chest, abdomen and pelvis showed no significant abnormality. PET/CT imaging highlighted an area of increased isotope uptake in the terminal spinal cord correlating with the abnormal area seen using MRI (arrow, Figure 81.2). No other areas of abnormal uptake were evident.

Flow cytometry

In view of the localised area of possible disease relapse and after considering the implications of neurological

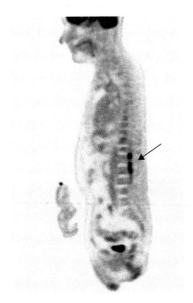

Figure 81.2 PET/CT.

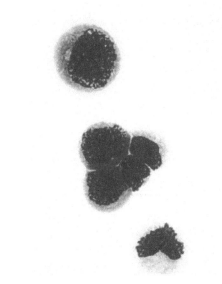

Figure 81.4 MGG, ×1000.

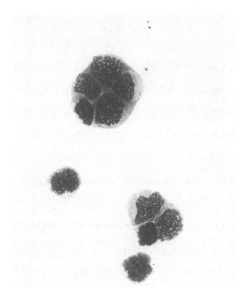

Figure 81.3 MGG, ×1000.

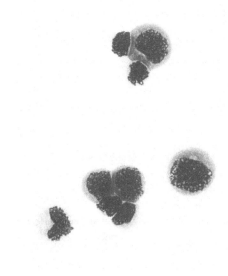

Figure 81.5 MGG, ×1000.

decompensation we proceeded to a radiologically guided L5 approach lumbar puncture to acquire a CSF specimen. No other tissue was available for a definitive diagnosis. A cytospin preparation showed a population of pleomorphic large cells with a minor reactive lymphocytic response. Flow analysis using a CD2/CD19 gated approach, focussing on the large cells, identified a significant excess of B cells. The total cell count was 0.16×10^9/L.

The B-cell population was abnormal, showing kappa surface light chain restriction; the phenotype was mature with expression of CD19, CD20, FMC7, CD22 and CD79b. The cell morphology was in keeping with a lymphomatous population (Figures 81.3–81.6).

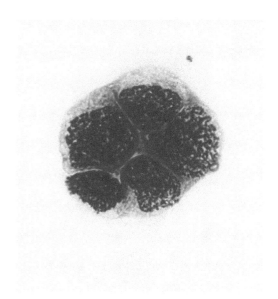

Figure 81.6 MGG, ×1000.

Discussion

This case illustrates the rare and unfortunate CNS relapse of diffuse large B-cell lymphoma. The case is even more unusual in that relapse occurred within the terminal part of the spinal cord. Despite the highly unusual features, a relapse was suspected in view of the prior history, the new neurological presentation and the findings on imaging. Morphological and flow cytometry analysis of CSF allowed a definitive confirmation which informed the subsequent treatment plan.

Final diagnosis

Isolated lower spinal cord and intraconal CNS relapse of diffuse large B-cell lymphoma.

82

Case 82

A 50-year-old female presented with a 6-week history of unexplained fever, night sweats and low back pain. Discrete renal infiltrates were noted on CT, but a renal biopsy was unsuccessful. There was a longstanding past medical history of mild psoriatic arthritis. Worsening pancytopenia prompted blood film and marrow examination.

Laboratory data

FBC: Hb 106 g/L, WBC 3.5×10^9/L and platelets 72×10^9/L.

U&Es, LFTs and bone profile were normal with a serum LDH of 2050 U/L.

Blood film

Blood film examination revealed 20% blast cells and granular myeloid precursors (Figures 82.1–82.3). The blasts were small to medium sized and lacked granules. They had a very high nuclear-cytoplasmic ratio and frequent irregular nuclear margins. A left shifted myeloid series was obvious (Figure 82.2), with nucleated red cells (not shown).

Bone marrow aspirate

The marrow aspirate was dry.

Flow cytometry (peripheral blood)

Blast gating was performed on CD45 dim/negative cells (Figure 82.4). These were CD19$^+$, CD10$^+$, CD79a$^+$, TdT$^+$

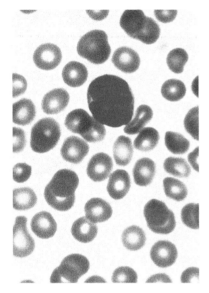

Figure 82.1 MGG, ×1000.

and partially MPO$^+$ (Figures 82.5–82.8). CD34 and cCD3 (Figure 82.8) were negative, with there being weak partial positivity for CD20 (Figure 82.6).

Trephine biopsy

H&E staining of trephine biopsy sections demonstrated extensive marrow necrosis (Figures 82.9) with occasional clusters of lymphoid cells, some of which were degenerate (Figure 82.10), in an amorphous pink background. Small 'islands' of viable cells were present, comprised of a diffuse infiltrate of blast cells with pleomorphic nuclei and small nucleoli but without cytoplasmic differentiation

Practical Flow Cytometry in Haematology: 100 Worked Examples, First Edition. Mike Leach, Mark Drummond, Allyson Doig, Pam McKay, Bob Jackson and Barbara J. Bain.

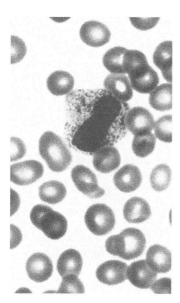

Figure 82.2 MGG, ×1000.

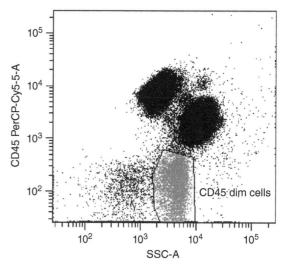

Figure 82.4 CD45/SSC.

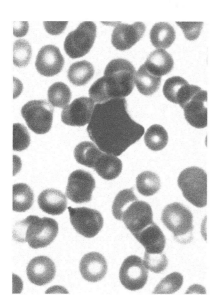

Figure 82.3 MGG, ×1000.

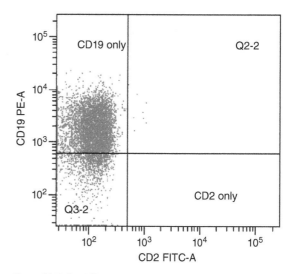

Figure 82.5 CD19/CD2.

blast cells (Figure 82.18). Note how this pattern of staining contrasts with the strong and homogeneous nuclear staining exhibited by TdT (Figure 82.17).

Cytogenetic analysis

Analysis of 200 nuclei following hybridisation of the cultured bone marrow sample with probes specific for *BCR-ABL1*, *MLL* and *ETV6-RUNX1* showed normal signal patterns. Loss

(Figures 82.11 and 82.12). Little remaining normal haemopoietic tissue was seen. Patchy osteosclerosis was noted throughout the sample.

Immunocytochemistry showed the infiltrating cells to be positive for CD79a, PAX5, CD10, CD20, TdT and MPO (Figures 82.13–82.18). With regards to the latter, granular cytoplasmic staining was noted in approximately 50% of

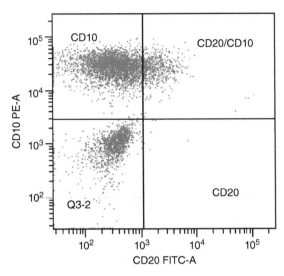

Figure 82.6 CD20/CD10.

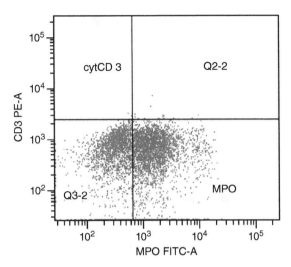

Figure 82.8 cCD3/MPO.

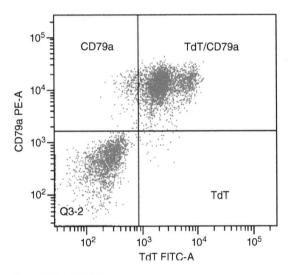

Figure 82.7 TdT/CD79a.

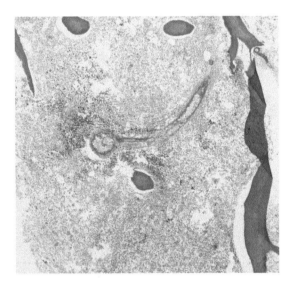

Figure 82.9 H&E necrosis, ×40.

of one copy of *ABL1*, however, was detected in 65% of cells indicating either loss of one copy of chromosome 9 or deletion of the long arm of chromosome 9 involving *ABL1* at 9q34. Unfortunately, a full metaphase chromosome analysis failed so the exact mechanism for this signal loss was not elucidated.

Discussion

This case proved a diagnostic dilemma at presentation, with no circulating blast cells in the early stages and initial

suspicion of a disseminated solid tumour or high-grade lymphoma. The worsening pancytopenia however indicated progressive marrow pathology. Bone pain in adult acute leukaemia is most frequently seen in ALL in the authors' experience and can often be severe enough to necessitate opiate analgesia. A dry tap is not infrequent as in this case, often necessitating diagnosis by trephine biopsy. If there are no circulating blast cells this can present a challenge to cytogenetic and molecular analyses; the authors' practice is to submit a separate trephine biopsy specimen in cell culture

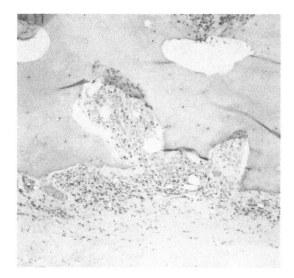

Figure 82.10 H&E degenerate cells, ×400.

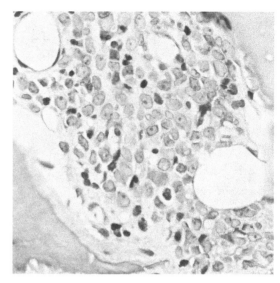

Figure 82.12 H&E viable, ×400.

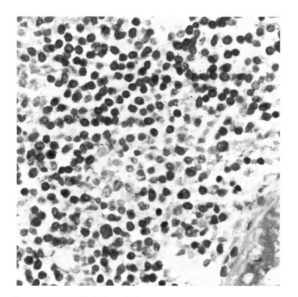

Figure 82.11 H&E viable, ×100.

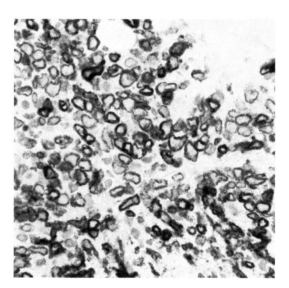

Figure 82.13 CD79a, ×400.

medium from which metaphase preparations and nucleic acid extraction are usually successful (1).

Bone marrow necrosis is a rare finding, being best described in sickle cell disease and primary or metastatic marrow malignancies. The mechanism is unknown but it seems likely that rapid bone marrow replacement by highly proliferative tumours lead to distortion and occlusion of normal marrow vessels and sinusoids. Necrosis is best appreciated on trephine biopsy sections (sometimes being

mistaken for artefact or the effects of trauma) and it may significantly hamper diagnosis if few viable cells are present. In acute leukaemia it is more common in lymphoid lineage leukaemias than in myeloid (2), and is often accompanied by fever, bone pain, a leucoerythroblastic film and failure to acquire a bone marrow aspirate, as in this case.

Co-expression of lymphoid- and myeloid-associated antigens is frequent in acute leukaemia and care should be taken that an incorrect lineage is not assigned to the

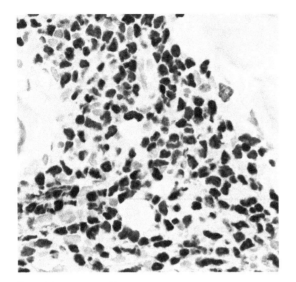

Figure 82.14 PAX5, ×400.

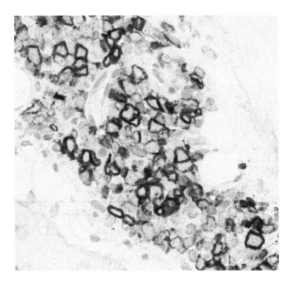

Figure 82.16 CD20, ×400.

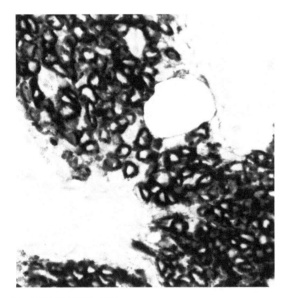

Figure 82.15 CD10, ×400.

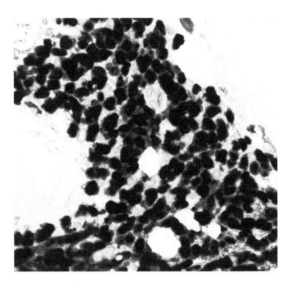

Figure 82.17 TdT, ×400.

blast population (with potentially serious treatment-related consequences). These patterns are well described (for example aberrant expression of CD13, CD33 or CD15 in B ALL or aberrant expression of CD7 or CD19 in AML) and should not lead to confusion. However the expression of the myeloid-specific antigen MPO alongside strongly expressed pan-B cell markers (in particular cCD79a and CD19, but in addition in this case PAX5 expression detected

by immunohistochemistry) indicates a mixed phenotype acute leukaemia, termed B/myeloid acute leukaemia as per WHO criteria. Both flow cytometry and IHC in this case showed the MPO expression. When WHO criteria are strictly applied these leukaemias are relatively rare, which has hampered their accurate characterisation and the development of specific treatment approaches. They are associated with marked cytogenetic and molecular diversity and generally have a poor outcome. It is particularly important to exclude *BCR-ABL1* or *MLL* translocations, which occur

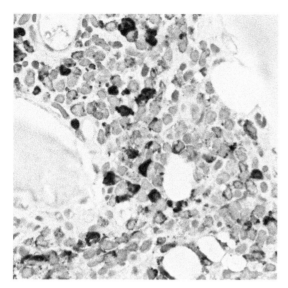

Figure 82.18 MPO, ×400.

at a high frequency in these disorders and are considered by the WHO as specific entities (3). Consensus on the best approach to management of mixed phenotype acute leukaemia is lacking, although recent reviews concluded that ALL-based treatment approaches demonstrate higher CR rates than AML-type approaches (4, 5). Allogeneic stem cell transplant is the only therapy reported to induce long-term remission. This patient was commenced on ALL induction therapy but failed to achieve CR. Two cycles of FLAG-IDA achieved a good CR and the patient proceeded to allogeneic transplant.

Final diagnosis

Mixed phenotype acute leukaemia: B/myeloid.

References

1 Fyfe, A.J., Morris, A. & Drummond, M.W. (2009) Successful routine cytogenetic analysis from trephine biopsy specimens following failure to aspirate bone marrow. *British Journal of Haematology*, **146** (**5**), 573. doi:10.1111/j.1365-2141.2009.07788.x-2141.2009.07788.x. Epub 2009 June, 29.

2 Invernizzi, R., D'Alessio, A., Iannone, A.M., Pecci, A., Bernuzzi, S. & Castello, A. (1995) Bone marrow necrosis in acute lymphoblastic leukemia. *Haematologica*, **80** (**6**), 572–573.

3 Swerdlow, S.H., Campo, E., Harris, N.L. et al. (2008) *WHO Classification of Tumours of Haematopoietic and Lymphoid Tissues*, 4th edn. IARC Press, Lyon, France.

4 Zheng, C., Wu, J., Liu, X., Ding, K., Cai, X. & Zhu, W. (2009) What is the optimal treatment for biphenotypic acute leukemia? *Haematologica*, **94** (**12**), 1778–1780; author reply 1780.

5 Heesch, S., Neumann, M., Schwartz, S. et al. (2013) Acute leukemias of ambiguous lineage in adults: molecular and clinical characterization. *Annals of Hematology*, **92** (**6**), 747–758.

83

Case 83

A previously well 81-year-old woman presented with a short history of profound fatigue, anorexia, weight loss, fevers and sweats. A small right groin lymph node and spleen tip were palpable but the examination was otherwise unremarkable.

Laboratory data

FBC: Hb 102 g/L, MCV 93 fl, WBC 1.1×10^9/L (neutrophils 0.5×10^9/L) and platelets 52×10^9/L.
   U&Es, LFTs and bone profile: normal.
   Serum LDH: 482 U/L.

Blood film

A number of blastoid lymphoid cells were noted; these had a high nuclear:cytoplasmic ratio and some had clear nucleoli.

Imaging

A CT scan of thorax, abdomen and pelvis with contrast showed widespread, moderate volume, lymphadenopathy in the mediastinum and in hilar, mesenteric, para-aortic and right inguinal regions. The spleen was enlarged at 15 cm.

Bone marrow aspirate

A relatively minor infiltrate of large, primitive cells was noted with a high nuclear to cytoplasmic ratio, convoluted nuclei, open chromatin and deep blue cytoplasm (Figures 83.1–83.3). Haemophagocytosis was readily seen.

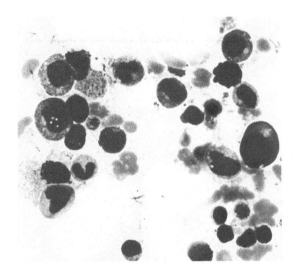

Figure 83.1 MGG, ×500.

In the light of the clinical presentation, the diagnosis was thought most likely to be bone marrow involvement by a T-lymphoblastic lymphoma. However, haemophagocytosis is not a common feature with T-precursor neoplasms so a peripheral T-cell lymphoma was also considered.

Flow cytometry (bone marrow aspirate)

An abnormal population of T cells was identified using a blast gate approach on the FSC/SSC profile. The cells expressed CD2, CD3 and HLA-DR (Figure 83.4). There was loss of the T-cell antigens, CD5 and CD7. There was no significant expression of CD4, CD8 (Figure 83.5), CD30,

Practical Flow Cytometry in Haematology: 100 Worked Examples, First Edition. Mike Leach,
Mark Drummond, Allyson Doig, Pam McKay, Bob Jackson and Barbara J. Bain.
© 2015 John Wiley & Sons, Ltd. Published 2015 by John Wiley & Sons, Ltd.

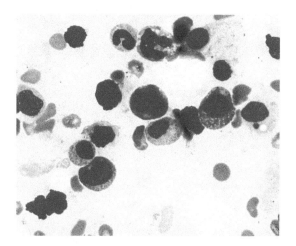

Figure 83.2 MGG, ×500.

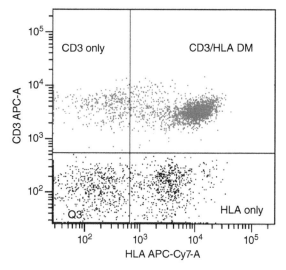

Figure 83.4 CD3/HLA-DR.

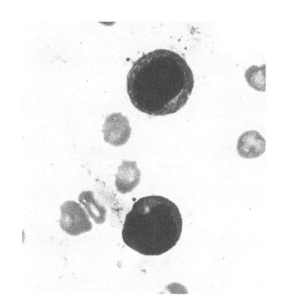

Figure 83.3 MGG, ×1000.

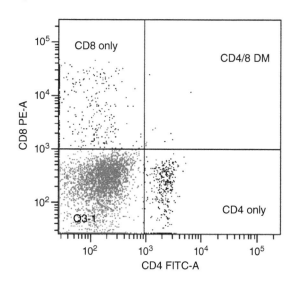

Figure 83.5 CD4/CD8.

CD56, TdT or CD1a. CD26 expression was abnormal being uniformly negative (Figure 83.6).

The loss of CD7 makes T-cell acute lymphoblastic leukaemia (T-ALL) unlikely as CD7 is almost universally expressed. CD7 is the earliest T-cell surface membrane antigen to be expressed. HLA-DR positivity normally indicates reactive T cells but it can be expressed on the cells of some neoplastic proliferations, notably mycosis fungoides, some peripheral T-cell lymphomas and, rarely, T-ALL (usually in pre-T ALL phenotypes).

Trephine biopsy

A 1.2 cm core was obtained, showing variable cellularity (5–40%). In addition to normal haemopoietic elements there were a small number of lymphoid nodules with atypical larger pleomorphic cells (Figure 83.7). At high power these cells appeared intermediate to large in size with irregular nuclei (Figure 83.8).

By immunohistochemistry they expressed CD2 and CD3 (Figures 83.9 and 83.10) with loss of CD5 and CD7 (Figures 83.11 and 83.12). The cells immunoreactive for

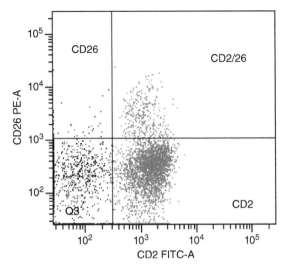

Figure 83.6 CD2/CD26.

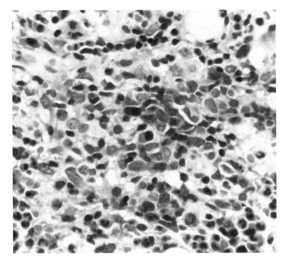

Figure 83.8 H&E, ×400.

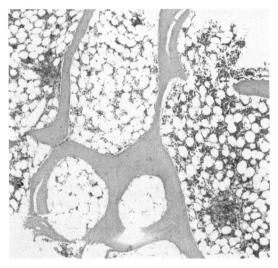

Figure 83.7 H&E, ×100.

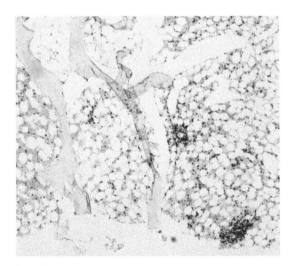

Figure 83.9 CD2, ×40.

the latter markers were considered to be reactive T cells. The abnormal T-cell population did not express CD4, CD8, CD30, TdT, ALK1, granzyme B, TIA, CD56, CD20 or CD34. The abnormal T-lymphoid population therefore had a phenotype identical to that identified using flow cytometry on the marrow aspirate.

Lymph node biopsy

A small fragmented 1 cm core was obtained from an inguinal lymph node.

Some cellular areas were present containing a mixed infiltrate of small and intermediate cells with vaguely nodular areas. At high power there was a population of intermediate sized to large cells, similar to those seen in the trephine biopsy, showing high mitotic activity. Appearances were suspicious of involvement by non-Hodgkin lymphoma but there was insufficient material for immunohistochemistry.

Discussion

The clinical picture and blood film appearances were in keeping with an aggressive condition, either acute leukaemia

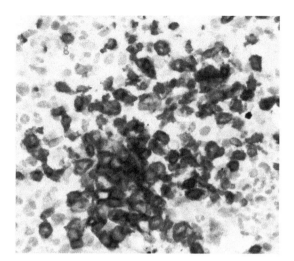

Figure 83.10 CD3, ×400.

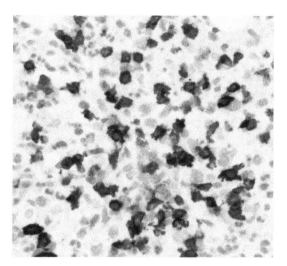

Figure 83.12 CD7, ×400.

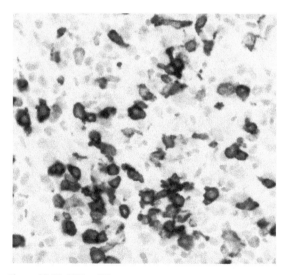

Figure 83.11 CD5, ×400.

or high-grade lymphoma with peripheral blood involvement. The prominent haemophagocytosis made the latter more likely. Normally non-Hodgkin lymphoma is best defined by histopathological assessment of nodal tissue. In this case analysis of the bone marrow using flow cytometry and histopathology allowed the identification of a neoplastic T-cell population. The accessible lymph nodes were small volume and the biopsy yielded a small amount of tissue insufficient to make a diagnosis in isolation. In such situations it is possible to make a definitive diagnosis when extranodal tissue is involved in the disease process.

The bone marrow findings were in keeping with a diagnosis of involvement by a peripheral T-cell lymphoma. Features supporting a diagnosis of lymphoma rather than ALL were the presence of generalised lymphadenopathy and splenomegaly, patchy low level bone marrow involvement, lack of expression of TdT and CD34 and the pattern of antigen loss, especially the loss of CD7. There was no expression of additional antigens, such as CD30, CD10 or CD56, which may be found in anaplastic large cell, angioimmunoblastic T-cell lymphoma and NK/T-cell lymphoma, respectively. By a process of exclusion the case was categorised as peripheral T-cell lymphoma, not otherwise specified (PTCL-NOS).

Peripheral T-cell lymphoma, NOS is the most common subtype of mature T-cell neoplasm representing approximately 25–30% of all T-cell lymphomas. It usually occurs in elderly patients who present with systemic upset, generalized disease and bone marrow involvement. Intramedullary haemophagocytosis often contributes to the peripheral cytopenias seen in these T-cell neoplasms. Treatment is usually with anthracycline-based combination chemotherapy such as the CHOP regimen but the outcome is poor compared with the responses seen in similarly aged patients with diffuse large B-cell lymphoma.

Final diagnosis

Peripheral T-cell lymphoma, NOS, with nodal, blood and bone marrow involvement.

Case 84

A 45-year-old man was referred for investigation of splenomegaly and thrombocytopenia. He had first been noted to have a mildly enlarged spleen 7 years previously at a routine medical examination for life insurance. For a few months prior to the current presentation he had become aware of discomfort in the left hypochondrium. On examination he had no significant lymphadenopathy but an easily palpable spleen (4–5 finger breadths below the costal margin).

Laboratory results

FBC: Hb 130 g/L, WBC 15 × 10^9/L (neutrophils 4 × 10^9/L, lymphocytes 9 × 10^9/L) and platelets 256 × 10^9/L.

U&Es, LFTs and LDH normal.

Immunoglobulins reduced. No paraprotein.

Imaging

CT imaging confirmed significant splenomegaly, the spleen measuring 27 cm in the long axis. No lymphadenopathy was demonstrated.

Peripheral blood morphology

The morphology of this case was interesting. A population of cells with irregular nuclei with small indistinct nucleoli and basophilic, sometimes vacuolated, irregular villous cytoplasm was noted (Figures 84.1–84.4). On the basis of this, and the clinical presentation, a splenic marginal zone lymphoma (SMZL) was felt to be the most likely diagnosis though hairy cell leukaemia variant was also considered.

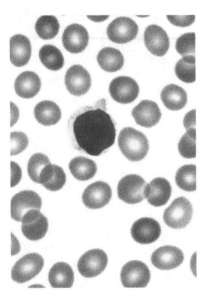

Figure 84.1 MGG, ×1000.

Flow cytometry (peripheral blood)

A kappa[bright] restricted, mature B-lymphoid population was identified. The cells co-expressed CD20[bright], CD5[dim], CD38, FMC7[dim to mod], CD23, CD79b and HLA-DR (Figures 84.5–84.7). They were negative for CD10, CD11c, CD25, CD103 and CD123. The CLL score here was thus 2/5 making this diagnosis unlikely. Note also the intensity of expression of CD20: most typical CLL patients will have a mean fluorescence intensity of around 10^4 in our laboratory, again not favouring a diagnosis of CLL. A splenic marginal zone lymphoma with peripheral blood spread and expression of CD5 and CD23 was therefore the favoured diagnosis from the morphology and immunophenotyping.

Practical Flow Cytometry in Haematology: 100 Worked Examples, First Edition. Mike Leach, Mark Drummond, Allyson Doig, Pam McKay, Bob Jackson and Barbara J. Bain.
© 2015 John Wiley & Sons, Ltd. Published 2015 by John Wiley & Sons, Ltd.

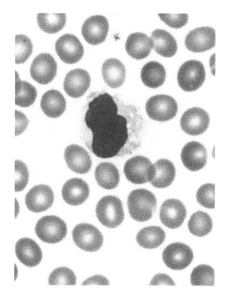

Figure 84.2 MGG, ×1000.

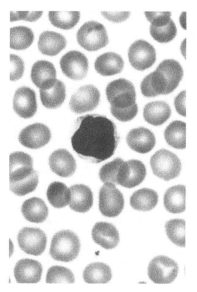

Figure 84.4 MGG, ×1000.

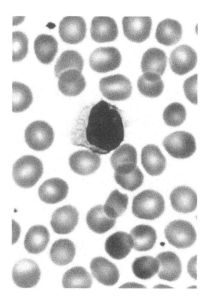

Figure 84.3 MGG, ×1000.

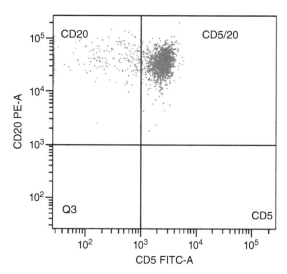

Figure 84.5 CD5/CD20.

Histopathology

Bone marrow trephine biopsy: the overall cellularity was within normal limits at 30–40%. There was a nodular lymphocytic infiltrate (not paratrabecular) composed of small cells. No intrasinusoidal infiltrate was detected. These cells were positive for CD20 (Figure 84.8) and CD5 and weakly positive for CD23 (Figure 84.9). CD10, BCL6, cyclin D1 and CD72 (DBA44) were negative.

There was no evidence of plasmacytic differentiation. Appearances were thought to be in keeping with marrow involvement by CLL/SLL.

This finding was in contrast to the working diagnosis of SMZL. In the absence of enlarged lymph nodes accessible for biopsy and because of the therapeutic implications in a 45-year-old male we proceeded to percutaneous splenic biopsy.

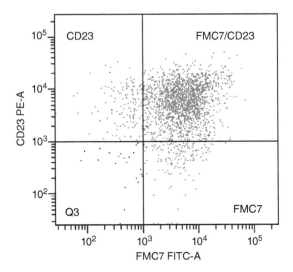

Figure 84.6 FMC7/CD23.

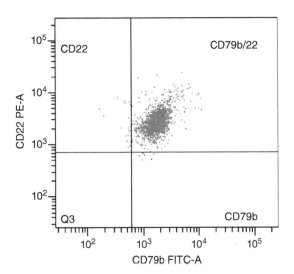

Figure 84.7 CD79b/CD22.

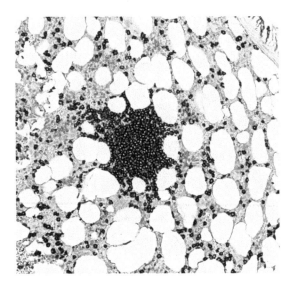

Figure 84.8 CD20, ×100.

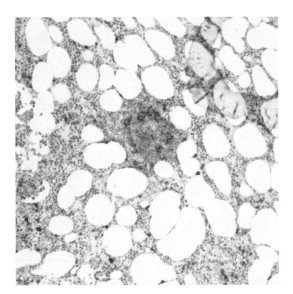

Figure 84.9 CD23, ×100.

Spleen: the adequate core biopsies showed prominent involvement of the white and red pulp by a lymphoid infiltrate (Figures 84.10 and 84.11). The abnormal cells were small and monomorphic and expressed CD20 (Figure 84.12), CD5 (Figure 84.13), BCL2, CD43 and CD23 (Figure 84.14). They were negative for CD3 (but showing background positive T cells) (Figure 84.15), CD10, BCL6 and cyclin D1.

Morphologically this was a low-grade lymphoma with predominant white pulp involvement. Immunohistologically this was most in keeping with CLL/SLL although a CD5+ SMZL was a less likely possibility. CD5 expression can occur

in marginal zone lymphoma but is seen in less than 5% of cases. CD43 is expressed in CLL but also sometimes in SMZL.

Molecular studies

FISH performed on peripheral blood showed trisomy 12 in approximately 25% of cells. There was no loss of 17p nor of 11q and no evidence of a t(11;14) translocation.

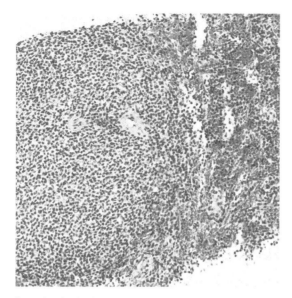

Figure 84.10 H&E, ×100.

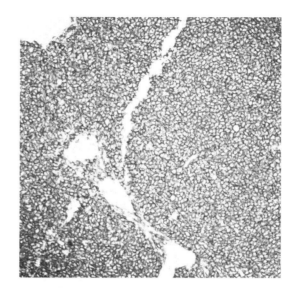

Figure 84.12 CD20, ×100.

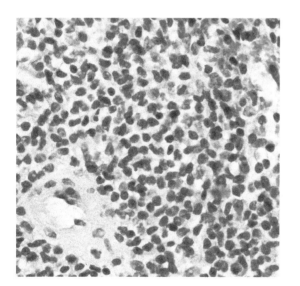

Figure 84.11 H&E, ×400.

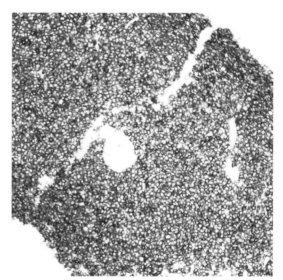

Figure 84.13 CD5, ×100.

Discussion

The diagnosis in this case caused some difficulty. The presentation, peripheral blood morphology and immunophenotyping data were suggestive of a diagnosis of splenic marginal zone lymphoma. The nodular bone marrow involvement without intrasinusoidal infiltration, red and white pulp splenic involvement and SLL/CLL phenotype

on immunohistochemistry, however, were suggestive of SLL/CLL. This case illustrates the value of a combined approach to diagnosis. The finding of trisomy 12 on cytogenetic analysis of peripheral blood was highly informative. Trisomy 12 CLL is associated with atypical morphology, increased circulating prolymphocytoid cells and low CLL scores on immunophenotyping due to expression of CD79b, FMC7 and surface Ig$^{mod/strong}$; this has been referred to as variant CLL (1). Furthermore, it may also be associated

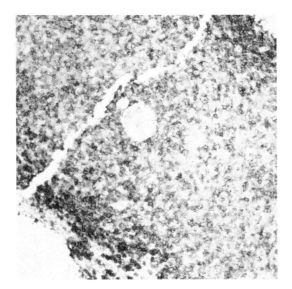

Figure 84.14 CD23, ×100.

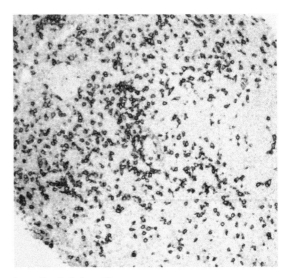

Figure 84.15 CD3, ×100.

with a less favourable prognosis particularly in cases with associated *NOTCH1* mutations (2).

In view of the nature of the presentation, the young age of the patient and the strong CD20 expression he was treated with single agent rituximab. There has been marked improvement in the degree of splenomegaly with clearance of circulating disease cells and full resolution of symptoms. Single agent rituximab would not normally be a therapeutic option for CLL but in this case, with an atypical immunophenotype and strong CD20 expression, it was an appropriate treatment. This is an example of how the use of flow cytometry and immunohistochemistry can assess the intensity of antigen expression, and alongside cytogenetic data, not just derive a sound diagnosis but also inform appropriate treatment.

Final diagnosis

Trisomy 12 chronic lymphocytic leukaemia with atypical morphology and low CLL score.

References

1 Cro, L., Ferrario, A., Lionetti, M. *et al.* (2010) The clinical and biological features of a series of immunophenotypic variant of B-CLL. *European Journal of Haematology*, **85** (**2**), 120–129. PubMed PMID: 20408870.

2 Balatti, V., Bottoni, A., Palamarchuk, A. *et al.* (2012) NOTCH1 mutations in CLL associated with trisomy 12. *Blood*, **119** (**2**), 329–331. PubMed PMID: 22086416.

Case 85

Some 3 years previously a 53-year-old female presented with symptoms and signs of superior vena cava obstruction. A large anterior mediastinal mass was identified by CT and biopsy demonstrated T-cell lymphoblastic lymphoma (TdT[+], CD1a[+], CD2[+], CD3[+], CD4[+], CD5[+], CD7[+], CD8[dim], CD10[+] and CD99[+] by flow cytometry and IHC). Bone marrow examination was normal. Treatment was commenced with an intensive ALL regimen (comprising steroids, vincristine, daunorubicin, cyclophosphamide, methotrexate, cytarabine, etoposide and asparaginase, as well as a prolonged maintenance phase with mercaptopurine and methotrexate plus pulsed steroids/vincristine). The patient entered remission (based upon serial re-imaging of the thymic mass) and completed maintenance therapy. Six months later a follow up FBC demonstrated significant pancytopenia.

Laboratory data

FBC: Hb 105×10^9/L, MCV 97.1 fl, WBC 2.54×10^9/L (neutrophils 0.88×10^9/L) and platelets 27×10^9/L.

Blood film

Blood film examination revealed medium-sized to large angular blast cells with basophilic cytoplasm and scant granules (Figures 85.1 and 85.2). Dysplastic changes were noted in residual neutrophils, with abnormal nuclear segmentation (Figures 85.3 and 85.4) and platelet granulation was reduced (Figure 85.2).

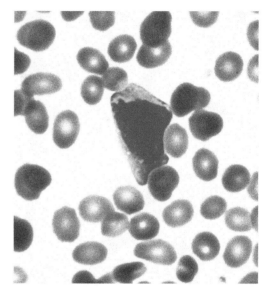

Figure 85.1 MGG, ×1000.

Imaging

In view of the previous history the patient was re-imaged. The CT performed at the time of original diagnosis had shown, in addition to a pleural effusion, a large anterior mediastinal mass surrounding the great vessels, typical of cortical type T-lymphoblastic lymphoma (Figure 85.5). The repeat CT showed no recurrence of a mediastinal mass (Figure 85.6).

Practical Flow Cytometry in Haematology: 100 Worked Examples, First Edition. Mike Leach, Mark Drummond, Allyson Doig, Pam McKay, Bob Jackson and Barbara J. Bain.

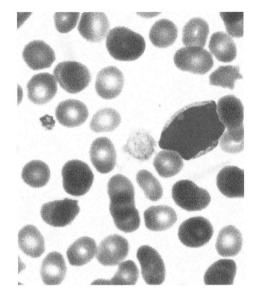

Figure 85.2 MGG, ×1000.

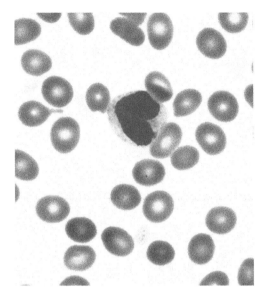

Figure 85.4 MGG, ×1000.

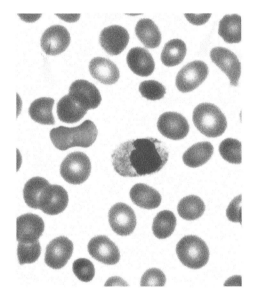

Figure 85.3 MGG, ×1000.

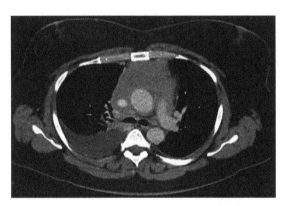

Figure 85.5 CT chest at original presentation.

Bone marrow aspirate

This confirmed 25% myeloblasts as well as trilineage dysplastic changes (not shown).

Flow cytometry (bone marrow aspirate)

Flow cytometry on bone marrow demonstrated 22% CD34+ cells (Figure 85.7). These were CD117+, CD13+, CD56+ (Figure 85.8) and HLA-DR+. TdT was negative. Despite the presence of granules in some blasts cells, MPO was also negative, as were monocytic, megakaryocytic, erythroid and lymphoid markers.

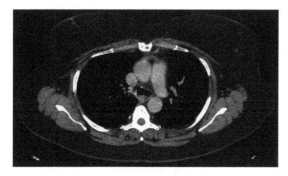

Figure 85.6 CT chest at second presentation.

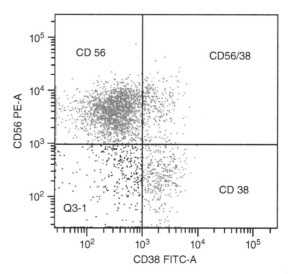

Figure 85.8 CD56/CD38.

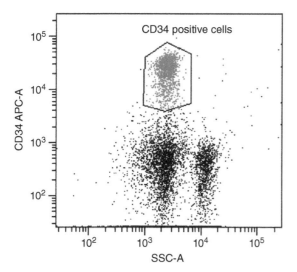

Figure 85.7 CD34/SSC.

Cytogenetic analysis and FISH

Del(7q) was detected in 10/10 cells on metaphase analysis. A deletion involving 7q22 and 7q36 was confirmed by FISH, in 78% of cells.

Discussion

This unfortunate case illustrates the relatively rare but well recognised late consequence of systemic chemotherapy, particularly of regimens containing alkylating agents. Monosomy 5/del(5q) and monosomy 7/del(7q) are the most commonly reported cytogenetic abnormalities in therapy-related MDS/AML (t-MDS/t-AML), being strongly associated with prior exposure to alkylating agents and poor outcome. Typically, alkylating agent-related t-MDS/t-AML presents late (5–10 years after original therapy) and is most commonly associated with an initial MDS phase and unbalanced loss of genetic material (most often involving chromosomes 5 and 7). Earlier presentations (1–5 years), often with a balanced chromosomal abnormality, are associated with topoisomerase II inhibitors (such as etoposide and doxorubicin) and usually present as AML without a prior MDS phase (1). This case, as with many others in our experience, did not quite fit with either of these classical scenarios since onset was early but the cytogenetic abnormalities were more suggestive of alkylating agent-related disease than t-AML resulting from topoisomerase II-interactive drugs.

There are no specific immunophenotype patterns in t-MDS/t-AML, although a high incidence of CD34, CD7 and/or CD56 positivity is reported. MPO-negativity is recognised in a minority of cases of AML, in particular in AML with minimal differentiation, acute monoblastic leukaemia (MPO is expressed from the promonocyte stage onwards), acute erythroid leukaemia, acute megakaryoblastic leukaemia and acute basophilic leukaemia. Thus, although MPO is indicative of myeloid differentiation, its absence does not preclude a diagnosis of AML and in this case it likely reflects the minimal differentiation of the blast population.

An interesting cytological feature in this patient is the indentation of blast cells by surrounding red cells. This is more often seen in reactive lymphocytes, as in infectious mononucleosis, but can also be seen in both ALL and AML, so is lacking in diagnostic specificity.

Prognosis in such cases is generally poor; resistance to induction chemotherapy is common, and allogeneic transplantation is the only hope for long-term survival. Our

patient failed to remit with intensive AML-type chemotherapy and also failed a further induction attempt with an
experimental agent. The patient died from progressive
disease 4 months from re-presentation.

Final diagnosis

Therapy-related AML.

Reference

1 Brunning, R.D., Matutes, E., Harris, N.L. *et al.* (2001) Acute
  myeloid leukaemia: introduction. In: Jaffe, E.S., Harris, N.L.,
  Stein, H. & Vardiman, J.W. (eds), *World Health Organization
  Classification of Tumours: Pathology and Genetics of Tumours
  of Haematopoietic and Lymphoid Tissues.* pp. 77–80, IARC
  Press, Lyon.

Case 86

A 54-year-old man with a myelodysplastic syndrome and associated monosomy 7 underwent an unrelated donor reduced intensity conditioning peripheral blood stem cell transplant. Two months later he developed fevers, sweats and neck pain. He had widespread peripheral lymphadenopathy and an increasing EBV viral load in his peripheral blood.

Laboratory results

FBC: Hb 93 g/L, WBC 5.7×10^9/L (neutrophils 3.5×10^9/L, lymphocytes 1.26×10^9/L) and platelets 118×10^9/L.

U&Es and LFTs normal. LDH: 479 U/L.

EBV PCR: log 5.42 copies/mL. This is a substantial peripheral blood EBV viral load that might be seen with primary EBV infection or proliferation of an EBV-driven lymphoma.

Blood film

Pleomorphic large lymphoid cells, with basophilic cytoplasm, and some nucleoli, were present in low numbers (Figures 86.1–86.3). There was no other significant abnormality.

Flow cytometry (peripheral blood)

A CD19 versus CD2 analysis showed normal proportions of T and B cells. In view of the history we were interested in analysing the B cells despite the fact that they did not appear in excess and represented only 6% of leucocytes.

The B cells expressed CD20, CD38, FMC7, CD79b and HLA-DR with surface membrane kappa restriction; a proportion of cells also expressed CD10.

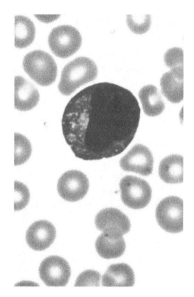

Figure 86.1 MGG, ×1000.

Histopathology

The trephine biopsy sections showed adequate engraftment with a variable cellularity up to 60% in some areas. There was good representation and maturation of erythroid, myeloid and megakaryocyte series with no excess blasts or abnormal lymphoid infiltrate.

Imaging

CT scan of neck, thorax, abdomen and pelvis showed extensive small volume lymphadenopathy in the chest and abdomen.

Practical Flow Cytometry in Haematology: 100 Worked Examples, First Edition. Mike Leach, Mark Drummond, Allyson Doig, Pam McKay, Bob Jackson and Barbara J. Bain.
© 2015 John Wiley & Sons, Ltd. Published 2015 by John Wiley & Sons, Ltd.

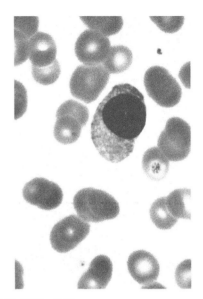

Figure 86.2 MGG, ×1000.

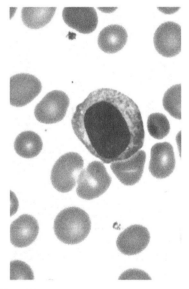

Figure 86.3 MGG, ×1000.

Discussion

The clinical (fevers and sweats) and laboratory features are in keeping with a post-transplant lymphoproliferative disorder (PTLD). These conditions occur in recipients of solid organ and bone marrow or other stem cell allografts and are a consequence of immunosuppression. They are lymphoid, usually B-cell or plasmacytic, proliferations and may be polyclonal or monoclonal. The majority are associated with EBV infection. Monomorphic PTLDs include B-cell lymphomas (usually diffuse large B-cell lymphoma, DLBCL) or Burkitt lymphoma, and T/NK-cell lymphomas. This case is an example of a B-cell PTLD of probable DLBCL subtype but is unusual in that the disease was involving the blood. A lymph node biopsy was not performed as there was adequate evidence for this diagnosis. The cells identified in the peripheral blood presumably originated in involved lymph nodes. The patient was managed by reduction in immunosuppression and with five weekly rituximab infusions. His symptoms settled, the lymphadenopathy resolved and he remains well on follow up 1 year later.

Final diagnosis

Monomorphic B-cell post-transplant lymphoproliferative disorder, identified in peripheral blood.

Case 87

A 5-year-old male child was referred with fatigue, sweats and pallor. He had no prior history of note and had met all normal developmental targets. He was referred to our city paediatric unit from another specialist centre. He was noted to have significant hepatosplenomegaly on clinical examination and the working diagnosis at the time of referral was acute myeloid leukaemia.

Laboratory data

Hb 45 g/L, MCV 101 fl, WBC 154×10^9/L and platelets 21×10^9/L.

U&Es: Na 132 mmol/L, K 3.6 mmol/L, urea 3.1 mmol/L, creatinine 68 μmol/L.

LFTs and bone profile: bilirubin 13 μmol/L, AST 71 U/L, ALT 13 U/L, ALP 123 U/L, calcium 2.24 mmol/L, phosphate 0.97 mmol/L and albumin 26 g/L.

Serum LDH was 3783 U/L and urate 0.61 mmol/L.

Coagulation profile: normal.

Imaging

The CXR showed a significant mediastinal mass (Figure 87.1). CT imaging confirmed an anterior mediastinal mass, hepatosplenomegaly and widespread lymphadenopathy (not shown).

Blood film

This was grossly abnormal with a marked leucocytosis, anaemia and thrombocytopenia (Figure 87.2). There was a pleomorphic population of lobulated, apparently lymphoid

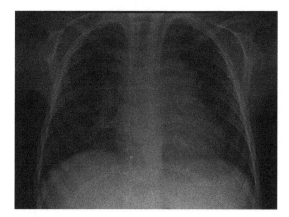

Figure 87.1 CXR.

cells with cytoplasmic vacuolation together with a marked myeloid proliferation with prominent abnormal basophils, eosinophils and probable mast cells (Figures 87.3–87.6). Some of the pleomorphic blast population with highly lobulated nuclei had cytoplasmic granules, suggesting a myeloid derivation (Figures 87.4–87.6).

Bone marrow aspirate

This was abnormal with an extensive infiltrate of pleomorphic blast cells as described above together with an abnormal myeloid population. The morphology was exactly as described in the peripheral blood.

Flow cytometry (bone marrow aspirate)

Flow cytometry studies were extremely informative in this case where normal boundaries and rules of morphological

Practical Flow Cytometry in Haematology: 100 Worked Examples, First Edition. Mike Leach, Mark Drummond, Allyson Doig, Pam McKay, Bob Jackson and Barbara J. Bain.
© 2015 John Wiley & Sons, Ltd. Published 2015 by John Wiley & Sons, Ltd.

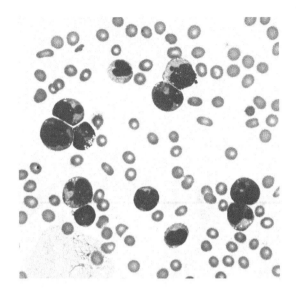

Figure 87.2 MGG, ×500.

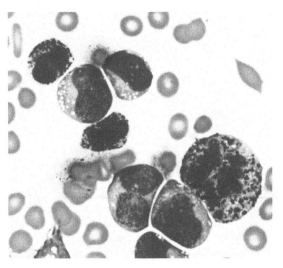

Figure 87.4 MGG, ×1000.

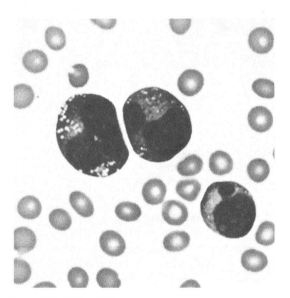

Figure 87.3 MGG, ×1000.

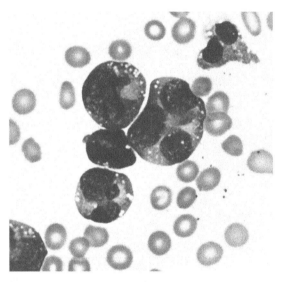

Figure 87.5 MGG, ×1000.

assessment were challenged to the extreme. Gating using a CD34 versus SSC strategy was employed and a CD34$^+$, TdT$^-$, CD117$^+$, CD56$^+$, CD38$^+$, CD33$^+$, HLA-DR$^-$, MPO$^-$, cCD3$^+$, cCD79a$^-$, CD7$^+$, CD5^{dim}, CD2$^+$, CD1a$^-$, CD3$^-$, CD4$^-$, CD8$^-$ population was identified and reported. WHO criteria for lineage specificity were applied, remembering that expression of CD34, CD38, CD56, CD117 and CD33 do not necessarily indicate myeloid derivation. MPO was

apparently not expressed on the blast population and there was no indication of monoblastic/monocytic differentiation (CD15, CD14 and CD64 negativity). Expression of cytoplasmic CD3 indicated T-lineage origin and the myeloid antigen expression was therefore classed as aberrant.

However, the presence of small population of granular blast cells together with the prominent eosinophils, basophils, apparent mast cells and bizarre immature granular cells of uncertain lineage raised the suspicion that this was actually a mixed phenotype acute leukaemia (MPAL).

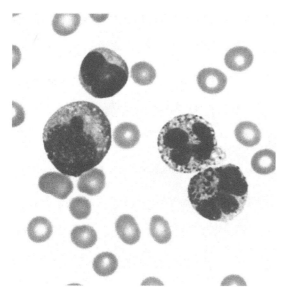

Figure 87.6 MGG, ×1000.

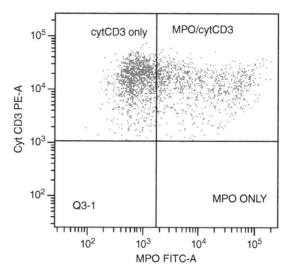

Figure 87.7 cCD3/MPO.

The flow cytometric data were therefore reassessed. The majority of cells expressed CD34 so a CD34 versus SSC gating strategy was appropriate. However, paying particular attention to the flow cytometry plots on the analyser it was clear that a sub-population of the blast cells (34%) did in fact co-express cytoplasmic CD3 and MPO (Figure 87.7). This result had been erroneously omitted from the data reported, the percentage of positive events expressing MPO only (without cCD3) being given; this figure was zero.

The only cells expressing MPO without cCD3 were the maturing myeloid cells, but these of course did not fall in the CD34+ gate. This episode illustrates the importance of actually reviewing primary data on the analyser database in puzzling cases, particularly where antigen co-expression will have a major impact on diagnosis.

Cytogenetic analysis

46,XY,add(1)(p12),add(2)(q33),?inv(2)(p13q21),+4,dic(4;6)(q11;q12),del(5)(q11.2),del(7)(p11.2),del(9)(p13),add(9)(q3?2),?inv(15)(q11.2q24),der(16)add(16)(p11.2)add(16)q2?2),del(18)(q11.2q21),add(19)(p13)[10].

Molecular studies

A *FLT3* ITD mutation was not identified.

Discussion

This case presented a diagnostic challenge both in terms of morphological and immunophenotypic assessment. Our initial interpretation was that this was a T-lineage disorder (cytoplasmic CD3+). Furthermore the presence of antigens of immaturity such as CD34, CD117, and CD38 with the weak expression of CD5 and CD2 and the lack of surface CD3 suggested an early precursor T-cell neoplasm. The presence of non-lineage specific myeloid antigens was interpreted as aberrant expression. Aberrant myeloid antigen expression is seen in some cases of B-precursor ALL, particularly in patients with t(9;22), t(12;21) and 11q23 translocations. Aberrant myeloid antigen expression in T-ALL is unusual except in cases now identified as early T-cell precursor ALL (ETP ALL). This is an aggressive T-precursor/stem cell neoplasm with a characteristic immunophenotype that was originally defined and characterised by Coustan-Smith *et al.* at St Jude's Research Hospital, Memphis, Tennessee, USA (1). This neoplasm is predominantly encountered in paediatric patients and differs from other 'typical' T-ALL cases, in that it shows a primitive T-precursor phenotype, expression of multiple early myeloid antigens, complex cytogenetics without regularly recurring aberrations, a different gene expression signature, reduced frequency of acknowledged genetic aberrations of T-ALL and the presence of *FLT3* mutations (2–4). The cell of origin shows arrest very early in T-cell differentiation, at a stage closely related to haemopoietic stem cells and myeloid progenitors (3). The prognosis is historically poor compared with the outcome in non-ETP

ALL with significantly reduced morphological and MRD based remissions, event free and overall survival (1).

Our initial suspicion was that this patient did indeed have ETP ALL. However we continued to be preoccupied by the remarkable myeloid features shown by the peripheral blood and bone marrow films. This led us to re-evaluate the primary flow cytometric data leading to a revision of the diagnosis to MPAL. We postulate that the leukaemic clone arose from an early T-cell precursor with bilineage potential and that, unusually, myeloid differentiation occurred. This case illustrates the fundamental role of morphology and the crucial importance of keeping in mind all aspects of a case rather than relying on a single technique in isolation. A number of members of the patient's family had a history of carcinoma and a paternal uncle had died in childhood of bone marrow failure. Chromosome fragility studies were undertaken and gave a positive result. Subsequent molecular studies identified the homozygous *BRCA2* sequence variant c.517-2A>G. *BRCA2* is now known to be identical to *FANCD1*, one of the genes involved in the pathogenesis of Fanconi anaemia (FA). Fanconi anaemia is a rare autosomal recessive disease associated with progressive bone marrow failure, acute leukaemia and cancer susceptibility. Many, but not all, patients have other congenital anomalies including skeletal abnormalities, short stature and abnormal skin pigmentation. The FA related proteins A, C, E, F and G are now known to function in an important pathway interacting with BRCA1 and BRCA2 (FANCD1) in the regulation of DNA repair in normal cells (reviewed in 5). Mutations in the genes involved in this pathway lead to chromosomal instability, drug and radiation sensitivity and predisposition to malignancy. The final diagnosis, is therefore a mixed phenotype acute leukaemia developing in a child with Fanconi anaemia. This is an important finding as such patients will ultimately require allogeneic stem cell transplantation. Additionally, such patients show excess toxicity to normal tissues following chemotherapy and bone marrow transplant conditioning so all treatment regimens will need to be carefully considered. The patient will need careful monitoring for late effects of such therapy and will need lifelong scrutiny with regard to the development of other tumours.

See also Case 42.

Final diagnosis

1. Mixed phenotype acute leukaemia, T/myeloid
2. Fanconi anaemia due to homozygous BRCA2 gene mutation

References

1 Coustan-Smith, E., Mullighan, C.G., Onciu, M. *et al.* (2009) Early T-cell precursor leukaemia: a subtype of very high-risk acute lymphoblastic leukaemia. *The Lancet Oncology*, **10** (2), 147–156. PubMed PMID: 19147408.

2 Haydu, J.E. & Ferrando, A.A. (2013) Early T-cell precursor acute lymphoblastic leukaemia. *Current Opinion in Hematology*, **20** (4), 369–373. PubMed PMID: 23695450.

3 Zhang, J., Ding, L., Holmfeldt, L. *et al.* (2012) The genetic basis of early T-cell precursor acute lymphoblastic leukaemia. *Nature*, **481** (7380), 157–163. PubMed PMID: 22237106.

4 Neumann, M., Heesch, S., Gokbuget, N. *et al.* (2012) Clinical and molecular characterization of early T-cell precursor leukemia: a high-risk subgroup in adult T-ALL with a high frequency of FLT3 mutations. *Blood Cancer Journal*, **2** (1), e55. PubMed PMID: 22829239.

5 D'Andrea, A.D. & Grompe, M. (2003) The Fanconi anaemia/BRCA pathway. *Nature Reviews Cancer*, **3** (1), 23–34. Pubmed PMID: 12509764.

Case 88

A 42-year-old female with a history of common B-cell acute lymphoblastic leukaemia was being monitored as an outpatient during the maintenance phase of treatment. She presented earlier than planned with the recent onset of a dry barking cough, dyspnoea and low-grade fever. A CXR did not show any notable abnormality but her full blood count was found to be abnormal.

Laboratory data

FBC: Hb 102 g/L, WBC 11.54 × 10^9/L (neutrophils 1.78 × 10^9/L, lymphocytes 7.16 × 10^9/L, 'monocytes' 2.32 × 10^9/L) and platelets 162 × 10^9/L.

U&Es, bone profile and LFTs were normal except AST 50 U/L and ALT 65 U/L.

Serum LDH was 190 U/L.

Blood film

This was carefully examined as the initial concern was that the patient might have developed relapsed disease with an associated immunosuppression-related infection. The film showed a population of large pleomorphic lymphoid cells with nuclear convolutions and deeply basophilic cytoplasm (Figures 88.1–88.4). Note that the automated instrument has classified some of these abnormal cells as monocytes. Although there were no real features of bone marrow failure (moderate cytopenias are common in well managed patients on maintenance chemotherapy) there was still concern that the findings might indicate relapse and immunophenotyping was therefore performed.

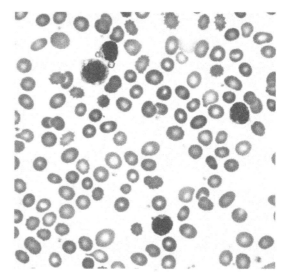

Figure 88.1 MGG, ×500.

Flow cytometry (peripheral blood)

Peripheral blood was examined using a blast gate approach, focussing on the large lymphoid cells seen in the film. The large cells were predominantly CD8$^+$ T cells expressing CD2, CD3, CD5, HLA-DR and CD7 with a normal distribution of CD26. There was no excess of B cells and those present had a mature polyclonal phenotype. This profile, showing activated (HLA-DR$^+$) T cells, is indicative of a reactive phenomenon, typically seen in patients with a viral infection.

Additional investigations

A throat gargle was taken for PCR studies. This proved negative for all the common upper respiratory tract viral

Practical Flow Cytometry in Haematology: 100 Worked Examples, First Edition. Mike Leach, Mark Drummond, Allyson Doig, Pam McKay, Bob Jackson and Barbara J. Bain.
© 2015 John Wiley & Sons, Ltd. Published 2015 by John Wiley & Sons, Ltd.

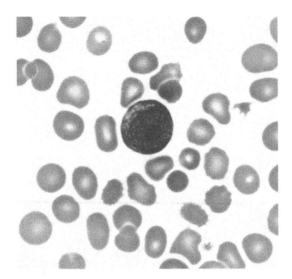

Figure 88.2 MGG, ×1000.

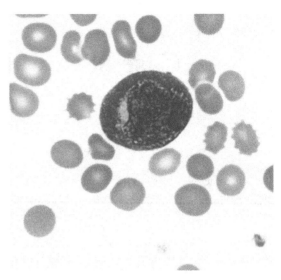

Figure 88.4 MGG, ×1000.

Discussion

The peripheral blood morphology was somewhat alarming in this case with the finding of large pleomorphic lymphoid cells in the circulation. The morphology of reactive T cells can be remarkably pleomorphic but to the experienced eye this variability can actually be reassuring and indicative of a T-cell reaction rather than relapse of a previous neoplasm. The intense basophilia of the reactive cell cytoplasm is a particular feature of note and is a frequent characteristic of viral induced T-cell lymphocytosis. Of course if the primary pathology had shown similar cell morphology then extra consideration needs to be taken.

The patient's symptoms subsequently resolved with symptomatic treatment and she was firmly reassured that her primary disease remained in remission.

Final diagnosis

Reactive T-cell lymphocytosis secondary to whooping cough in a patient on maintenance therapy for common B-cell acute lymphoblastic leukaemia.

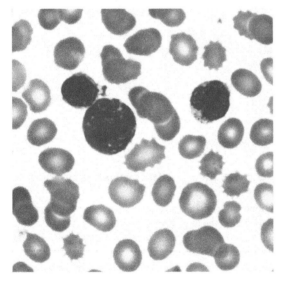

Figure 88.3 MGG, ×1000.

pathogens. In view of the nature of the cough with a degree of stridor (or whoop), the clinical haematologist caring for the patient was convinced that this was a case of whooping cough due to *Bordetella pertussis*. A specific PCR on the gargle specimen gave negative results for *B. pertussis* and *B. parapertussis* but subsequent serology proved positive for recent *B. pertussis* infection.

89

Case 89

A 72-year-old female attended her GP because of a purpuric rash and a short history of worsening fatigue. Clinical examination confirmed purpura on her abdomen and lower limbs but no organomegaly or lymphadenopathy. She was otherwise clinically stable and was able to give a clear history. An FBC was analysed.

Laboratory data

FBC: Hb 92 g/L, WBC 71 × 10^9/L and platelets 17 × 10^9/L.

Coagulation: PT 18 s, APTT 35 s, TT 15 s, fibrinogen 3.0 g/L, D-dimer 15,000 ng/mL.

U&Es, LFTs and bone profile: normal. Serum LDH: 500 U/L.

Blood film

Considerable numbers of medium sized blast cells were noted. Some had large cytoplasmic inclusions, so-called 'pseudo-Chédiak-Higashi' granules (Figure 89.1), with occasional finer granules also observed. The most striking abnormality was the presence of 'cup-like' indentations of the nuclei, resulting in an area of pallor often at the periphery of the nuclear membrane (Figures 89.2–89.4, arrows). When sited more centrally, they simulated an abnormally large nucleolus (Figure 89.2).

Bone marrow aspirate

A substantial blast cell infiltrate was noted (>90% of cells) but 'cup-like' morphology was less easy to appreciate than in the blood (not shown).

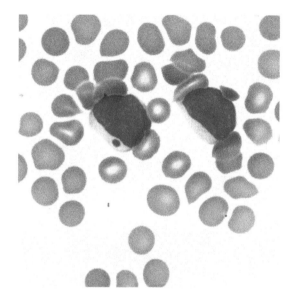

Figure 89.1 MGG, ×1000.

Flow cytometry

A distinctive blast immunophenotype was noted: CD34$^-$, CD56$^+$, CD117$^+$, CD33$^+$, CD13$^+$, HLA-DR$^-$ and MPO$^+$.

Histopathology

A cellular bone marrow aspiration was obtained so no bone marrow trephine biopsy was performed.

Cytogenetic analysis

Analysis of 20 metaphases demonstrated a normal female karyotype (46,XX) in 20 cells.

Practical Flow Cytometry in Haematology: 100 Worked Examples, First Edition. Mike Leach, Mark Drummond, Allyson Doig, Pam McKay, Bob Jackson and Barbara J. Bain.
© 2015 John Wiley & Sons, Ltd. Published 2015 by John Wiley & Sons, Ltd.

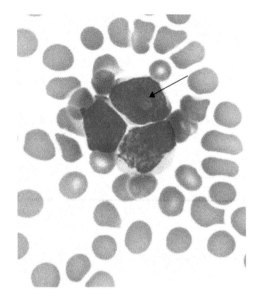

Figure 89.2 MGG, ×1000.

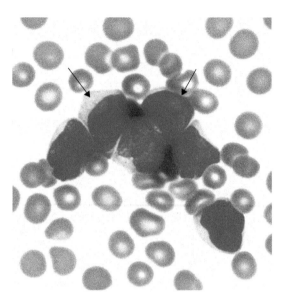

Figure 89.4 MGG, ×1000.

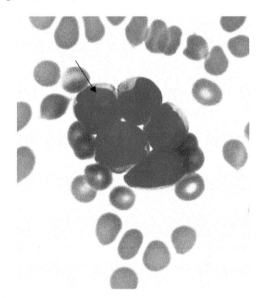

Figure 89.3 MGG, ×1000.

Molecular studies

The presence of a *FLT3* ITD and a co-existing *NPM1* mutation was detected.

Discussion

AML with cup-like morphology is now a well recognised pathological entity having typical (and remarkably

consistent) morphological, flow cytometric and cytogenetic findings. Estimates of its incidence vary significantly: according to two recent studies it would appear to comprise somewhere between 1% and 21% of newly diagnosed AML cases (1, 2). Differences in morphological definition probably account for the bulk of variation here. Markedly raised D-dimers also appear to be a feature of this disorder, emphasising that this feature is not (as is commonly assumed) synonymous with APL. Indeed in a recent study in our department there was no significant difference between D-dimer levels in APL or non-APL AML (personal communication): there was however a statistically significant association of lower fibrinogen levels with APL as compared to other AML cases.

Initial morphologic assessment of 'cup-like' AML may raise suspicion of APL or AML of monocytic lineage, as the nuclear indentations can give the appearance of nuclear lobation and/or indentation. Suspicion of APL may be further compounded by flow cytometric results, which confirm the blasts to be CD34$^-$ and HLA-DR$^-$. In one large study comprising 800 cases of *de novo* AML, a total of 15% of cases were HLA-DR$^-$ (3), with approximately half of these being confirmed as APL. Of the remainder, >80% were CD34$^-$, NPM1$^+$ and >35% exhibited cup like blasts and *FLT3* ITD positivity. A normal karyotype is usual. Subsequent studies have demonstrated that almost 80% of cup-like cases are *FLT3* ITD and *NPM1* mutated and that the HLA-DR$^-$, CD34$^-$ phenotype is consistently present (1). Recognition of this entity by morphological and flow cytometric assessment should certainly prompt appropriate genetic studies, if not carried out routinely, particularly since cup-like morphology has also been reported in association with *FLT3* ITD without *NPM1* mutation (4) and these two molecular abnormalities differ in their prognostic significance. For AML as a whole, the *NPM1* mutation confers a favourable prognostic impact across all age groups, but in younger patients this is predominantly in *FLT3* ITD-negative patients (5) whereas in older patients it is an independent predictor of better outcome, particularly in patients ≥70 years of age (6).

Final diagnosis

AML without maturation, with cup-like morphology and co-existing *NPM1* and *FLT3* ITD mutations.

References

1 Chen, W., Konoplev, S., Medeiros, L.J. *et al.* (2009) Cuplike nuclei (prominent nuclear invaginations) in acute myeloid leukemia are highly associated with FLT3 internal tandem duplication and NPM1 mutation. *Cancer*, **115**, 5481–5489.

2 Park, B.G., Chi, H.S., Jang, S. *et al.* (2013) Association of cup-like nuclei in blasts with FLT3 and NPM1 mutations in acute myeloid leukemia. *Annals of Hematology*, **92**, 451–457.

3 Oelschlaegel, U., Mohr, B., Schaich, M. *et al.* (2009) HLA-DRneg patients without acute promyelocytic leukemia show distinct immunophenotypic, genetic, molecular, and cytomorphologic characteristics compared to acute promyelocytic leukemia. *Cytometry Part B: Clinical Cytometry*, **76**, 321–327.

4 Kroschinsky, F.P., Schäkel, U., Fischer, R. *et al.* (2008) On behalf of the DSIL (Deutsche Studieninitiative Leukämie) Study Group. Cup-like acute myeloid leukemia: new disease or artificial phenomenon? *Haematologica*, **93**, 283–286.

5 Dohner, K., Schlenk, R.F., Habdank, M. *et al.* (2005) Mutant nucleophosmin (NPM1) predicts favorable prognosis in younger adults with acute myeloid leukemia and normal cytogenetics: interaction with other gene mutations. *Blood*, **106**, 3740–3746.

6 Becker, H., Marcucci, G., Maharry, K. *et al.* (2010) Favorable prognostic impact of NPM1 mutations in older patients with cytogenetically normal de novo acute myeloid leukemia and associated gene- and microRNA-expression signatures: a Cancer and Leukemia Group B study. *Journal of Clinical Oncology*, **28**, 596–604.

90

Case 90

A 48-year-old male with a known diagnosis of chronic lymphocytic leukaemia had received a number of different therapies over the previous 4 years, the disease having proved fludarabine refractory. The clinical course had been complicated by recurrent viral and bacterial infections. His leukaemic cells did not appear to harbour an 11q22 or 17p13 deletion but he was classed as poor risk in view of the refractoriness to fludarabine. His therapy was being directed toward a possible allogeneic stem cell transplant and he had completed two cycles of rituximab with high dose methylprednisolone. There had been a substantial improvement in his bulky nodal disease and blood indices but he presented early with a rapid development of a mass over his left submandibular and parotid region. On examination, a large warm nodal mass was evident in this region. All the other previously enlarged nodes had regressed. He had no new night sweats or systemic upset and no obvious focus of infection.

Laboratory data

FBC: Hb 105 g/L, WBC 2.5×10^9/L (neutrophils 1.0×10^9/L, lymphocytes 1.1×10^9/L, 'monocytes' 9.8×10^9/L) and platelets 80×10^9/L.

U&Es, LFTs and bone profile: normal. CRP was 12 mg/L and LDH 300 U/L.

Blood film

This did not show any notable features but the CLL cells were large with a moderate amount of cytoplasm. This explains the apparent monocytosis from the automated analyser.

Flow cytometry

Previous flow cytometric studies at diagnosis had shown a typical CLL immunophenotype with a CLL score of 5/5.

Bone marrow aspirate and trephine biopsy

This showed an extensive diffuse involvement by CLL with substantial reduction in normal haemopoietic activity. No additional abnormal infiltrate was identified.

Imaging

CT imaging showed a substantial improvement in all previously involved nodal areas but confirmed the presence of a new nodal mass over the left parotid region measuring 5.5 cm × 6 cm. There was no radiological evidence of necrosis and an ultrasound-guided biopsy of this mass was performed.

A PET/CT was performed to fully assess the distribution of a possible Richter transformation with a view to guiding decisions on management. This showed two patterns of nodal uptake with a large cluster of strongly FDG-avid nodes in the left neck whilst the other nodal regions showed low level uptake. This is best seen by comparing the intensity of signal in the left neck (long arrow) with that seen in the right neck and both axillae (short arrows) in Figure 90.1. (Note the normal uptake in the heart, liver and intestine).

Histopathology

The two 20 mm core biopsies showed effaced lymph node architecture (Figure 90.2) with a polymorphous infiltrate

Practical Flow Cytometry in Haematology: 100 Worked Examples, First Edition. Mike Leach, Mark Drummond, Allyson Doig, Pam McKay, Bob Jackson and Barbara J. Bain.
© 2015 John Wiley & Sons, Ltd. Published 2015 by John Wiley & Sons, Ltd.

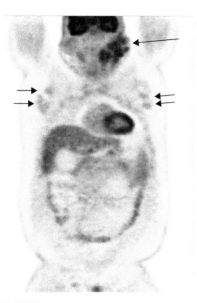

Figure 90.1 PET/CT.

Figure 90.2 H&E, ×40.

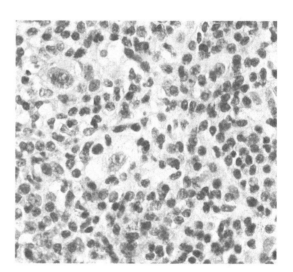

Figure 90.3 H&E, ×400.

containing lymphoid cells, eosinophils, plasma cells and large atypical cells (Figures 90.3 and 90.4). Some of the latter had typical binucleate morphology of Reed – Sternberg (RS) cells nicely highlighted by positive staining for CD30 (Figure 90.5) and CD15 (Figure 90.6). Expression of MUM1, EBV (EBER) (Figure 90.7) and PAX5 (Figure 90.8, large cells positive but CLL cells also positive) was seen but CD45 and CD20 were negative. In the background there were areas of diffuse involvement with small B cells expressing CD20, PAX5, CD23, CD5 (Figure 90.9) and BCL6, in keeping with the known CLL, in addition to reactive T cells (Figure 90.10). Note the voids left by the unstained Hodgkin and RS cells using CD5 in Figure 90.9 and the T-cell rosettes around similar voids using CD3 in Figure 90.10.

These features were diagnostic of Hodgkin lymphoma (HL) developing on a background of CLL.

Discussion

Transformation to a high grade B-cell lymphoma occurs in 5 – 10% of patients with CLL. These lymphomas have diverse genetic and molecular characteristics and may arise directly from the CLL clone or develop from a residual non-clonal B cell, possibly as a result of immunosuppressive treatment and the T-cell depletion that results; in the latter instance the term 'transformation', although conventional, is not strictly speaking correct; Richter syndrome covers both types of event. The Hodgkin variant of Richter syndrome is a rare but well recognised development (1) and is perhaps some 10 fold less common than a high-grade B-cell lymphoma. The disease shows typical morphology and immunophenotype of HL and EBV is often positive. It is presumed to occur as a result of T-cell depletion, particularly following fludarabine therapy, as a result of transformation of an EBV-infected cell. The disease outcome is generally poor as the response to standard therapies is not nearly as favourable as that seen in *de novo* HL. In addition, the ongoing management of the

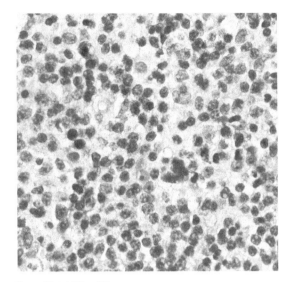

Figure 90.4 H&E, ×400.

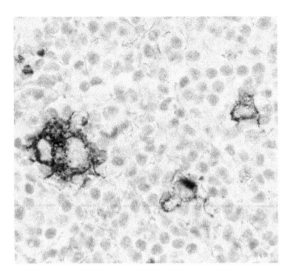

Figure 90.6 CD15, ×400.

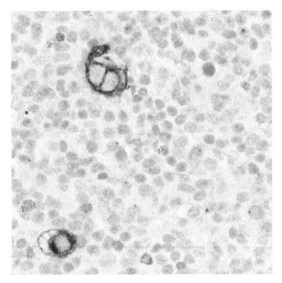

Figure 90.5 CD30, ×400.

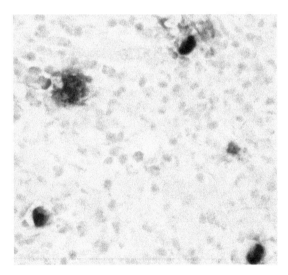

Figure 90.7 EBV (EBER), ×400.

CLL alongside the established immune-compromised state, poses a major challenge.

This case illustrates the importance of considering a second pathology in any patient presenting with new onset nodal disease in the setting of a documented response to therapy. The new nodal mass in this case was clinically obvious and easily biopsied. A Richter transformation should be considered in any CLL patient who develops a rapid onset of lymphadenopathy or of an extranodal mass.

Flow cytometry was important with regard to establishing the initial CLL diagnosis but had little to contribute with regard to the transformation. In this situation we rely on histopathological assessment with immunohistochemistry. Hodgkin and RS cells can be defined using flow cytometry (2) but there are inherent difficulties due to their size, adherence to T cells and difficulties in freeing them from the fibrous reactive stroma that they have induced. This disease is therefore not routinely investigated in most diagnostic flow laboratories.

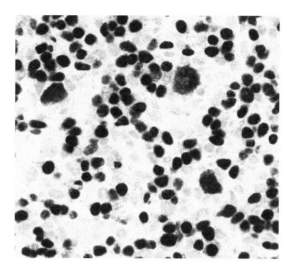

Figure 90.8 PAX5, ×400.

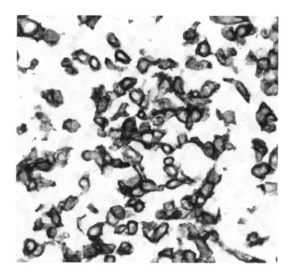

Figure 90.10 CD3, ×400.

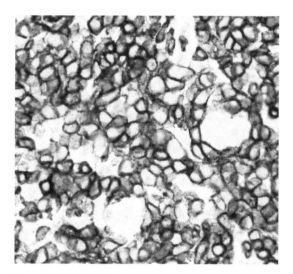

Figure 90.9 CD5, ×400.

use of radiotherapy in due course particularly if the early response to chemotherapy appears incomplete.

Final diagnosis

Hodgkin lymphoma as Richter transformation/Richter syndrome in CLL following fludarabine therapy.

References

1 Bockorny, B., Codreanu, I. & Dasanu, C.A. (2012) Hodgkin lymphoma as Richter transformation in chronic lymphocytic leukaemia: a retrospective analysis of world literature. *British Journal of Haematology*, **156** (**1**), 50–66. PubMed PMID: 22017478.

2 Fromm, J.R. & Wood, B.L. (2014) A six-color flow cytometry assay for immunophenotyping classical Hodgkin lymphoma in lymph nodes. *American Journal of Clinical Pathology*, **141** (**3**), 388–396. PubMed PMID: 24515767.

3 Papajik, T., Myslivecek, M., Urbanova, R. *et al.* (2014) 2-[18F]fluoro-2-deoxy-D-glucose positron emission tomography/computed tomography examination in patients with chronic lymphocytic leukemia may reveal Richter transformation. *Leukemia & Lymphoma*, **55** (**2**), 314–319. PubMed PMID: 23656196.

PET/CT scanning provided interesting images demonstrating the differential uptake of FDG by the nodes involved by CLL and those involved by HL. This imaging technique is proving valuable in assessing patients with CLL with possible transformed or other associated high-grade disease (3). As treatment of this condition presents substantial difficulty the localised nature of the HL transformation might merit the

91

Case 91

A 42-year-old man was admitted via his GP after attending the practice for investigation of a 4-week history of weight loss and bruising. On examination, there was extensive superficial bruising and buccal blood blisters. An FBC was taken and a blood film was promptly examined.

Laboratory data

FBC: Hb 138 g/L, WBC 19.9×10^9/L and platelets 23×10^9/L.
   Coagulation screen including fibrinogen: normal.
   U&Es, LFTs and bone profile were normal. Serum LDH was 550 U/L.

Blood film

Myeloblasts were noted (Figures 91.1 and 91.2) with some exhibiting fine Auer rods (Figure 91.2). Dysplasia was evident in later myeloid stages with neutrophils showing hypogranularity and pseudo-Pelger nuclei (Figure 91.1).

Bone marrow aspirate

Frequent myeloblasts were present, many displaying maturation in the form of cytoplasmic granules (type 2 blasts); hypogranular segmented myeloid forms were again easily seen (Figures 91.3 and 91.4). No significant dysplastic changes were noted in the erythroid or megakaryocytic lineages.

Flow cytometry at diagnosis

CD117 and discordant CD15 co-expression was noted on almost all CD34+ blast cells (Figures 91.5 and 91.6), as well as

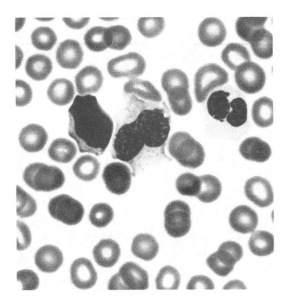

Figure 91.1 MGG, ×1000.

aberrant CD7 expression (Figure 91.7). Otherwise the blasts were CD13+, HLA-DR+, MPO+ and negative for T- and B-lineage markers.

Cytogenetic analysis

Normal male karyotype.

Molecular studies

FLT3 ITD and *NPM1* mutations were not detected.

Practical Flow Cytometry in Haematology: 100 Worked Examples, First Edition. Mike Leach, Mark Drummond, Allyson Doig, Pam McKay, Bob Jackson and Barbara J. Bain.

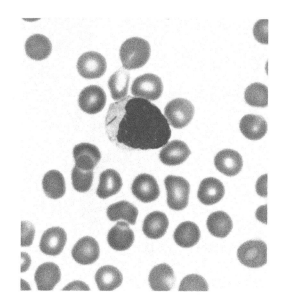

Figure 91.2 MGG, ×1000.

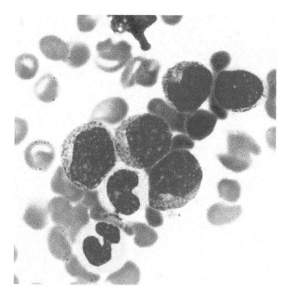

Figure 91.4 MGG, ×1000.

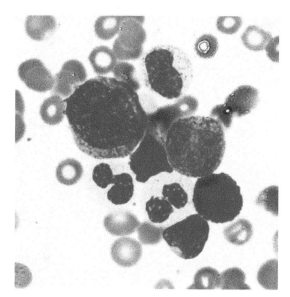

Figure 91.3 MGG, ×1000.

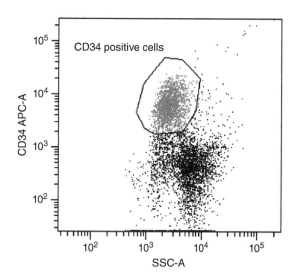

Figure 91.5 CD34/SSC baseline.

Treatment course

The patient was treated with standard induction chemotherapy and showed prompt recovery of peripheral blood counts at day 28. The marrow aspirate was reassessed for remission status. The morphology showed good recovery of all lineages with clearance of blasts (not shown). Flow cytometric assessment was greatly assisted by the aberrant blast phenotype. The flow plots following induction course 1 are shown in Figures 91.8–91.10.

A normal myeloid precursor phenotype (1% of events) is demonstrated, namely CD34+, CD117+/−, with no evidence of the previous asynchronous CD15 or aberrant CD7 expression.

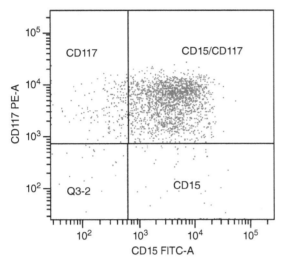

Figure 91.6 CD15/CD117 baseline.

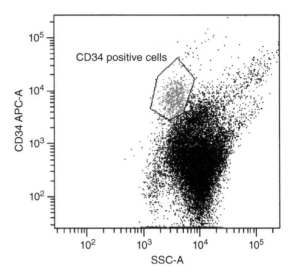

Figure 91.8 CD34/SSC post-induction.

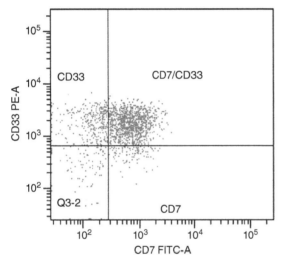

Figure 91.7 CD7/CD33 baseline.

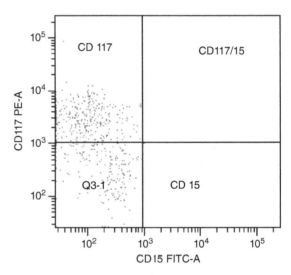

Figure 91.9 CD15/CD117 post-induction.

Discussion

Expression of precursor cell antigens is seen in a majority of cases of AML, with 60–70% expressing CD34 and 70–90% expressing CD117. Asynchronous co-expression of CD15 (an antigen associated with a mature myeloid phenotype) or aberrant expression of CD7 (a T-cell associated antigen) is common in AML. This serves both to highlight the neo-plastic nature of the cells at diagnosis and to facilitate flow cytometric tracking of small populations in the marrow after

therapy. Identification of a leukaemia-associated phenotype (LAP) is possible in the majority of patients and is variable in terms of the technical difficulty involved in tracking small populations of cells. At diagnosis of AML, the leukaemic cells may comprise heterogeneous populations (e.g. AML M4 Eo, comprising myeloblasts, eosinophilic cells and a monocytic component) meaning any one population may not be fully representative of the disease. Furthermore LAPs may change at relapse, and the original pattern of antigen expression cannot be assumed to be consistent. Notwithstanding these

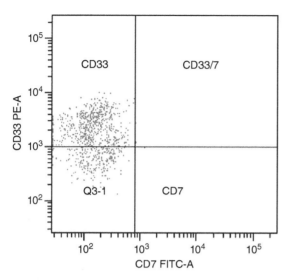

Figure 91.10 CD33/CD7 post-induction.

challenges, follow up of AML with flow cytometry is a powerful technique and tracking cells with the LAP allows accurate assessment of minimal residual disease (MRD) levels.

The patient in this case was treated with a total of four cycles of intensive chemotherapy and remains in continued remission.

Final diagnosis

Acute myeloid leukaemia with maturation with a leukaemia-associated phenotype that allowed accurate MRD assessment.

92

Case 92

A 58-year-old Chinese woman, who had recently returned from Eastern China, presented with a short history of dry cough, dyspnoea, fevers, weight loss and sweats. She was thoroughly investigated by an Infectious Disease Unit but a causative organism was not found.

Laboratory results

FBC: Hb 57 g/L, WBC 8.6×10^9/L and platelets 175×10^9/L. Reticulocytes were raised at 101×10^9/L. Direct Coombs test was positive (IgG^{++}).

Ferritin 1299 ng/mL.

U&Es and bone profile normal. LFTs: AST 120 U/L, ALT 70 U/L, ALP 110 U/L, GGT 60 U/L, bilirubin 50 μmol/L, albumin 20 g/L.

LDH was raised at 1413 U/L.

Blood and bone marrow examination

The initial blood films showed features of haemolysis with polychromasia and spherocytes with rouleaux. No abnormal leucocytes were seen. The initial bone marrow aspirate was hypocellular but did show prominent macrophages and haemophagocytosis.

Imaging

Extensive imaging was undertaken in an attempt to identify an infective focus. As part of this series, a CT scan identified marked splenomegaly and a degree of hepatomegaly, whilst

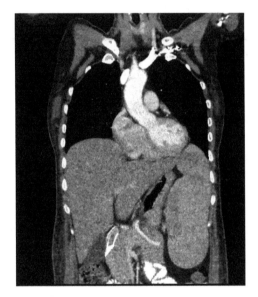

Figure 92.1 CT.

no lymphadenopathy was apparent (Figure 92.1). The spleen was of uniform texture without focal abnormality.

Clinical course

The working diagnosis at this stage was an idiopathic autoimmune haemolytic anaemia with a reactive haemophagocytic syndrome. No viral or bacterial pathogens had been identified but an extensive serological panel had shown positivity for epidemic scrub typhus. It was suspected that this might be the primary pathogen so a course of doxycycline with dexamethasone was commenced with some symptomatic improve-

Practical Flow Cytometry in Haematology: 100 Worked Examples, First Edition. Mike Leach, Mark Drummond, Allyson Doig, Pam McKay, Bob Jackson and Barbara J. Bain.
© 2015 John Wiley & Sons, Ltd. Published 2015 by John Wiley & Sons, Ltd.

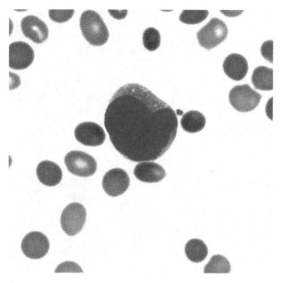

Figure 92.2 MGG, ×1000.

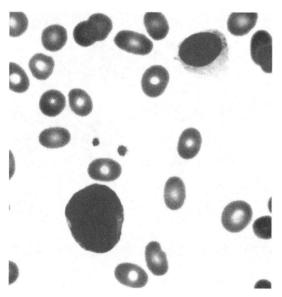

Figure 92.3 MGG, ×1000.

ment and resolution of fever. Within 1 week of discontinuing steroids, however, her symptoms returned. The patient was now showing progressive thrombocytopenia and renal impairment. The blood film at this point showed a population of large lymphoid cells with irregular nuclei and basophilic cytoplasm (Figures 92.2 and 92.3).

This finding was now suggestive of a neoplastic process so a fresh peripheral blood specimen was requested for flow cytometry studies.

Flow cytometry (peripheral blood)

The large lymphoid cells seen in the blood film occupied the upper part of the blast gate on the FSC versus SSC profile. These cells accounted for only 5.5% of leucocytes but a clear clonal B-cell population could be identified with the following immunophenotype: $CD19^+$, $CD20^+$, $CD79b^+$, $CD22^+$, partial FMC7, partial $CD5^+$ and $CD23^+$, HLA-DR$^+$ and surface membrane kappa^{dim}. CD10 was not expressed. This profile indicated a mature B-cell disorder with partial aberrant expression of CD5. A repeat bone marrow aspirate and a trephine biopsy were taken. The aspirate was again hypocellular and unhelpful.

Bone marrow trephine biopsy

Cellularity was increased at 60–70% with all haemopoietic lineages identified. The sinusoids appeared to be focally dilated (Figures 92.4 and 92.5, long arrows) and contained a small number of large cells, some of which were spindle shaped (Figures 92.6 and 92.7, short arrows).

Immunocytochemistry for CD20 identified a scattered large cell population, with many of these cells located within the dilated sinusoids and some within the interstitium (Figure 92.8). The $CD20^+$ cells co-expressed PAX5, BCL2 and MUM1 but were negative for CD10, BCL6, CD5, CD30 and CD56. Note the spindled morphology of the intra-sinusoidal B cells in Figure 92.9. The intravascular location of the lymphoma cells is nicely illustrated using PAX5 staining in Figures 92.10 and 92.11 (long arrows): note the red cell ghosts also within these vessels (short arrows).

Discussion

At initial presentation this woman was found to have haemophagocytosis thought to be secondary to scrub typhus (an illness resulting from *Orientia tsutsugamushi* infection and occurring in China). Criteria for an infection-related haemophagocytic syndrome were not fully satisfied however and other underlying diagnoses needed to be excluded. Identification of a small abnormal B-cell population in the peripheral blood by flow cytometry and the localisation of these cells within the sinusoids on the bone marrow biopsy sections yielded the diagnosis of intravascular large B-cell lymphoma (IVBCL). This is a rare type of extranodal large B-cell lymphoma where the malignant cells can be found within the lumina of small or intermediate blood vessels in various organs. Two types are described, Western and

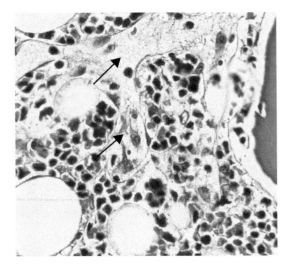

Figure 92.4 H&E, ×400.

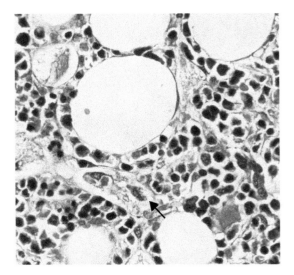

Figure 92.6 H&E, ×400.

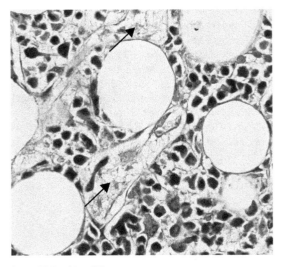

Figure 92.5 H&E, ×400.

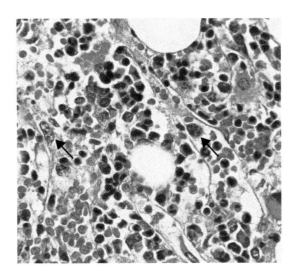

Figure 92.7 H&E, ×400.

Asian. This case is an example of the Asian sub-type in which patients typically present with fever, pancytopenia, haemophagocytic syndrome, hepatosplenomegaly and multi-organ failure (1). Sinusoidal involvement occurs in the liver, spleen and bone marrow and abnormal cells may be seen in the peripheral blood. Lymphadenopathy is frequently absent and the diagnosis is often delayed and prognosis poor. The diagnosis might even be missed on the trephine biopsy as the interstitial and sinusoidal B cells might not be obvious without the use of B-cell markers. The neoplastic cells often show an activated B-cell phenotype; MUM1 is expressed in

70% and CD5 in 15% of cases. In this case the administration of steroids obscured the disease features, contributing to the delay in diagnosis. Subsequent commencement of treatment with R-CHOP led to rapid clinical improvement and the patient achieved complete remission with six cycles of therapy. Anthracycline-based chemotherapy can be effective in this condition and rituximab improves outcome (2). A prompt diagnosis and early introduction of chemotherapy is key if the patient is to be offered the best opportunity of a successful outcome.

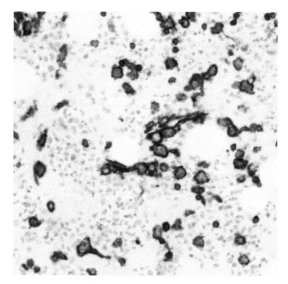

Figure 92.8 CD20, ×200.

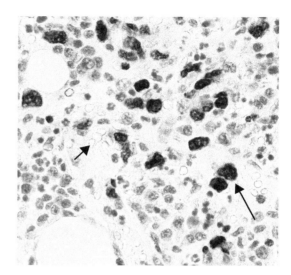

Figure 92.10 PAX5, ×400.

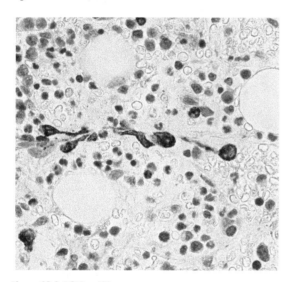

Figure 92.9 BCL2, ×400.

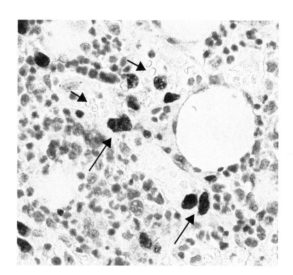

Figure 92.11 PAX5, ×400.

Final diagnosis

Intravascular B-cell lymphoma of Asian sub-type, with an associated Coombs-positive haemolytic anaemia and reactive haemophagocytosis.

See also Case 48, Western sub-type intravascular B-cell lymphoma.

References

1 Saab, J., Nassif, S. & Boulos, F. (2013) Asian-type intravascular large B-cell lymphoma of the spleen and bone marrow with Hodgkin-like morphology and immunophenotype. *British Journal of Haematology*, **163** (**3**), 294. PubMed PMID: 23961992.

2 Hong, J.Y., Kim, H.J., Ko, Y.H. *et al.* (2014) Clinical features and treatment outcomes of intravascular large B-cell lymphoma: a single-center experience in Korea. *Acta Haematologica*, **131** (**1**), 18–27. PubMed PMID: 24021554.

Case 93

A 20-year-old male presented with a 3-month history of pain in the upper left tibia. He had attributed this to a previous football injury but the pain was getting progressively worse. On examination there was no clearly definable abnormality but he was in pain on standing. There appeared to be some minor erythema just below the left knee joint. The remainder of the general examination was normal.

Laboratory data

FBC: Hb 130 g/L, WBC 7.5 × 10^9/L (neutrophils 4.5 × 10^9/L, lymphocytes 2.1 × 10^9/L, monocytes 0.8 × 10^9/L) and platelets 351 × 10^9/L.

U&Es, LFTs and bone profile were normal. CRP 2 mg/L, LDH 190 U/L.

Blood film

The film was unremarkable.

Imaging

Plain X-rays showed an alteration in the bone texture of the upper left tibia (long arrows) with an associated periosteal reaction (short arrows) (Figures 93.1 and 93.2).

The abnormal area was further assessed by MRI where it was now apparent that the upper tibia was replaced by abnormal tissue extending through the periosteum and into the soft tissues (Figures 93.3 and 93.4). The knee joint was not involved. The findings were typical of a primary bone tumour and a series of core biopsies were taken.

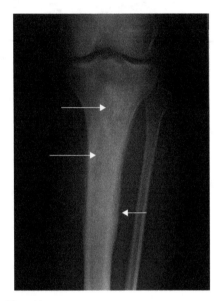

Figure 93.1 Plain X-ray.

Histopathology

The cores showed extensive necrosis but the viable areas showed infiltration by a small round 'blue cell tumour' (Figures 93.5 and 93.6) with abundant cytoplasmic glycogen highlighted by staining with periodic acid-Schiff (PAS) (Figure 93.9). Immunohistochemistry showed the tumour cells to be negative for CD45 (Figure 93.7) and also for various markers of non-haemopoietic tumours, S100, AE1/3, NB84, SMA, MyoD1 and desmin. There was positive membranous staining for CD99 (Figure 93.8) and CD56. The morphological features, together with cytoplasmic PAS positivity (Figure 93.9) and CD99 positivity, in conjunction

Practical Flow Cytometry in Haematology: 100 Worked Examples, First Edition. Mike Leach, Mark Drummond, Allyson Doig, Pam McKay, Bob Jackson and Barbara J. Bain.
© 2015 John Wiley & Sons, Ltd. Published 2015 by John Wiley & Sons, Ltd.

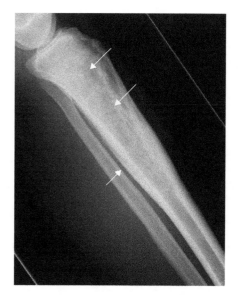

Figure 93.2 Plain X-ray.

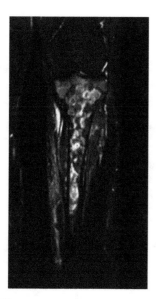

Figure 93.4 MRI.

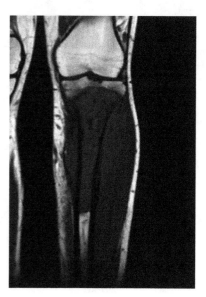

Figure 93.3 MRI.

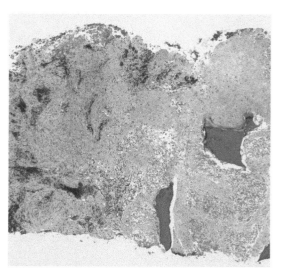

Figure 93.5 H&E, ×40.

with the age of the patient and site of disease, were diagnostic of a Ewing sarcoma family tumour (ESFT).

Cytogenetic analysis

Cytogenetic studies identified a t(11;22)(q24;q12) which results in a *EWSR1-FLI1* fusion gene. This reciprocal

translocation is characteristic of ESFT and confirmed the histological diagnosis.

Bone marrow aspirate

Bilateral bone marrow aspirates were obtained for staging purposes. The aspirate was hypercellular with good preservation of normal haemopoietic activity but small

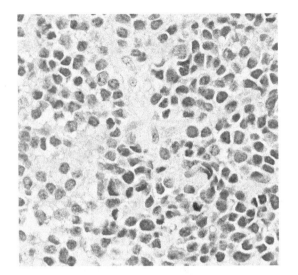

Figure 93.6 H&E, ×400.

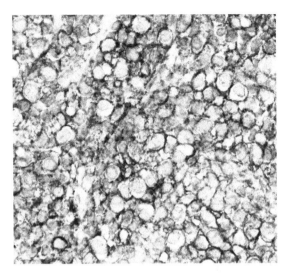

Figure 93.8 CD99, ×400.

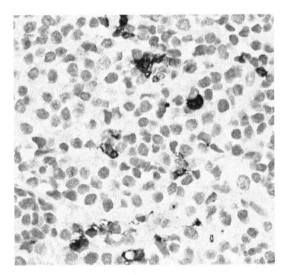

Figure 93.7 CD45, ×400.

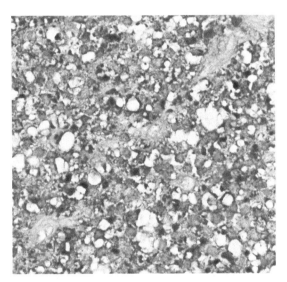

Figure 93.9 PAS, ×400.

clumps of abnormal cells were noted (Figures 93.10 and 93.11). On closer scrutiny these had round or oval nuclei, some with nucleoli, and pale blue wispy cytoplasm (Figures 93.12 and 93.13).

Flow cytometry (bone marrow aspirate)

A population of CD45$^-$, CD56$^+$ cells was identified. No lineage-specific haemopoietic markers were expressed.

This was indicative of marrow involvement by a non-haemopoietic CD56$^+$ tumour which, in the knowledge of the primary tumour histology, was in keeping with a diagnosis of Ewing sarcoma.

Trephine biopsies

Bilateral trephine biopsy specimens, examined at multiple levels and with immunocytochemistry, showed no histological evidence of involvement by tumour.

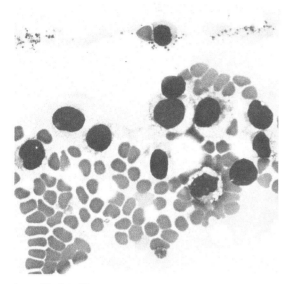

Figure 93.10 MGG, ×500.

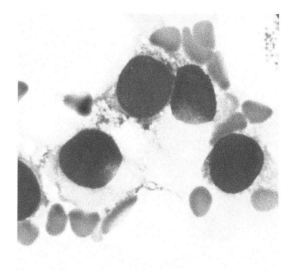

Figure 93.12 MGG, ×1000.

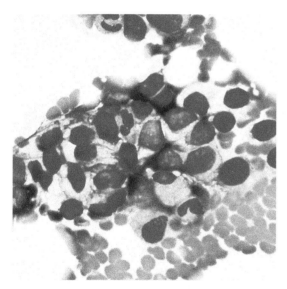

Figure 93.11 MGG, ×500.

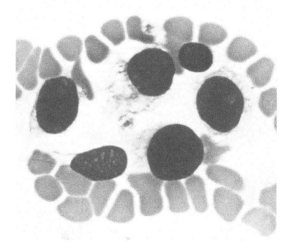

Figure 93.13 MGG, ×1000.

Discussion

Ewing sarcoma (ES), primitive neuroectodermal tumours (PNET) and Askin tumours are a group of small round 'blue cell tumours' occurring in the bone and soft tissues of children, adolescents and young adults. Together they are known as the Ewing sarcoma family tumours (ESFT) and are thought to have a mesenchymal stem cell origin (1). Ewing sarcoma and other ESFT are characterised by balanced chromosome translocations affecting the Ewing sarcoma gene (*EWSR1*) on chromosome 22 and *FLI1* gene on chromosome 11 in 85% of cases. Other cases can have a variant translocation also involving *EWSR1*. This is the second most common primary tumour of bone after osteosarcoma. It causes pain and inflammation at the primary site and is characterised by aggressive clinical behaviour with extensive local growth and a tendency for haematogenous metastasis to distant tissues. Bone marrow involvement is not uncommon and staging bone marrow biopsies are routinely performed at diagnosis (3). The described case is unusual in that the aspirate and flow cytometry sample contained tumour but the trephine biopsies specimens were negative. This can be explained by the focal nature of bone marrow involvement in this condition. The reverse, a normal aspirate but infiltrated trephine biopsy specimen, is a more common observation in metastatic tumours. CD56 positivity is seen in a proportion of ESFT, particularly in the PNET variant where neural differentiation is more pronounced, and can be used as a target for flow cytometry as in this case. CD56 is by no means specific for ESFT but in the clinical context and coupled with CD45 negativity, can be used as a relatively robust marker of marrow involvement. CD56 positivity detected by flow cytometry in the bone marrow of patients with ESFT has been associated with predisposition to relapse (2). Accurate staging is important because distant spread, affecting approximately 25% of patients at the outset, has a major influence on prognosis, reducing survival significantly below the 70% at 5 years expected in localised disease (3). Treatment is with neoadjuvant chemotherapy, radiation therapy and surgical resection of the primary tumour.

Final diagnosis

Ewing sarcoma of tibia with bone marrow micrometastases.

References

1 Riggi, N. & Stamenkovic, I. (2007) The biology of Ewing sarcoma. *Cancer Letters*, **254** (**1**), 1–10. PubMed PMID: 17250957.

2 Ash, S., Luria, D., Cohen, J. *et al.* (2011) Excellent prognosis in a subset of patients with Ewing sarcoma identified at diagnosis by CD56 using flow cytometry. *Clinical Cancer Research*, **17** (**9**), 2900–2907.

3 Potratz, J., Dirksen, U., Jurgens, H. & Craft, A. (2012) Ewing sarcoma: clinical state-of-the-art. *Pediatric Hematology and Oncology*, **29** (**1**), 1–11. PubMed PMID: 22295994.

Case 94

A 1-year-old girl was brought for medical assessment by her mother who was concerned that her child was ill; she reported her to be irritable with abdominal bloating, erratic sleep and altered feeding patterns. On examination the child was pale and unwell with moderate hepato-splenomegaly.

Laboratory data

FBC: Hb 80 g/L, WBC 14.4 × 10⁹/L (neutrophils 2.9 × 10⁹/L, lymphocytes 7 × 10⁹/L, large unidentified cells 4 × 10⁹/L) and platelets 100 × 10⁹/L.

U&Es, LFTs and bone profile: normal. LDH: 340 U/L.

Blood film

A number of large blasts cells were seen at the Base hospital and acute lymphoblastic leukaemia was suspected.

Bone marrow aspirate

This was cellular but aparticulate. A population of large blast cells with basophilic cytoplasm and areas of paranuclear pallor, resembling abnormal Golgi zones, were seen (Figures 94.1–94.3). Cytoplasmic granules and Auer rods were not seen. Some blast cells showed nuclear clefts and some were extremely large, approaching 25 μm in diameter (Figure 94.4). There was some residual myeloid activity.

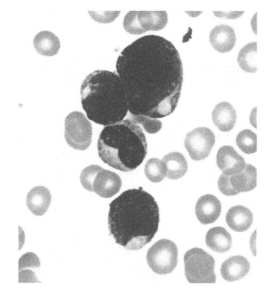

Figure 94.1 MGG, ×1000.

Flow cytometry (marrow aspirate)

The blast cells were readily apparent high in the blast gate in the FSC/SSC plot (Figure 94.5) and in the CD45^{dim} zone (Figure 94.6). These cells were CD34⁻, CD117⁻, CD15⁻, CD64⁻ and MPO⁻ (Figure 94.7) but expressed CD13, CD33, CD7, HLA-DR and CD10. Furthermore cCD79a, TdT, CD19 and cCD3 were all negative. This case therefore presented some difficulty as all the lineage-specific markers were negative. A number of myeloid antigens were expressed but the negativity for CD34 and CD117 suggested some degree of maturation. This was not toward monoblastic

Practical Flow Cytometry in Haematology: 100 Worked Examples, First Edition. Mike Leach, Mark Drummond, Allyson Doig, Pam McKay, Bob Jackson and Barbara J. Bain.
© 2015 John Wiley & Sons, Ltd. Published 2015 by John Wiley & Sons, Ltd.

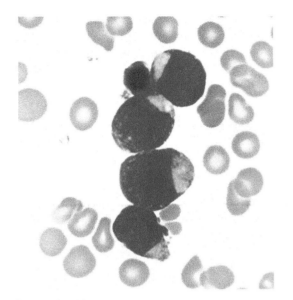

Figure 94.2 MGG, ×1000.

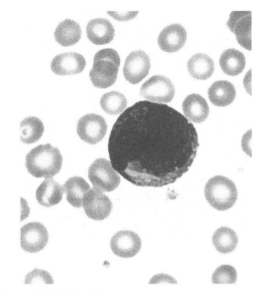

Figure 94.4 MGG, ×1000.

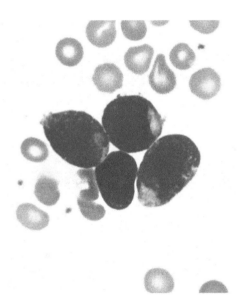

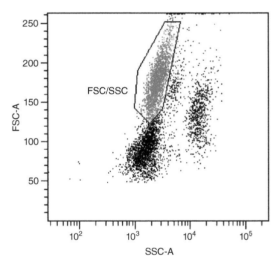

Figure 94.5 FSC/SSC.

Figure 94.3 MGG, ×1000.

differentiation as the cells were negative for CD14, CD15 and CD64.

The morphology was not in keeping with an ery-throleukaemia (which is a rare diagnosis in this age group) but megakaryoblastic differentiation was a possibility. Cyto-plasmic marking for CD41 and CD61 was partially positive in keeping with this diagnosis (Figures 94.8 and 94.9). The

expression of CD7 and CD10 in this case was therefore aberrant.

Histopathology

A small fragmented trephine specimen consisting largely of bone and cartilage was obtained. It was unsuitable for diag-nostic purposes.

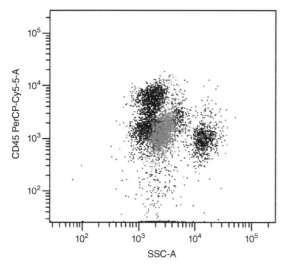

Figure 94.6 CD45/SSC.

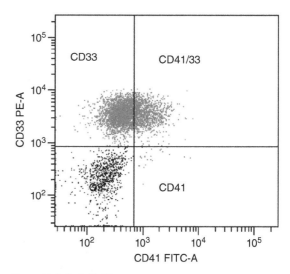

Figure 94.8 CD41/CD33.

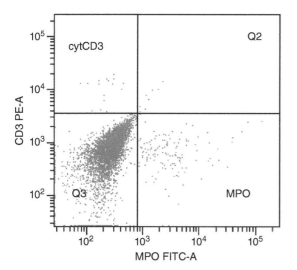

Figure 94.7 cCD3/MPO.

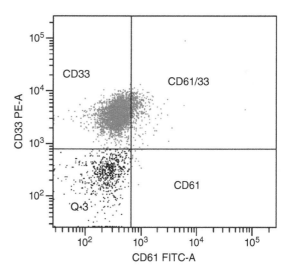

Figure 94.9 CD61/CD33.

Cytogenetics

A t(1;22)(p13;q13) translocation was identified in a 46,XX female. No trisomy 21 was seen.

Discussion

In the adult population megakaryoblastic leukaemia most often occurs as a transformation of a pre-existing myeloproliferative neoplasm. In children the disease occurs *de novo* and often presents as an infantile leukaemia particularly in those with Down syndrome (1) or in young children without Down syndrome in association with t(1;22)(p13;q13). The diagnosis can present some difficulty in terms of morphology and immunophenotype as myeloid lineage-specific markers may be absent. The presence of a recurring cytogenetic translocation, as in this case, is highly informative and supports the diagnosis. Morphologically megakaryoblasts can have a varied appearance, from large undifferentiated blast cells at one extreme to blasts resembling immature micromegakaryocytes with cytoplasmic blebbing at the other. The morphology in this patient with prominent paranuclear pallor is quite unusual. Diagnosis by immunophenotyping can also present some difficulty as cases are MPO$^-$ and often CD34$^-$, show varying degrees of CD13 and CD33 positivity and commonly displaying aberrant expression of CD7. Expression of CD10 is seen in some cases. An immunophenotypic diagnosis relies on the demonstration of cytoplasmic CD41 or CD61 expression. These antigens are also expressed on the cell membrane but we prefer to demonstrate them in the cytoplasm as platelet adherence to blasts can cause false positive results with blast cells that are not megakaryoblasts.

A number of cytogenetic abnormalities have been described in childhood megakaryoblastic leukaemia (2) but t(1;22)(p13;q13), generating a *RBM15-MKL1* fusion gene, is particularly characteristic of this disease affecting non-Down syndrome patients under 3 years. These patients generally respond well to chemotherapy with a long disease-free survival.

Final diagnosis

Infantile acute megakaryoblastic leukaemia with t(1;22)(p13;q13).

References

1 Hama, A., Yagasaki, H., Takahashi, Y. *et al.* (2008) Acute megakaryoblastic leukaemia (AMKL) in children: a comparison of AMKL with and without Down syndrome. *British Journal of Haematology*, **140** (5), 552–561. PubMed PMID: 18275433.

2 Hama, A., Muramatsu, H., Makishima, H. *et al.* (2012) Molecular lesions in childhood and adult acute megakaryoblastic leukaemia. *British Journal of Haematology*, **156** (3), 316–325. PubMed PMID: 22122069.

95

Case 95

A 53-years-old female attended her GP because of fatigue and easy bruising. Prior medical history was unremarkable. An FBC was taken.

Laboratory data

FBC: Hb 69 g/L, WBC 11.4×10^9/L (neutrophils 7.1×10^9/L) and platelets 36×10^9/L.

Coagulation screen: normal.

U&Es, LFTs and bone profile: normal.

Blood film

This showed profoundly dysplastic neutrophils with hypogranularity and abnormal nuclear segmentation together with blasts, some of which were granular (Figures 95.1–95.5). There were some giant platelets (Figure 95.2). Nucleated red cells were frequent with some showing dysplastic features (Figure 95.6).

Flow cytometry (peripheral blood)

Due to their hypogranularity, neutrophils were impossible to separate from blast cells which were superimposed using a FSC/SSC analysis (Figure 95.7, red events). CD45^{dim} CD10$^-$ blasts (blue events) were easily separated from CD45$^+$ CD10$^+$ neutrophils however (green events, Figures 95.8 and 95.9), with back gating highlighting the original juxtaposition of these cells on FSC/SSC (Figure 95.10). The full myeloblast phenotype (using CD45^{dim} gating) was: CD34$^-$, CD117$^+$, CD13$^+$, CD15$^+$, CD33$^+$, MPO$^+$ and HLA-DR$^-$.

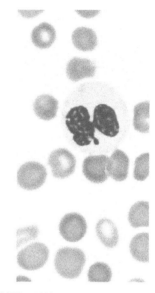

Figure 95.1 MGG, ×1000.

Bone marrow aspirate

Profound trilineage dysplasia was present, with 34% myeloblasts.

Cytogenetic analysis

46,XX. Normal female karyotype.

Molecular studies

NPM1 mutation and *FLT3* ITD positive.

Practical Flow Cytometry in Haematology: 100 Worked Examples, First Edition. Mike Leach, Mark Drummond, Allyson Doig, Pam McKay, Bob Jackson and Barbara J. Bain.
© 2015 John Wiley & Sons, Ltd. Published 2015 by John Wiley & Sons, Ltd.

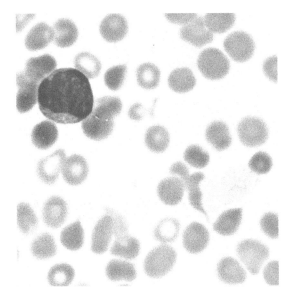

Figure 95.2 MGG, ×1000.

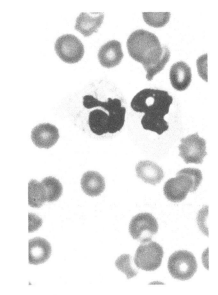

Figure 95.4 MGG, ×1000.

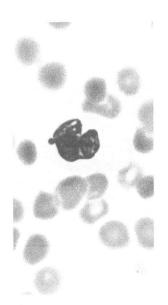

Figure 95.3 MGG, ×1000.

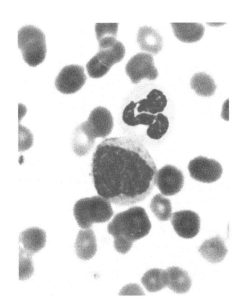

Figure 95.5 MGG, ×1000.

Discussion

This case is a good illustration of the importance of full cytogenetic and molecular profiling. Initial morphological assessment noted striking dysplastic features, raising legitimate initial concern with regards the potential presence of poor risk, myelodysplasia-related cytogenetic abnormalities

in a relatively young patient. Cytogenetic analysis was however normal; indeed conventional chromosome banding techniques fail to demonstrate a cytogenetic abnormality in approximately 50% of AML patients (so called cytogenetically normal AML, or CN-AML). There is great heterogeneity of clinical outcome within this group of patients and much of this is now known to be due to the

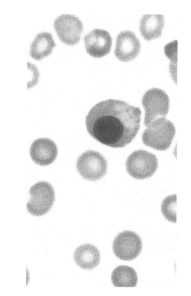

Figure 95.6 MGG, ×1000.

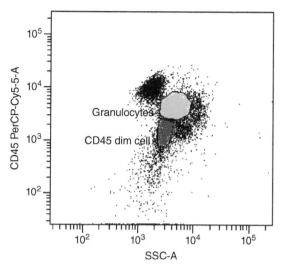

Figure 95.8 CD45/SSC.

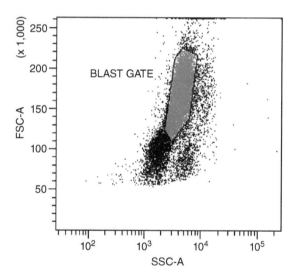

Figure 95.7 FSC/SSC basic.

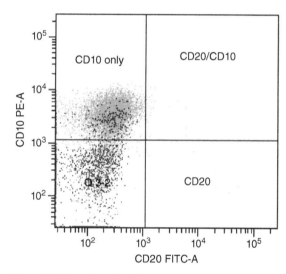

Figure 95.9 CD10/CD20 from blast gate.

presence of particular mutations. In particular, mutations in *NPM1* and *CEBPA* appear to confer a good outcome, whereas *FLT3* internal tandem duplication (ITD) is associated with a poor outcome due to high risk of relapse. It should be noted that combinations of mutations are possible, appearing to confer an intermediate prognosis (e.g. *NPM1* and *FLT3* ITD, detected in approximately 17–18% of CN-AML) (1, 2). Particular phenotypes may be associated with some of these abnormalities, in particular the association of *NPM1*

mutation with myelomonocytic or monocytic morphology and low CD34 expression and also cup-like morphology (+/− *FLT3* ITD, see Case 89).

Integrating results of molecular typing into clinical treatment pathways, particularly with regards prognostic scoring, is important. The European Leukaemia Net has incorporated *FLT3* ITD, *NPM1* and *CEBPA* mutations together with conventional cytogenetic risk groups to generate a proposed standardized reporting system (2). Historical prognostic parameters that may retain validity in the molecular era

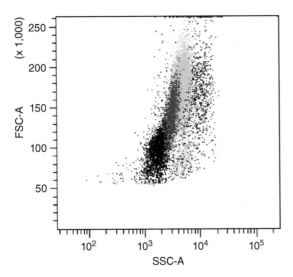

Figure 95.10 FSC/SSC back gated from CD45 plot.

(such as age, performance status and white cell count), should not be ignored however, and a recent publication has integrated these three clinical variables with mutation status to generate three risk groups for CN-AML (low, intermediate and high risk with 5-year survival rates of 74%, 28% and 3% respectively) (3). It seems highly likely that such scores will prove useful for future risk-adapted patient management.

Final diagnosis

Acute myeloid leukaemia with *NPM1* mutation and *FLT3* ITD.

References

1 Dohner, K., Schlenk, R.F., Habdank, M. *et al.* (2005) Mutant nucleophosmin (NPM1) predicts favorable prognosis in younger adults with acute myeloid leukemia and normal cytogenetics: interaction with other gene mutations. *Blood*, **106** (12), 3740–3746.

2 Dohner, H., Estey, E.H., Amadori, S. *et al.* (2010) Diagnosis and management of acute myeloid leukemia in adults: recommendations from an international expert panel, on behalf of the European LeukemiaNet. *Blood*, **115** (3), 453–474.

3 Pastore, F., Dufour, A., Benthaus, T. *et al.* (2014) Combined molecular and clinical prognostic index for relapse and survival in cytogenetically normal acute myeloid leukemia. *Journal of Clinical Oncology*, **32** (15), 1586–1594.

96

Case 96

A 67-year-old man was referred by the general medical team on account of splenomegaly and mild peripheral blood cytopenias. He was essentially asymptomatic and these findings had become apparent following clinical examination at the hypertension clinic. There was no palpable lymphadenopathy.

Laboratory data

FBC: Hb 134 g/L, WBC 2.4 × 10⁹/L (neutrophils 1.0 × 10⁹/L, lymphocytes 1.1 × 10⁹/L, monocytes 0.1 × 10⁹/L) and platelets 88 × 10⁹/L.

$$FBC: Hb\ 134\,g/L,\ WBC\ 2.4 \times 10^9/L$$

U&Es, LFTs and bone profile: normal.

Immunoglobulins: normal with no paraprotein.

Blood film

This showed a population of medium to large lymphoid cells with prominent pale blue cytoplasm with irregular frond-like margins. These cells had the typical morphology of hairy cells (Figures 96.1 and 96.2).

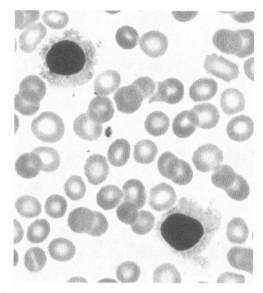

Figure 96.1 MGG, ×1000.

Flow cytometry (peripheral blood)

Peripheral blood was examined using a CD2 versus CD19 analysis. This identified a significant B-cell excess (T cells 14% and B cells 35% of leucocytes) and these were therefore the target of subsequent analysis. The B cells showed a mature pan-B phenotype, CD19⁺, CD20^{bright}, FMC7⁺, HLA-DR⁺, CD79b⁺, CD22⁺ and CD23^{dim} but without expression of CD5 or CD10. The B cells were surface kappa^{strong} restricted.

Additionally they expressed CD11c, CD25, CD103 and CD123 confirming a diagnosis of hairy cell leukaemia (hairy cell score 4/4).

Histopathology

The marrow trephine biopsy sections had a cellularity of approximately 50% (Figure 96.3) with an interstitial infiltrate of medium sized lymphoid cells that contrasted with the erythroid precursors with their more densely staining nuclei (Figure 96.4). The voluminous hairy cell cytoplasm generates space between the nuclei of individual cells, which is a prominent feature in trephine biopsy sections.

Practical Flow Cytometry in Haematology: 100 Worked Examples, First Edition. Mike Leach, Mark Drummond, Allyson Doig, Pam McKay, Bob Jackson and Barbara J. Bain.
© 2015 John Wiley & Sons, Ltd. Published 2015 by John Wiley & Sons, Ltd.

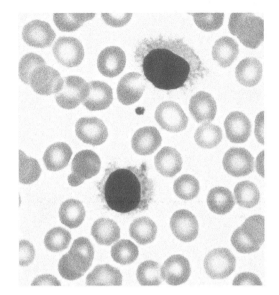

Figure 96.2 MGG, ×1000.

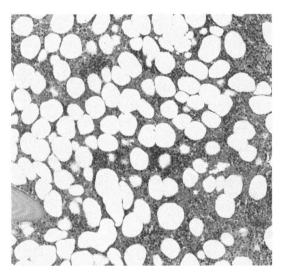

Figure 96.3 H&E, ×40.

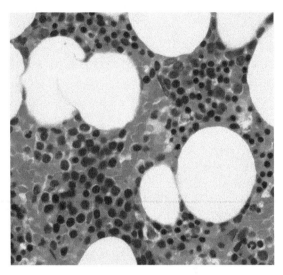

Figure 96.4 H&E, ×400.

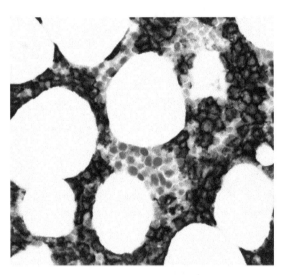

Figure 96.5 CD20, ×400.

The immunohistochemical profile was typical for hairy cell leukaemia showing positivity for CD20, CD11c, CD72 (DBA44), TRAP and annexin 1 with notable interstitial reticulin deposition (Figures 96.5–96.10).

Discussion

This patient had a classical presentation of hairy cell leukaemia. This rare B-cell disorder, which is more common in males, is largely asymptomatic until the later stages when cytopenias cause symptoms or result in opportunistic infections. Splenomegaly is almost universal and contributes to the cytopenias. Bone marrow infiltration can be subtle in

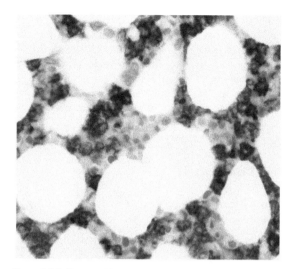

Figure 96.6 CD11c, ×400.

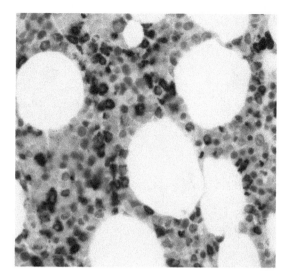

Figure 96.8 TRAP, ×400.

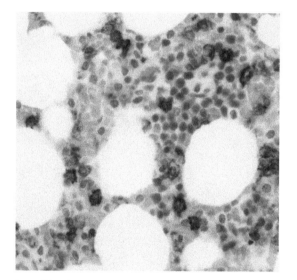

Figure 96.7 CD72, ×400.

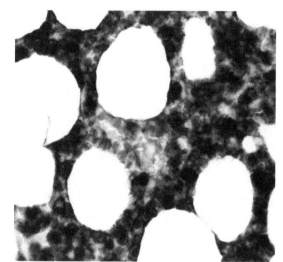

Figure 96.9 Annexin 1, ×400.

the early stages and need immunohistochemistry to outline the disease population. Note that in this case the overall trephine biopsy cellularity was only 50% and erythroid activity was well preserved so the hypersplenism must have contributed substantially to the peripheral blood cytopenias. The diagnosis should be straightforward as long as all features of the presentation are considered, including the peripheral blood film, which should be closely examined

(compare with Case 6). Otherwise the diagnosis can be missed or delayed. Note also the expected monocytopenia in this patient, which can be diagnostically useful. Although annexin 1 positivity in paraffin-embedded sections is highly specific for a diagnosis of HCL, it must be stressed that the antibody is less useful in early stages of involvement when interpretation is hampered by the large number of immunoreactive background myeloid precursors.

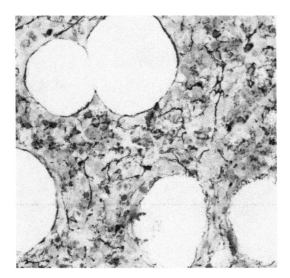

Figure 96.10 Reticulin, ×400.

With current treatment, hairy cell leukaemia carries an excellent prognosis with a near normal age-corrected life expectancy. The diagnosis is often missed at the first opportunity, due to the lack of symptoms and indolent disease progression. As in many clinical circumstances, careful scrutiny of the peripheral blood film, in the knowledge of the medical history and full blood count, can very be informative.

Final diagnosis

Hairy cell leukaemia.

97

Case 97

A 55-year-old man presented with fatigue, night sweats and a dry cough. He had no past medical history of note and physical examination was unremarkable.

Laboratory data

FBC: Hb 102 g/L, WBC 17.1 × 10^9/L (neutrophils 5.7 × 10^9/L, lymphocytes 5.5 × 10^9/L, monocytes 4.4 × 10^9/L, myeloid precursors 1.7 × 10^9/L), nucleated red blood cells 2.44 × 10^9/L and platelets 35 × 10^9/L.

U&Es, LFTs and bone profile were normal except albumin 30 g/L. LDH was 560 U/L.

Blood film

This showed an abnormal population of large lymphoid cells with folded, cleft and indented nuclei, which had hyperchromatic chromatin and prominent nucleoli (Figures 97.1–97.3). There was also a substantial

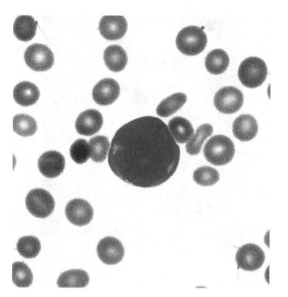

Figure 97.1 MGG, ×1000.

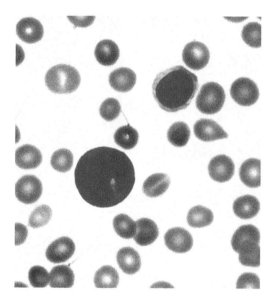

Figure 97.2 MGG, ×1000.

Practical Flow Cytometry in Haematology: 100 Worked Examples, First Edition. Mike Leach, Mark Drummond, Allyson Doig, Pam McKay, Bob Jackson and Barbara J. Bain.
© 2015 John Wiley & Sons, Ltd. Published 2015 by John Wiley & Sons, Ltd.

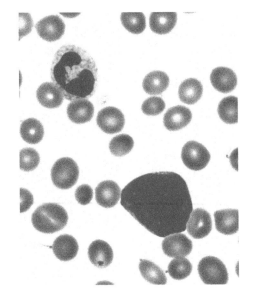

Figure 97.3 MGG, ×1000.

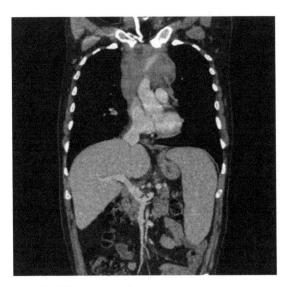

Figure 97.5 CT, anteroposterior.

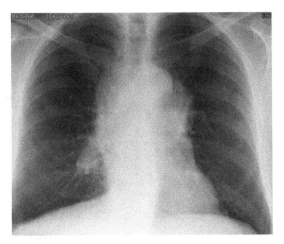

Figure 97.4 CXR.

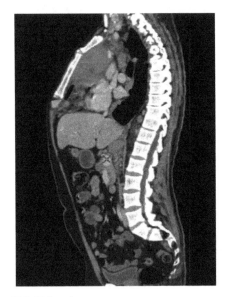

Figure 97.6 CT, lateral.

population of nucleated red cells and a left shift in the myeloid series.

Imaging

In view of the troublesome cough, a CXR was performed (Figure 97.4). This showed a prominent mediastinal mass which prompted CT imaging to better define the lesion (Figures 97.5–97.7). This confirmed a bulky anterior mediastinal mass with encroachment on the major vessels. In addition, scanning of the abdomen identified a mass infiltrating the left kidney (arrow, Figure 97.8).

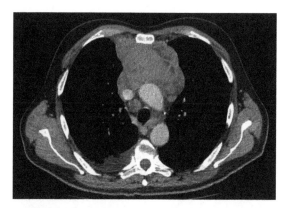

Figure 97.7 CT, upper chest.

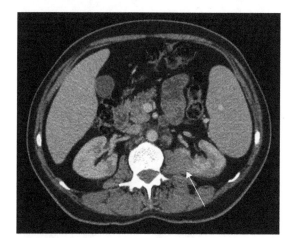

Figure 97.8 CT, abdomen.

Marrow aspirate

These findings were in keeping with an aggressive neoplastic process with involvement of blood, mediastinum and kidney.

Flow cytometry (bone marrow aspirate)

The aspirate was heavily involved by cells similar to those described in peripheral blood. These cells showed a heterogeneous CD45 expression varying between that seen in acute leukaemia and approaching that of normal lymphocytes (Figure 97.9). These cells were shown to be of T-cell lineage expressing cCD3, CD5, CD7 and TdT

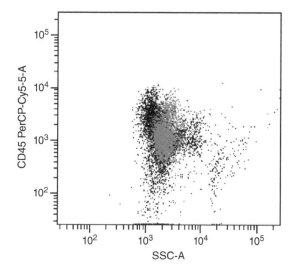

Figure 97.9 CD45/SSC.

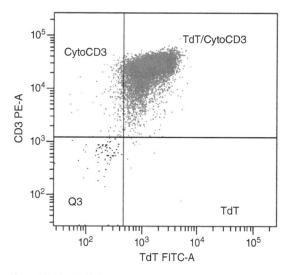

Figure 97.10 cCD3/TdT.

(Figures 97.10–97.12) with CD1a indicating a cortical T-cell acute lymphoblastic leukaemia. There was aberrant CD10 expression (Figure 97.11).

Bone marrow trephine biopsy

The trephine biopsy was reported independently. This is good practice in terms of approaching the pathology without

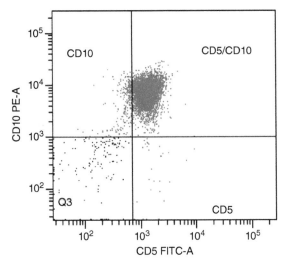

Figure 97.11 CD5/CD10.

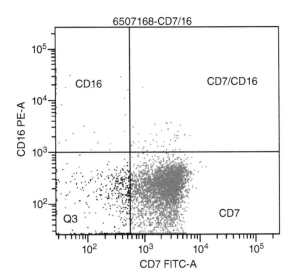

Figure 97.12 CD7/CD16.

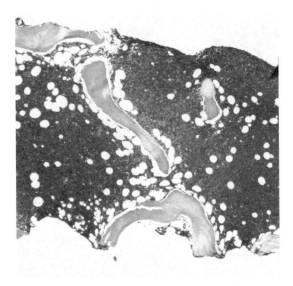

Figure 97.13 H&E, ×40.

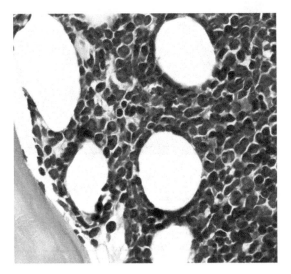

Figure 97.14 H&E, ×400.

preconceived ideas regarding the diagnosis. Once a diagnosis is formulated it is important to see how this correlates with the clinical presentation, flow cytometric studies and cytogenetic and molecular analyses. The trephine biopsy specimen was heavily infiltrated by a lymphoid tumour expressing CD3, TdT, CD10 and CD1a (Figures 97.13–97.18). The phenotype was identical to that noted using flow cytometry. The tumour was inducing marrow fibrosis at WHO grade 1–2 (Figure 97.19).

Cytogenetic analysis

Standard metaphase preparations failed but FISH studies indicated near tetrasomy.

Discussion

The presentation here is typical of a cortical type (CD1a⁺) T-cell acute lymphoblastic leukaemia/lymphoma.

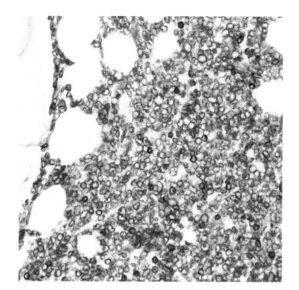

Figure 97.15 CD3, ×200.

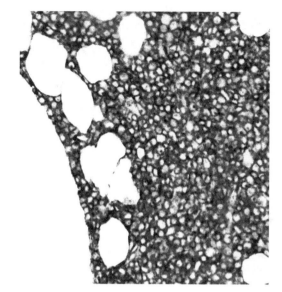

Figure 97.17 CD10, ×200.

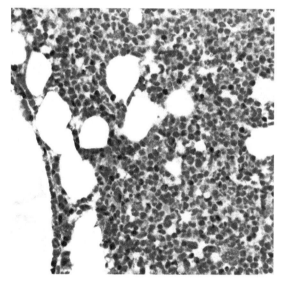

Figure 97.16 TdT, ×200

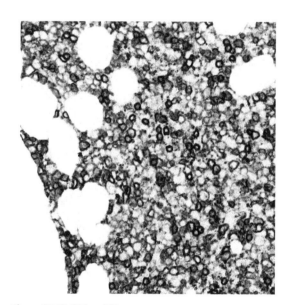

Figure 97.18 CD1a, ×200.

Importantly the disease was showing leukaemic (bone marrow and blood involvement) and lymphomatous (mediastinal and renal tumour) characteristics. Cortical type T-lymphoblastic lymphoma frequently generates an anterior mediastinal mass; the cell of origin is understood to be a thymic T-cell (thymocyte) that acquires a mutation at the point of differentiation to T-helper and T-suppressor cells. It therefore has a relatively unique phenotype in expressing

CD1a, this being a transient characteristic of cells at this maturation stage. Some clones (in different patients) show differentiation toward CD4, some toward CD8 and some co-express the two antigens.

The prognosis in T-lymphoblastic leukaemia/lymphoma is determined by patient age and fitness, disease behaviour and cytogenetic data. This is a highly curable tumour in

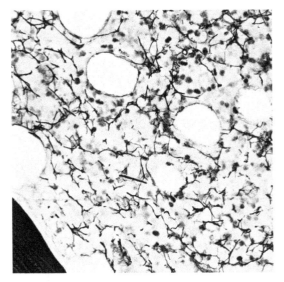

Figure 97.19 Reticulin, ×200.

childhood (though see Case 70) but the prognosis is mixed in adults as the treatment is toxic and protracted and often difficult to deliver. The presence of a near tetrasomy karyotype in this case alongside an aggressive clinical presentation with multiple sites of extranodal disease was felt to be a poor prognostic indicator. Complete remission was achieved with ALL-type induction chemotherapy with clearance of marrow disease and resolution of the mediastinal and renal tumours. A sibling donor was available so an allogeneic transplant was performed in first complete remission. The patient remains well at follow up some 18 months later.

Final diagnosis

Cortical type T-cell lymphoblastic leukaemia/lymphoma.

98

Case 98

A 64-year-old man presented with a rapid onset of fever, night sweats and right flank pain. An infective aetiology was suspected.

Laboratory investigations

FBC: Hb 120 g/L, WBC 7.5 $\times 10^9$/L (neutrophils 4.0 $\times 10^9$/L, lymphocytes 2.0 $\times 10^9$/L) and platelets 164 $\times 10^9$/L.

U&Es: creatinine 146 μmol/L on admission rising within a few days to 522 μmol/L.

Bone profile: calcium 2.4 mmol/L, phosphate 1.8 mmol/L, ALP 185 U/L.

LFTs: normal except albumin 18 g/L. Urate was raised at 1.3 mmol/L.

LDH grossly elevated at 8554 U/L.

Blood film

The blood film was leucoerythroblastic but also showed small numbers of medium-sized undifferentiated cleft lymphoid cells (Figure 98.1); a proportion had vacuolation of the cytoplasm.

Imaging

Imaging was undertaken with some urgency to identify the cause of abdominal pain and to assess the kidneys. A CT scan showed diffuse thickening of the walls of the collecting system in the left kidney but no focal discrete mass and no evidence of hydronephrosis. In addition there was extensive abnormal perirenal shadowing and a large

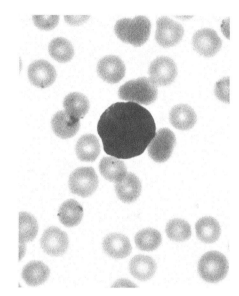

Figure 98.1 MGG, ×1000.

mass at the renal hilum encasing the renal vessels. There was lymphadenopathy in the mesenteric and para-aortic regions. While a biopsy of the perirenal mass was being planned a bone marrow aspiration and trephine biopsy were performed.

Bone marrow aspirate

The bone marrow aspirate showed an abnormal infiltrate of small, medium sized and large nucleolated lymphoid cells (Figures 98.2 and 98.3).

Practical Flow Cytometry in Haematology: 100 Worked Examples, First Edition. Mike Leach,
Mark Drummond, Allyson Doig, Pam McKay, Bob Jackson and Barbara J. Bain.
© 2015 John Wiley & Sons, Ltd. Published 2015 by John Wiley & Sons, Ltd.

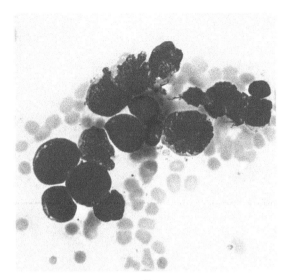

Figure 98.2 MGG, ×500.

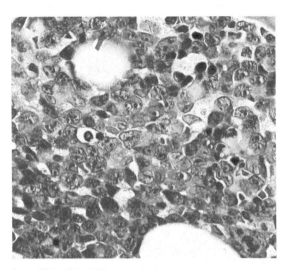

Figure 98.4 H&E, ×500.

keeping with a precursor neoplasm. Burkitt lymphoma, which was clinically suspected, would normally have a fully mature CD10$^+$, CD20$^+$, FMC7$^+$, Sig$^+$ phenotype (as well as somewhat different cytological features).

Histopathology

Bone marrow trephine biopsy: the trephine biopsy sections showed extensive diffuse involvement by pleomorphic blastoid lymphoid cells with intermediate to large vesicular nuclei with prominent nucleoli; little residual normal haemopoiesis was evident (Figure 98.4).

Core biopsy of the perirenal mass: this showed diffuse sheets of lymphoid cells, identical to those noted in the trephine biopsy sections, infiltrating adipose tissue (Figures 98.5 and 98.6). Areas of necrosis were present.

Immunohistochemistry demonstrated the cells to be positive for CD79a (Figure 98.7), CD20 weak/focal (Figure 98.8), CD10 (Figure 98.9), BCL2 (Figure 98.10), MUM1 (Figure 98.11), PAX5 and p53. The proliferation fraction was high at 90% (Figure 98.12).

The tumour cells were negative for CD5, CD138, CD30, cyclin D1, ALK1, TdT, CD23 and CD21.

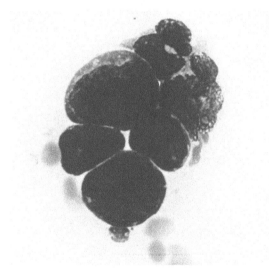

Figure 98.3 MGG, ×1000.

Flow cytometry

Studies on peripheral blood and bone marrow identified the abnormal cells as clonal B cells expressing surface kappa^{dim}, CD20^{dim}, CD10, CD38, HLA-DR, CD22 and CD79b whilst FMC7 was negative. This was therefore an aggressive CD10$^+$ B-cell disorder but the phenotype was unusual in that the presence of surface immunoglobulin suggested a mature neoplasm whilst the absence of FMC7 and partial positivity for CD20 would have been more in

FISH and cytogenetics

Rearrangement of *BCL6*, *BCL2* and *MYC* was detected by FISH studies on the core biopsy specimen. Classical

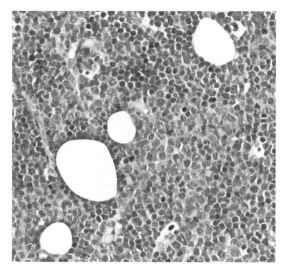

Figure 98.5 H&E, ×200.

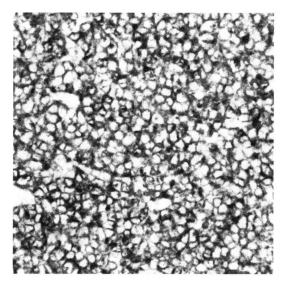

Figure 98.7 CD79a, ×200.

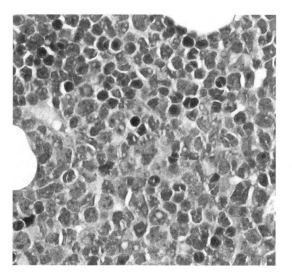

Figure 98.6 H&E, ×400.

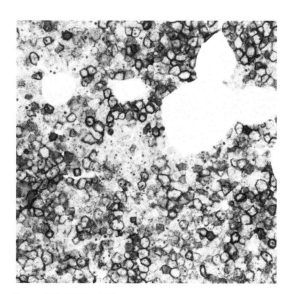

Figure 98.8 CD20, ×200.

cytogenetic studies performed on the bone marrow aspirate identified a triple translocation, t(8;14;18)(q24;q32;q22), involving *MYC* (8q24), *IGH* (14q32) and *BCL2* (18q22).

Discussion

This patient had a highly proliferative CD10$^+$ B-cell tumour with a rapid onset of symptoms due to extranodal

tissue invasion with involvement of the kidneys, bone marrow and blood. There was also a high serum LDH and features of spontaneous tumour-lysis. A diagnosis of B-lymphoblastic lymphoma was excluded by the presence of surface immunoglobulin and lack of TdT expression. Despite some morphological similarities, this is not classical Burkitt lymphoma (BL) as weak CD20 and loss of FMC7 are not typical and the proliferation fraction, although high, was not as high as expected in BL. More importantly the tumour

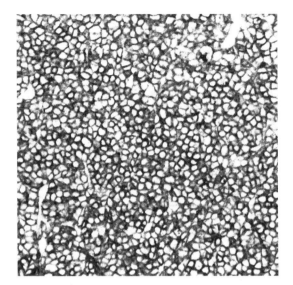

Figure 98.9 CD10, ×200.

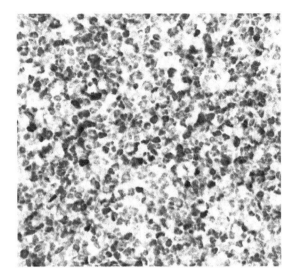

Figure 98.11 MUM1, ×200.

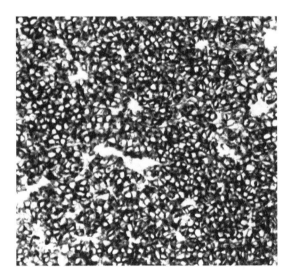

Figure 98.10 BCL2, ×200.

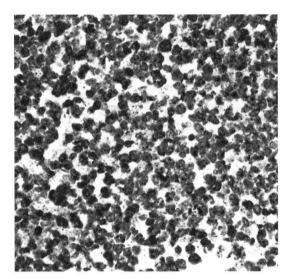

Figure 98.12 Ki-67, ×200.

expressed BCL2 protein which is characteristically negative in BL. Although a translocation involving *MYC* is typically found in BL this is usually a single translocation. This case was found to have a complex three-way translocation involving *MYC*, *IGH* and *BCL2* genes. BCL2 expression in this case is likely due to juxtaposition of the promoter region of the *IGH* gene (14q32) and the *BCL2* locus (18q21) resulting in upregulation of the latter. BCL6 protein was expressed and *BCL6* (3q27) translocations are found commonly in DLBCL and occasionally in follicular lymphoma. As this case has

morphological and genetic features of both DLBCL and BL it is best described, using the WHO terminology, as a B-cell lymphoma, unclassifiable, with features intermediate between diffuse large B-cell lymphoma (DLBCL) and Burkitt lymphoma (BL).

The optimal treatment of this lymphoma subtype, sometimes referred to as a double hit lymphoma (involvement of *MYC* and *BCL2*), or a triple hit lymphoma (involvement of *MYC*, *BCL2* and *BCL6* as in this case), is unknown. Results with standard R-CHOP therapy are poor and primary refractoriness to chemotherapy is common (1). This patient received rasburicase and intravenous fluids in addition to intensive chemotherapy (two cycles of CODOX-M-IVAC plus rituximab). Despite an early response the disease progressed before planned treatment was completed.

Final diagnosis

B-cell lymphoma, unclassifiable, with features intermediate between DLBCL and BL, with blood and bone marrow involvement.

Reference

1 Green, T. M., Young, K. H., Visco, C. *et al.* (2012) Immunohistochemical double-hit score is a strong predictor of outcome in patients with diffuse large B-cell lymphoma treated with rituximab plus cyclophosphamide, doxorubicin, vincristine, and prednisone. *Journal of Clinical Oncology*, **30** (**28**), 3460–3467. PubMed PMID: 22665537.

99

Case 99

A 12-year-old boy presented with a short history of abdominal pain, lethargy and vomiting. On examination he had a distended abdomen but no clear abdominal mass. Ultrasound examination showed an abnormal but poorly defined mass in the right iliac fossa and on CXR there was a large right pleural effusion.

Laboratory data

FBC: Hb 130 g/L, WBC 12×10^9/L (neutrophils 8×10^9/L, lymphocytes 2.1×10^9/L, monocytes 0.8×10^9/L) and platelets 312×10^9/L.

U&Es: Na 135 mmol/l, K 4.2 mmol/L, bicarbonate 13 mmol/L, urea 11.9 mmol/L, creatinine 65 μmol/L.

CRP 293 mg/L. Urate 1.36 mmol/L.

Bone profile: calcium 2.48 mmol/L, phosphate 1.41 mmol/L, ALP 85 U/L.

LFTs: normal except albumin 29 g/L.

Serum LDH 3075 U/L.

Blood film

The film appeared normal without leucoerythroblastosis or circulating abnormal cells.

CT imaging

There was a poorly defined right flank mass measuring 8.6 cm ×8.1 cm ×7.3 cm (Figure 99.1, arrow). The mass was surrounded by small bowel allowing no suitable percutaneous

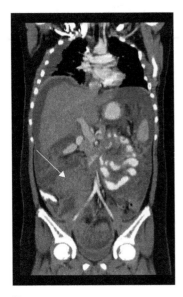

Figure 99.1 CT.

window for biopsy. The bowel appeared thickened and infiltrated, the spleen was enlarged and the kidneys showed patchy enhancement in keeping with infiltration by tumour (Figure 99.2, arrows). The peritoneum appeared grossly thickened (long arrow) and there was extensive ascites (short arrow) (Figure 99.3). There were no significantly enlarged cervical, axillary or inguinal lymph nodes suitable for biopsy.

The patient had a right chest drain inserted and pleural fluid was taken for analysis. Under the same anaesthetic a bone marrow aspirate and trephine biopsy were taken and a mini-laparoscopy was performed to acquire an omental biopsy.

Practical Flow Cytometry in Haematology: 100 Worked Examples, First Edition. Mike Leach, Mark Drummond, Allyson Doig, Pam McKay, Bob Jackson and Barbara J. Bain.
© 2015 John Wiley & Sons, Ltd. Published 2015 by John Wiley & Sons, Ltd.

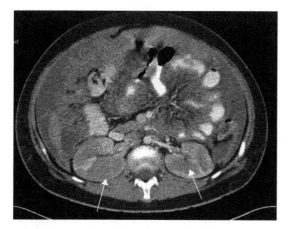

Figure 99.2 CT.

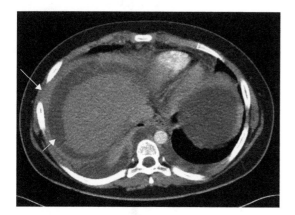

Figure 99.3 CT.

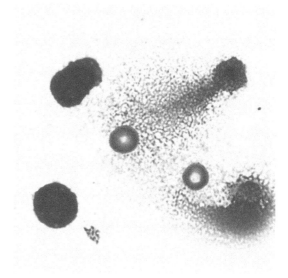

Figure 99.4 MGG, ×1000.

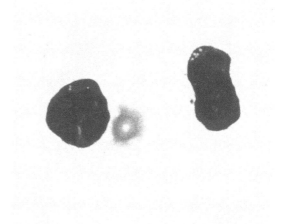

Flow cytometry (pleural fluid)

The pleural fluid was cellular (WBC 34×10^9/L) with a high protein content and high LDH. A population of large nucleolated lymphoid cells with basophilic cytoplasm and vacuoles was present (Figures 99.4–99.7). There was considerable cell debris and mitotic figures were seen (Figures 99.4 and 99.7, respectively). The findings were those of a high-grade lymphoma and the features would be consistent with Burkitt lymphoma.

The large lymphoid cells were characterised further by immunophenotyping, gating on the CD19+ cells that appeared to be in excess. The CD19bright cells were selected and these showed a CD20+, CD10+, CD38+, HLA-DR+, FMC7dim CD22+, CD79b+, surface kappadim phenotype (Figures 99.8–99.10).

This mature CD10+ B-cell phenotype was consistent with Burkitt lymphoma as suggested by the clinical presentation.

Figure 99.5 MGG, ×1000.

Clonally-restricted surface light chains and FMC7 are normally expressed in Burkitt lymphoma though surface Ig is sometimes lost from cells in effusions and ascites.

Bone marrow aspirate and trephine biopsy

These both showed reactive features but without a neoplastic infiltrate.

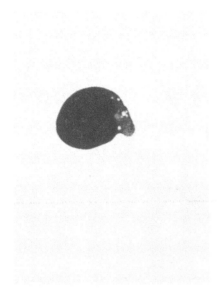

Figure 99.6 MGG, ×1000.

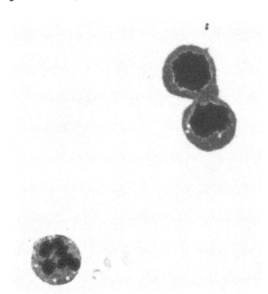

Figure 99.7 MGG, ×1000.

Omental biopsy

The omental fat showed extensive infiltration by a monotonous population of medium-sized tumour cells. They had hyperchromatic nuclei with multiple mainly peripheral small nucleoli and scanty cytoplasm (Figures 99.11 and 99.12). There were scattered tingible body macrophages giving rise to a starry sky appearance. Scattered mitoses

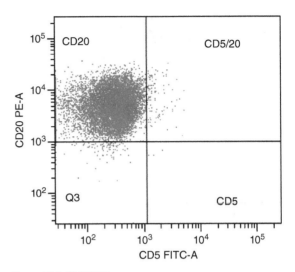

Figure 99.8 CD5/CD20.

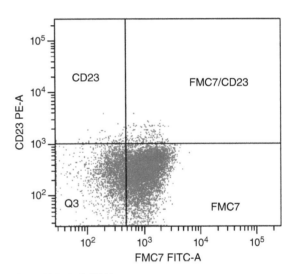

Figure 99.9 FMC7/CD23.

and frequent apoptoses were seen. Immunohistochemistry showed tumour positivity for CD45, CD20 (Figure 99.13), BCL6 and CD10 (Figure 99.14). BCL2 (Figure 99.15) and TdT were negative. The proliferation fraction was above 95% (Ki-67, Figure 99.16).

Cytogenetic analysis

Standard metaphase preparations showed t(8;14)(q24;q32).

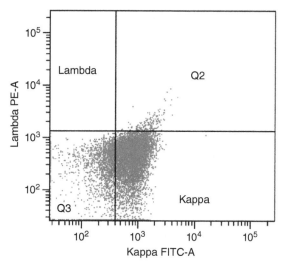

Figure 99.10 Kappa/lambda.

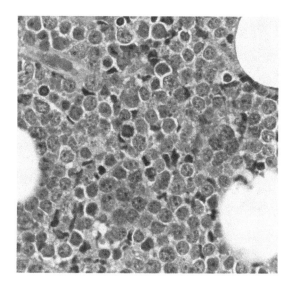

Figure 99.12 H&E, ×400.

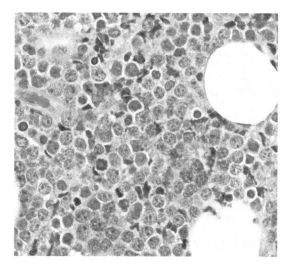

Figure 99.11 H&E, ×400.

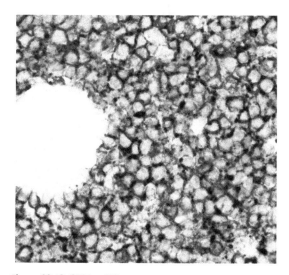

Figure 99.13 CD20, ×400.

FISH studies

These confirmed a *MYC-IGH* translocation.

Discussion

This patient presented with a high grade B-cell neoplasm with extensive bulky extra-nodal disease, advanced stage, high serum LDH and laboratory features of spontaneous tumour-lysis. A Burkitt lymphoma should always be suspected with this constellation of features. Analysis of pleural fluid by morphology and immunophenotyping supported this diagnosis, which was later confirmed on omental biopsy and cytogenetic studies. The rapidity with which flow cytometric analysis can be performed makes it a very useful early investigation when a formal tissue biopsy needs careful planning and the assistance of a surgeon. It allows an early management plan to be initiated that is clearly important in this emergency scenario.

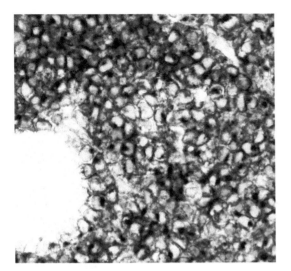

Figure 99.14 CD10, ×400.

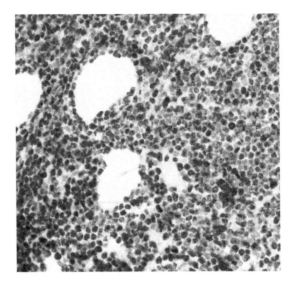

Figure 99.16 Ki-67, ×200.

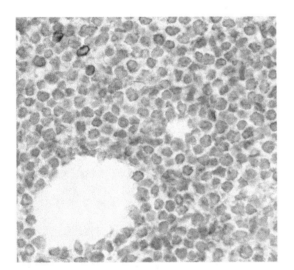

Figure 99.15 BCL2, ×400.

Burkitt lymphoma is one of the most aggressive B-cell tumours encountered in haematology practice. Patients typically present with a short history, marked B symptoms and rapidly evolving tumours that often involve multiple extranodal sites. The terminal ileum often appears to be the primary site of disease. A high serum LDH is almost universal and tumour-lysis is common as a result of spontaneous apoptosis seen in this highly proliferative tumour. Lymphoma cells have a mature CD10+ B-cell phenotype and express BCL6 but not BCL2. Cytogenetic studies should show the classic findings of t(8;14)(q24;q32) involving *MYC*

and *IGH* or one of the less common variant translocations t(2;8)(p12;q24) involving *IGK* and *MYC* or t(8;22)(q24;q11) involving *IGL* and *MYC*. Additional cytogenetic abnormalities may occasionally be present but these tend to be associated with a less favourable outcome (1) the presence of complex abnormalities and in particular t(14;18) should lead to consideration of B-cell lymphoma, unclassifiable, intermediate between Burkitt lymphoma and diffuse large B-cell lymphoma. Burkitt lymphoma is an important disease to identify early as the early use of intense hydration with rasburicase together with appropriate chemotherapy regimens with rituximab can yield rapid clinical responses and a high probability of long-term survival.

Reference

1 Poirel, H. A., *et al.* (2009) Specific cytogenetic abnormalities are associated with a significantly inferior outcome in children and adolescents with mature B-cell non-Hodgkin's lymphoma: results of the FAB/LMB 96 international study. *Leukemia*, (2009) **23** (**2**), 323–331.

Final diagnosis

Burkitt lymphoma with multiple sites of extranodal disease but without bone marrow involvement.

100

Case 100

A 41-year-old man who had undergone a cadaveric renal transplant for renal failure due to systemic lupus erythematosus some 10 years earlier, presented with the acute onset of general debility, fever, anorexia and night sweats. His graft function was well preserved but his immunosuppressive medications, tacrolimus and low dose prednisolone, were still required.

Laboratory data

FBC: Hb 54 g/L, WBC 18.5×10^9/L, platelets 42×10^9/L.

U&Es: Na 136 mmol/L, K 4.1 mmol/L, urea 24.3 mmol/L, creatinine 371 μmol/L. Urate 1.25 mmol/L. CRP 136 mg/L. Lactate 11.1 mmol/L.

Bone profile: calcium 2.5 mmol/L, phosphate 2.5 mmol/L, ALP 74 U/L.

LFTs: AST 115 U/L, ALT 54 U/L, albumin 23 g/L, total protein 55 g/L.

Immunoglobulins: normal with no paraprotein.

Blood film

The leucocytosis was due to a population of large pleomorphic plasmacytoid cells with intensely blue cytoplasm and some vacuolation (Figures 100.1–100.4). The differential diagnosis lay between a plasma cell neoplasm and a high-grade lymphoma with plasmablastic morphology.

Flow cytometry (peripheral blood)

These large cells were gated using a variety of strategies including size on the FSC/SSC plot, CD45 expression and

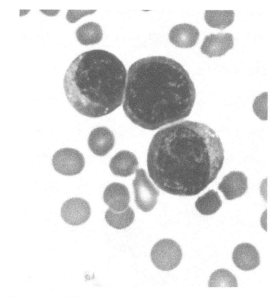

Figure 100.1 MGG, ×1000.

CD138 expression. Flow cytometry often comes to the rescue of even the most able morphologist, but not in this case. These large cells had a CD45$^+$, CD138^{dim}, CD38$^+$, HLA-DR$^+$ phenotype with absence of all B-cell, T-cell and myeloid lineage antigens. Weak and heterogeneous CD138 positivity was noted in the large cells but these did not show the strong discrete positivity typically seen in plasma cell neoplasms (Figure 100.5, P1, red events). The size of the malignant cells (P1, red events) can be appreciated in Figure 100.6. Clonality was demonstrated using cytoplasmic kappa/lambda; the tumour was lambda restricted (Figures 100.7 and 100.8).

Practical Flow Cytometry in Haematology: 100 Worked Examples, First Edition. Mike Leach, Mark Drummond, Allyson Doig, Pam McKay, Bob Jackson and Barbara J. Bain.
© 2015 John Wiley & Sons, Ltd. Published 2015 by John Wiley & Sons, Ltd.

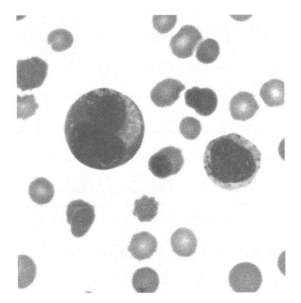

Figure 100.2 MGG, ×1000.

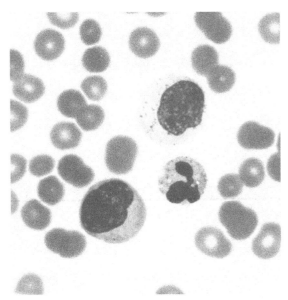

Figure 100.4 MGG, ×1000.

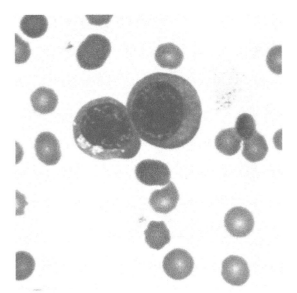

Figure 100.3 MGG, ×1000.

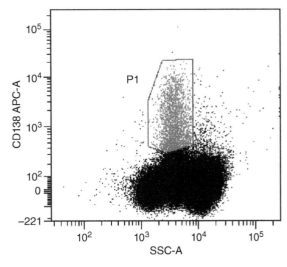

Figure 100.5 CD138/SSC.

Bone marrow aspirate

The marrow aspirate was heavily involved by the large cells described above. The cytoplasmic vacuolation was more prominent and some cells had multiple nuclei (Figures 100.9–100.12). We were curious as to the origin of these cells and were concerned that this could represent an immunosuppression-related neoplasm, possibly a plasmablastic lymphoma.

Histopathology

Examination of bone marrow trephine biopsy sections with a carefully chosen immunohistochemistry panel was

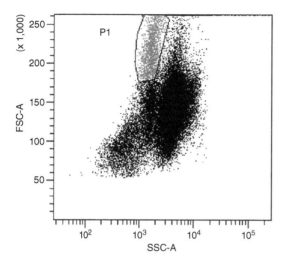

Figure 100.6 FSC/SSC.

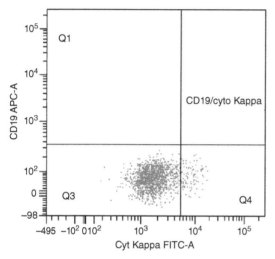

Figure 100.7 CD19/cytoplasmic kappa.

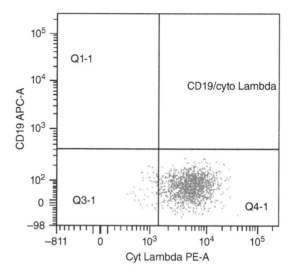

Figure 100.8 CD19/cytoplasmic lambda.

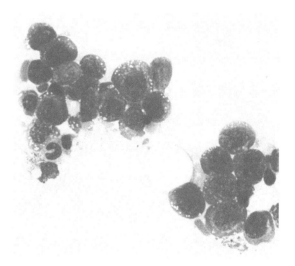

Figure 100.9 MGG, ×500.

highly informative in this case. The H&E-stained sections showed a clear interstitial infiltrate of large pleomorphic neoplastic cells (Figure 100.13) which had variable CD138 expression (Figure 100.14) but no CD20 or CD30 expression (Figures 100.15 and 100.16). This was therefore confirmed as a haemopoietic tumour with differentiation toward plasma cells albeit with high-grade behaviour. Staining for MUM1, which is expressed in post-germinal centre activated B-cell neoplasms and normal plasma cells, was positive (Figure 100.17). *In situ* hybridisation for EBV EBER was negative. Finally, ALK (anaplastic lymphoma kinase) was very strongly expressed in the tumour cell cytoplasm (Figure 100.18).

The findings therefore are of an aggressive haemopoietic neoplasm with immunoblastic/plasmablastic morphology, without B-lineage markers but with strong expression of ALK.

Cytogenetics

Metaphase preparations of cells from the marrow aspirate identified the following karyotype:

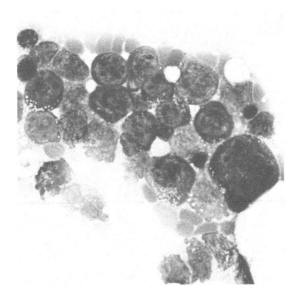

Figure 100.10 MGG, ×500.

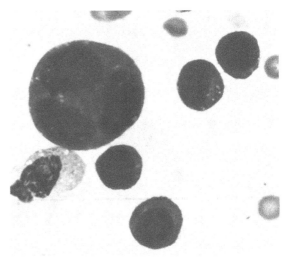

Figure 100.12 MGG, ×1000.

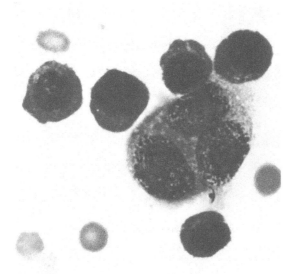

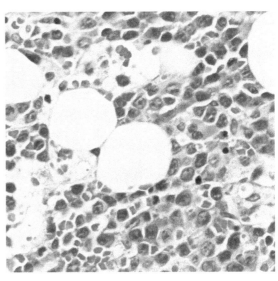

Figure 100.13 H&E, ×400.

Figure 100.11 MGG, ×1000.

46,XY,add(2)(p23),t(8;14)(q24;q32) plus complex additional non-specific abnormalities.

FISH studies

Studies using an *ALK* (2p23) break-apart probe showed no evidence of a translocation but the 2p23 locus was very

strongly amplified (Figure 100.19, long arrow). The normal copy of chromosome 2 showed two fusion signals on its short arm (one on each chromatid) as expected (Figure 100.19, short arrow).

Discussion

This is an interesting clinical case that generates a whole series of questions relating to the classification of disease

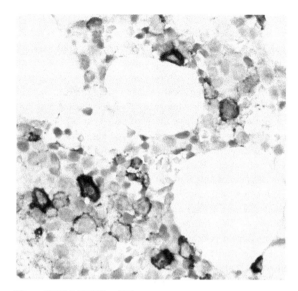

Figure 100.14 CD138, ×400.

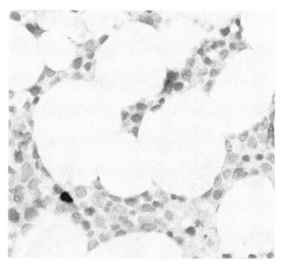

Figure 100.16 CD30, ×400.

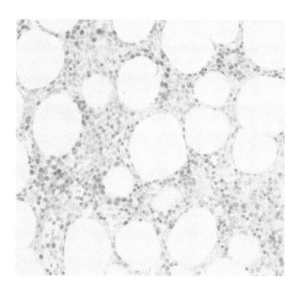

Figure 100.15 CD20, ×200.

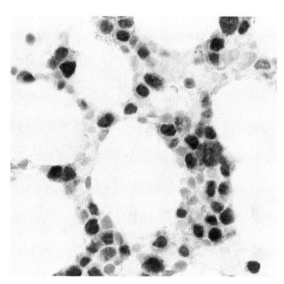

Figure 100.17 MUM1, ×400.

and the definition of the cell of origin. The clinical presentation had an acute onset with the rapid accumulation of immunoblastic cells in the peripheral blood and bone marrow in a patient on immunosuppressive therapy. The phenotype of the neoplastic cells most closely resembled that of plasma cells but was not typical of plasmablastic lymphoma as EBV EBER is expressed in the majority of such cases alongside CD30; whilst ALK typically is not expressed. The finding of strong ALK protein expression was

highly informative and this again illustrates the importance of correlation of multiple approaches to a diagnosis (morphology, immunophenotype, immunohistochemistry and cytogenetic/molecular profiling).

On identification of strong ALK expression in a lymphomatous infiltrate there are three entities to consider. Firstly, CD30+ ALK+ T/null anaplastic large cell lymphoma is a high-grade neoplasm composed of pleomorphic large cells. It usually has the classic t(2;5)(p23;q35) translocation rearranging *ALK* with the nucleophosmin gene (*NPM1*)

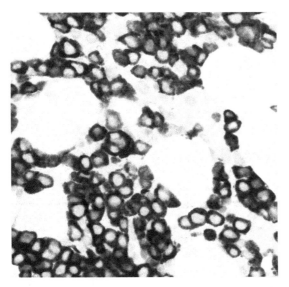

Figure 100.18 ALK, ×400.

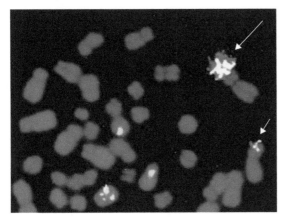

Figure 100.19 FISH for ALK at 2p23.

resulting in both nuclear and cytoplasmic expression of ALK protein. ALK⁺ ALCL is always positive for CD30 unlike the above case which was negative. The second lymphoma displaying ALK positivity is ALK-positive diffuse large B-cell lymphoma, which is characterised by immunoblastic/plasmablastic morphology, negativity for B- and T-lineage markers and CD30, expression of plasma cell markers and strong, usually granular cytoplasmic, positivity for ALK protein. This is most commonly associated with a t(2:17)(p23;q23) translocation generating an ALK-clathrin fusion protein. This abnormality was suspected but not confirmed in this case; overexpression of ALK protein seems to have been related to marked amplification of the *ALK* locus on the short arm of chromosome 2 rather than a translocation. Finally, a translocation involving *MYC* and *IGH* was identified and this may have contributed to the highly proliferative behaviour of this tumour though the exact role of this finding is not currently delineated in the biology of this very rare entity.

The third lymphoma with plasmablastic morphology that requires consideration is the EBV⁺ plasmablastic lymphoma associated, although not exclusively, with HIV infection. This lacks B-lineage markers but usually expresses CD30, is negative for ALK1 and is often positive for EBV EBER. Prognosis for patients with this rare tumour is very poor although some long survivals are recorded in patients with limited stage disease. This diagnosis is excluded in this case since EBER was negative. Our patient showed an extremely rapid clinical decline through a combination of disease proliferation, spontaneous tumour lysis and progressive renal failure and he died shortly after diagnosis. Our current understanding is that the described disease entity cannot be explained as a consequence of his post-transplant immunosuppressive therapy.

Final diagnosis

ALK-positive diffuse large B-cell lymphoma.

Antibodies Used in Immunohistochemistry Studies

Antibody	Target	Reactivity in tumours
ALK1 (CD246)	Recognises an epitope within the NPM-ALK chimeric and normal human ALK proteins. Expressed in some normal CNS cells.	Positivity is seen in a proportion of ALCL, ALK+DLBCL and inflammatory myofibroblastic tumour.
Annexin1	Annexin1 belongs to a family of calcium-dependent phospholipid-binding proteins and is involved in the innate and adaptive immune responses. It was found to be up-regulated in HCL by gene expression profiling. Stains myeloid precursors, macrophages and a subset of normal T cells.	Highly specific for HCL but is difficult to interpret in early marrow involvement as normal myeloid precursors stain strongly. Is negative in HCL-V, SMZL and other low-grade lymphomas.
BCL2	Integral inner mitochondrial protein which acts as an inhibitor of apoptosis. Expressed by many cells including normal B and T cells. Reactive germinal centre cells are negative.	Useful in distinguishing reactive from neoplastic follicles. Expressed by many lymphomas. Negative in the majority of BL. Also positive in many carcinomas.
BCL6	Zinc finger transcriptional repressor involved in B-cell activation and proliferation. Normally expressed within nuclei of germinal centre B cells.	Immunoreactivity is seen in the majority of FL and DLBCL, L&H cells of NLPHL and some T-cell lymphomas. Weak expression may be seen in a variety of other lymphomas.
Cam5.2	Identifies low-molecular-weight cytokeratins CK7 and CK8.	Stains a variety of epithelial cells and many but not all carcinomas.
CD1a	A non-polymorphic MHC class I-related cell surface glycoprotein normally expressed by medullary thymocytes and Langerhans cells	LCH and precursor-T-cell lymphoma. The lymphocytes in thymoma are positive for CD1a.
CD2	Transmembrane glycoprotein and pan-T-cell antigens expressed by almost all T lymphocytes and NK cells	Identifies precursor and mature T-cell lymphomas and NK-cell lymphomas.
CD3 epsilon	The antibody recognises the intracytoplasmic epsilon chain of CD3 which is present in all peripheral T cells, precursor T lymphocytes in the thymus and NK cells.	A useful pan-T-cell marker used in the diagnosis of T-cell lymphomas. NK-cell lymphomas are usually positive for CD3 epsilon (using immunohistochemistry) though the same cells are negative for surface CD3 when examined by flow cytometry.
CD4	A transmembrane glycoprotein which acts as a co-receptor in MHC class II-restricted antigen-mediated activation of T cells. Expressed by helper T cells, some suppressor/cytotoxic T cells, 60% of mature peripheral blood T lymphocytes, monocytes and Langerhans cells.	Used as part of a panel in subtyping of T-cell lymphomas particularly in the diagnosis of MF and AITL. Histiocytic and dendritic cells also stain strongly in histological sections, sometimes complicating interpretation.

Antibody	Target	Reactivity in tumours
CD5	A transmembrane glycoprotein involved in signal transduction. Expressed strongly by most T cells and by a small subset of normal B cells. Some epithelial cells may be positive.	This is a reliable pan-T-cell antigen, loss of which by a T-cell population is a strong indicator of neoplasia. Aberrant expression of CD5 is seen in B cells of CLL, MCL, 5% of DLBCL and in occasional MZL.
CD7	A membrane-bound glycoprotein which is the earliest T-cell antigen to be expressed and is found on most peripheral T and NK cells.	Used as pan-T-cell antigen in panels. Loss of CD7 expression, although seen in mature T-cell neoplasms, may also be found in reactive T-cell populations.
CD8	A dimeric membrane glycoprotein which binds to MHC class I protein.	Expressed by cytotoxic/suppressor T cells (20–30% of peripheral blood T lymphocytes), some NK cells and splenic sinusoidal lining cells.
CD10	Surface metalloendopeptidase expressed by a wide variety of cell types including lymphoblasts, normal germinal centre cells, fibroblasts, some epithelial cells and myoepithelial cells.	Expressed by ALL, FL, BL, some DLBCL and follicular T-helper cell lymphomas. A proportion of epithelium-derived tumours and endometrial stromal cell sarcomas may also be positive.
CD11c	CD11c is a member of the integrin family of adhesion proteins and is expressed strongly by normal monocytes and weakly by myeloid cells.	HCL is characterised by relatively high expression of CD11c in paraffin-embedded sections. Macrophages are also highlighted. Normal myeloid cells are usually negative in paraffin-embedded materials.
CD15	Identifies X-hapten, a membrane-related carbohydrate antigen expressed on normal mature granulocytes, promyelocytes and a subset of macrophages/monocytes but not by lymphoid cells. Is also expressed by some epithelial cells.	Expressed on Reed-Sternberg cells in the majority of cases of classical HL, some leukaemias and occasionally by other lymphomas. Is difficult to interpret in marrow due to the staining of normal myeloid cells. Adenocarcinomas are also commonly positive for CD15.
CD20	A non-glycosylated phosphoprotein expressed on B cells (late precursor and most mature B cells but not normal plasma cells). It is the target for rituximab and other anti-CD20 directed therapies.	Immunoreactivity is seen in B-cell lymphomas although there may be loss of positivity following treatment with CD20-directed therapy. L&H cells are uniformly positive. Weak expression may be seen in classical HL and aberrant expression may be identified in T-cell lymphomas and MM.
CD21	Membrane glycoprotein which acts as the C3d complement receptor	Stains follicular dendritic cells strongly and B cells in some B-cell lymphomas weakly.
CD23	Low-affinity IgE receptor, which stains a proportion of follicular dendritic cells and normal mantle zone lymphocytes.	Positive in CLL/SLL although expression may be weak and confined to proliferation centres in some cases. Also stains a minority of FL, MZL and mediastinal DLBCL.
CD30	Membrane glycoprotein which acts as receptor for a TNF-like cytokine, CD30 ligand, and has a role in control of cell growth. Normally expressed by activated T and B cells. Up-regulated by EBV infection.	Reed-Sternberg cells in classical HL and cells of ALCL are strongly immunoreactive. May also be positive focally in a proportion of DLBCL, plasmablastic lymphoma and peripheral T-cell lymphoma. CD30-positive reactive immunoblasts may be mistaken for mononuclear Hodgkin cells.
CD33	A glycosylated transmembrane protein that is a member of the sialic acid-binding immunoglobulin-like lectin (Siglec). This antigen is expressed in the earliest myeloid progenitor cells and is present during myeloid and monocytic differentiation as well as in granulocytes and monocytes at low levels.	Helpful in distinguishing ALL from AML and in the diagnosis of myeloid sarcoma in tissue sections. A subgroup of ALL may however express CD33, and, therefore, this antibody should always be used as part of an extended panel of antibodies.

Antibody	Target	Reactivity in tumours
CD34	A transmembrane glycoprotein of unknown function expressed by haemopoietic stem cells, vascular endothelial cells and normal perivascular stromal dendritic cells.	Highlights blast cells in MDS and stains the cells of most cases of acute leukaemia. Also allows assessment of vascularity in the bone marrow. Many other tumours are immunoreactive for CD34 including Kaposi sarcoma and gastrointestinal stromal tumours (GIST).
CD42b	A glycoprotein co-factor involved in ristocetin-induced aggregation of platelets and in the binding of platelets to blood vessel walls. Expressed by normal megakaryocytes.	Useful for identifying megakaryocytes in extramedullary haemopoiesis and detecting micromegakaryocytes in trephine biopsy sections from patients with MDS.
CD45	Leucocyte common antigen. A high-molecular-weight glycoprotein present on the surface of most human leucocytes.	Useful in screening an undifferentiated tumour to confirm a haemopoietic origin. Some lymphomas, such as plasmablastic lymphoma, may be negative. CD45 is characteristically negative in classical HL although interpretation is often difficult due to surrounding positive lymphocytes.
CD56	A membrane glycoprotein, neural cell adhesion molecule (NCAM). Many normal cells stain with this antibody including neural cells and neuroendocrine cells throughout the body.	NK/T-cell lymphoma, some PTCL and gamma delta T-cell lymphoma are positive. Plasma cells in myeloma although positive on flow cytometry may be negative or show only weak positivity in trephine biopsy specimens. Neuroendocrine tumours such as small cell anaplastic carcinoma of lung and many other tumour types, for example, neuroblastoma, carcinoid tumours and endocrine tumours are positive.
CD57	A glycoprotein expressed by a subset of T cells and NK cells. Also expressed by neural (myelin-associated protein) and neuroendocrine tissues.	CD57 is expressed in approx. 80% of cases of T-LGL leukaemia. It also highlights the specialised T lymphocytes that form rosettes around the L&H cell of NLPHL. Usually negative in NK-cell neoplasms.
CD79a/b	The CD79 complex is a disulphide-linked heterodimer which is non-covalently linked to membrane-bound Ig on B cells. The CD79a component is expressed on pre-B cells, whilst CD79b is expressed by mature B lymphocytes and plasma cells.	Stains the majority of B-cell lymphomas including precursor lymphomas and some plasmacytomas. Is useful in establishing B lineage when CD20 is negative following anti-CD20 therapy. Aberrant expression may be seen in T-ALL.
CD99	Transmembrane glycoprotein encoded by the *MIC2* gene involved in regulation of interactions between intercellular adhesion molecules, T-cell aggregation and apoptosis. Is expressed by many different cell types including lymphocytes, stromal and epithelial cells.	CD99 is strongly expressed in a variety of malignant tumours including Ewing's sarcoma, T-ALL, myeloid sarcoma, small cell anaplastic carcinoma of lung and peripheral neuroectodermal tumours. Its main use is in the diagnosis of Ewing's sarcoma family of tumours in which there is strong cytoplasmic and surface positivity.
CD117	A transmembrane receptor with tyrosine kinase activity encoded by the *KIT* proto-oncogene and involved in haemopoiesis, gametogenesis and melanogenesis. It is expressed by normal melanocytes, early myeloid precursors, mast cells and various epithelial cells.	Useful in identifying the spindle-shaped mast cells in systemic mastocytosis and blast cells in some cases of MDS and AML. Gastrointestinal stromal tumours and a proportion of melanomas are also strongly positive.

Antibody	Target	Reactivity in tumours
CD123	Identifies the alpha subunit of the interleukin-3 receptor. Expressed by many normal haemopoietic cells.	Positive in 95% of HCL. Not expressed by the majority of cases of HCL-V. Is also useful in identifying plasmacytoid dendritic cells in tissue sections (e.g. in CMML) and in the diagnosis of cases of BPDCN.
CD138	A transmembrane glycoprotein expressed by immature B cells and plasma cells in addition to squamous and other epithelia.	Useful for identifying plasma cells in trephine biopsy specimens. CD138 however is not lineage specific and some carcinomas and melanomas are positive. The combination of CD138 immunoreactivity and plasmacytoid morphology in metastatic melanoma may lead to an erroneous diagnosis of myeloma.
CyclinD1	One of a family of proteins which function by regulating the activity of cyclin-dependent kinases in the G1 phase of the cell cycle. Stains the basal nuclei of normal epithelium and nuclei of vascular endothelial cells.	Nuclear immunoreactivity is seen in MCL and a proportion of cases of HCL and MM. Also positive in some undifferentiated carcinomas.
DBA44 (CD72)	An antibody raised against an unknown antigen on a centroblastic cell line which stains normal mantle zone B lymphocytes in reactive lymph nodes.	Positive, often only focally, in HCL but not specific as it also may be positive in HCL-V and SMZL. Useful when used as part of a panel of antibodies in the diagnosis of HCL.
Desmin	A 53 kDa intermediate filament protein which is a structural component of the sarcomeres in muscle cells.	Positive in tumours displaying muscle differentiation including leiomyoma, leiomyosarcoma and rhabdomyosarcoma.
EBV LMP-1	This antibody recognises EBV latent membrane protein-1 which is expressed in the cytoplasm and on the membrane of EBV-infected cells exhibiting latency pattern II or III.	Stains the HRS cells in most cases of EBV+ classical HL and PTLPD. Does not stain EBV+ BL as the latter displays latency program I. Staining may be focal and weak. *In situ* hybridisation for EBV-encoded RNAs (EBERs) is more sensitive and is positive in all latency patterns.
Glycophorin C (CD236R)	A red cell membrane glycoprotein important for maintaining red cell mechanical stability.	Helpful for identifying erythroid precursors in trephine biopsy specimens. Also useful for identifying foci of extramedullary erythropoiesis in spleen and lymph nodes.
Granzyme B	A serine protease present in the cytotoxic granules of NK cells and cytotoxic T cells.	Granzyme B immunoreactivity is seen in extranodal NK/T-cell lymphomas, some PTCLs and T-LGL leukaemia.
Ki-67	A nuclear antigen expressed by cells in all active parts of the cell cycle but not by resting cells (G0). Is expressed by all human cell types.	Useful for the determination of the proliferation fraction in a population of tumour cells. Higher Ki-67 positivity is correlated with the clinical behaviour of various lymphomas and approaches 100% in Burkitt lymphoma.
MUM1	Multiple Myeloma Oncogene-1 is a member of the interferon regulatory factor family (IRF4) and plays a role in gene expression in response to interferons. Normally expressed (in the nucleus) by late germinal centre B cells, plasma cells, activated T cells and some melanomas.	Is used alongside CD10 and BCL6 in the classification of germinal centre and activated B-cell sub-classification of DLBCL (positive in the latter but not in the former). Is expressed strongly by HRS cells in classical HL but not usually by the L&H cells of NLPHL. Is strongly positive in plasmacytoma/myeloma and also in some PTCL and ALCL.

Antibody	Target	Reactivity in tumours
MyoD1	MyoD1 encodes a nuclear phosphoprotein transcription factor that induces myogenesis. Nuclear expression is seen only in tissue of skeletal muscle derivation. Mature skeletal muscle cells are usually negative.	The detection of nuclear positivity for MyoD1 is a useful pointer to myogenic differentiation and helps differentiate rhabdomyosarcomas from precursor lymphomas and other small round 'blue cell tumours'. Cytoplasmic staining is a non-specific finding and does not imply a myogenic origin.
NB84a	Anti−neuroblastoma is a monoclonal antibody produced by using neuroblastoma tissue as a source of antigen. This antigen is present in a variety of normal epithelial and endothelial cells.	Positive in 90% of all neuroblastomas and 50% of cases of Ewing sarcoma, 20–40% of Ewing sarcoma family tumours, but not other tumour types, such as leukaemia and other childhood sarcomas.
NSE	Neurone-specific enolase is a glycolytic enzyme found in both central and peripheral neural cells, neuroendocrine cells and their tumours. The antibody is directed against R−enolase.	Sensitive marker of neuroendocrine cells but lacks specificity as it is expressed by a large number of cell types due to cross-reactivity with other more widely distributed enolases. Strongly expressed by neuroblastoma, small cell carcinoma and carcinoid tumours.
PD-1 (CD279)	Programmed death-1 is a co-inhibitory receptor involved in lymphocyte activation. Is normally expressed in pro-B cells and germinal centre-associated T helper cells.	Is expressed in some T-cell lymphomas (particularly AITL), CLL/SLL, T cells in T-cell-rich B-cell lymphoma and the T cells of NLPHL.
S100	A family of low-molecular-weight proteins expressed by Schwann cells, melanocytes, chondrocytes, adipocytes, Langerhans cells and interdigitating reticulum cells of lymph nodes.	Useful for recognition of metastatic melanoma in marrow or nodes and is also positive in LCH, interdigitating reticulum cell sarcoma and sarcomas of neural derivation. It also stains the histiocytes of Rosai-Dorfman disease.
TRAP	Antibody directed against tartrate-resistant alkaline phosphatase, an enzyme normally expressed at high level by osteoclasts, activated macrophages and neurones.	Histochemical techniques were initially used for assessment of TRAP activity in HCL but this has been superseded by immunohistochemistry. Although high levels are seen in HCL, the stain is not specific as SMZL and HCL-V may be positive. Histiocytes and osteoclasts in tissue sections are also strongly positive. Should be used as part of a panel of antibodies.

AITL, angioimmunoblastic T-cell lymphoma; ALCL, anaplastic large cell lymphoma; ALL, acute lymphoblastic leukaemia/lymphoma; AML, acute myeloid leukaemia; BL, Burkitt lymphoma; BPDCN, blastic plasmacytoid dendritic cell neoplasm; CMML, chronic myelomonocytic leukaemia; CNS, central nervous system; DLBCL, diffuse large B-cell lymphoma; EBV, Epstein-Barr virus; FL, follicular lymphoma; HCL, hairy cell leukaemia; HCL-V, hairy cell leukaemia variant; HL, Hodgkin lymphoma; HRS, Hodgkin Reed-Sternberg; Ig, immunoglobulin; L&H cells, 'lymphocytic and histiocytic cells' − the neoplastic cells of NLPHL; LCH, Langerhans cell histiocytosis; MCL, mantle cell lymphoma; MDS, myelodysplastic syndrome/s; MF, mycosis fungoides; MM, multiple myeloma; MZL, marginal zone lymphoma; NK, natural killer; NLPHL, nodular lymphocyte predominant Hodgkin lymphoma; PTCL, peripheral T-cell lymphoma; PTLPD, post-transplant lymphoproliferative disorder; SLL, small lymphocytic lymphoma; SMZL, splenic marginal zone lymphoma; T-LGL, T-cell large granular lymphocytic leukaemia; TNF, tumour necrosis factor.

Flow Cytometry Antibodies

Monoclonal and other antibodies used in flow cytometric immunophenotyping of cells in peripheral blood, bone marrow, cerebrospinal fluid or effusions, showing specificity of reactions though some reference to expression in related tissues is described.

Antibody	Expression
FLAER	Fluorochrome-linked proaerolysin; detects glycosylphosphatidylinositol (GPI) anchor in normal blood cells; is not able to bind to PNH neutrophils
FMC7	An antibody detecting a conformational epitope of CD20; expression therefore tends to correlate with intensity of CD20; CD20^{dim} or negative neoplasms tend to be FMC7 negative; expressed by normal mature B cells and most neoplastic mature B cells but not by CLL cells or precursor B-cell neoplasms
HLA-DR	Human leucocyte antigen DR; expressed by haemopoietic stem cells, myeloblasts, B cells, activated T cells, NK cells, monocytes and plasmacytoid dendritic cells; expressed in some cases of myeloma and plasmacytomas but not by normal mature plasma cells; expressed by neoplastic cells of most AML, all B-lineage ALL and a minority of T-lineage ALL; some mature T-cell neoplasms are positive; activated T-cells seen as a reaction to viral infection are frequently HLA-DR positive
CD1a	Expressed by normal cortical thymocytes, dendritic cells and Langerhans cells. Expressed by some T-lineage ALL, indicating a cortical thymocyte phenotype
CD2	Expressed by T cells including neoplastic T cells and by most NK cells; may be aberrantly expressed in AML and mature B-cell neoplasms; expressed in systemic mastocytosis and in some cases of blastic plasmacytoid dendritic cell neoplasm

Antibody	Expression
CD3	Expressed by T cells, T-lineage ALL, mature T-cell lymphomas and MPAL and is highly lineage specific; expression may be cytoplasmic or surface membrane
CD4	Expressed by a normal T-cell subset, monocytes/macrophages, some T-ALL, most T-lineage lymphomas, blastic plasmacytoid dendritic cell neoplasm, systemic mastocytosis and some AML subtypes
CD5	Expressed by T cells including neoplastic T cells and a subpopulation of normal B cells; usually expressed by neoplastic cells in CLL and mantle cell lymphoma and rarely in marginal zone lymphomas and diffuse large B-cell lymphoma
CD7	Expressed by normal T cells and in T-ALL; expression is often lost in neoplasms of mature T cells but is usually retained in T-prolymphocytic leukaemia; expression may be lost or weak in activated reactive T cells.
CD8	Expressed by a T-cell subset, some T-ALL, most LGLLs and a minority of other T-lineage lymphomas
CD10	Germinal centre B Cells, pre B cells and neutrophils. Expressed in many cases of B-lineage ALL (hence 'common ALL antigen'), more weakly expressed in some T-lineage ALL; expressed in follicular lymphoma, germinal centre-derived diffuse large B-cell lymphoma and most cases of Burkitt lymphoma; expressed by T cells of angioimmunoblastic T-cell lymphoma.
CD11c	Expressed by neutrophils, monocytes, NK cells, hairy cells, SMZL and neoplastic mast cells
CD13	Expressed on granulocytes and granulocyte and monocyte progenitors; expressed in most AML and aberrantly in some ALL

Antibody	Expression
CD14	Expressed on mature monocytes and more weakly by neutrophils; expressed in AML with monocytic differentiation; being GPI anchored, expression is lost in PNH
CD15	Expressed by many monocytes and more weakly by most neutrophils; often expressed in M2 AML and AML with monocytic differentiation; expressed by Hodgkin and Reed-Sternberg cells; can be expressed by non-haemopoietic cells
CD16	Expressed by NK cells, monocytes, neutrophils and some T cells; not expressed by PNH neutrophils; expressed in some AML, particularly with monocytic differentiation; expressed in aggressive NK-cell leukaemia/lymphoma and some cases of nasal-type NK-cell leukaemia lymphoma
CD19	Expressed by B cells and normal plasma cells but typically not myeloma cells; expressed in most B-ALL and neoplasms of mature B cells; aberrantly expressed in some AML subtypes
CD20	Expressed by normal and neoplastic mature B cells, expression is weak in CLL; expressed in a proportion of B-lineage ALL; not usually expressed by plasma cells but may be expressed in cyclin D1-positive myeloma
CD21	Expressed by a subset of mature B cells, in most cases of CLL and in some B-lineage NHL
CD22	Expressed as a surface membrane antigen by mature B cells and in the cytoplasm of some B-cell precursors; cytoplasmic expression is seen in most B-lineage ALL; membrane expression is seen in mature B-cell lymphomas but expression in CLL is weak
CD23	Weakly expressed by less than half of normal mature B cells; expressed by CLL cells and much less often expressed in B-NHL
CD24	Expressed on B lymphocytes and precursors and by neutrophils and eosinophils; expressed in B-NHL and ALL; being GPI anchored, expression is lost in PNH
CD25	Expressed by activated T and B cells and in hairy cell leukaemia, ATLL and systemic mastocytosis
CD26	Expressed by some T cells, B cells and NK cells; on normal T cells there is a range of expression, whereas neoplastic T cells can show uniform expression or lack of expression
CD30	Expressed by activated B and T cells, by Reed-Sternberg and Hodgkin cells and in anaplastic large cell lymphoma, some peripheral T-cell lymphomas, plasmablastic lymphoma and primary effusion lymphoma
CD33	Expressed on myeloblasts, promyelocytes and myelocytes; expressed in most cases of AML; may be aberrantly expressed in ALL
CD34	Expressed by haemopoietic stem cells, lymphoid stem cells, myeloblasts and proerythroblasts; usually expressed in AML and B-lineage ALL and often in T-lineage ALL
CD38	Expressed on haemopoietic stem cells and early B and T cells, monocytes; an activation marker in many cell types; often expressed in AML and ALL; expressed by plasma cells and myeloma cells
CD41	Platelet glycoprotein IIb/IIa, expressed on platelets and megakaryocytes
CD42	Platelet glycoprotein Ib/IXa, expressed on platelets and megakaryocytes
CD45	Common leucocyte antigen; usually expressed on all leucocytes, both normal and neoplastic; weak expression is often a feature of AML and ALL; occasionally there is failure of expression in ALL; non-haemopoietic tumours are CD45 negative
CD56	Normally expressed by NK cells and a small subset of T cells; expressed in NK-cell and some mature T-cell neoplasms and in some T-ALL; often expressed by neoplastic monocytes, both in AML and, particularly, in CMML; not expressed by normal plasma cells, usually expressed by myeloma cells but not expressed by circulating cells in plasma cell leukaemia; expressed in plasmacytoid dendritic cell neoplasm; may be expressed in non-haematological neoplasms such as neuroblastoma and small cell carcinoma of the lung
CD57	Expressed on NK cells and subsets of T and B cells; usually expressed in T-cell LGLL and sometimes in NK-cell LGLL
CD64	Expressed by monocytes and their progenitors; expressed in AML with monocytic differentiation
CD66b	Expressed by normal neutrophils, but being GPI anchored, expression is lost in PNH
CD79b	Expressed by mature B cells including most neoplastic mature B cells but expression is lost or very weak in CLL
CD103	Expressed by intraepithelial T lymphocytes and a very low percentage of circulating T cells; expressed in hairy cell leukaemia, enteropathy-associated T-cell lymphoma and ATLL
CD117	Expressed by haemopoietic precursors, myeloblasts, promyelocytes and mast cells (typically strong expression); expressed in AML, systemic mastocytosis and in some cases of multiple myeloma; can be expressed by non-haemopoietic tumours

Antibody	Expression
CD123	Variably expressed on haemopoietic stem cells, eosinophils, monocytes, megakaryocytes and B-lymphocytes but not T-lymphocytes or neutrophils; expressed in hairy cell leukaemia, most cases of AML, blastic plasmacytoid dendritic cell neoplasm and B-lineage ALL
CD138	Expressed by plasma cells including myeloma cells, by the cells of primary effusion lymphoma, plasmablastic lymphoma and in some cases of NHL
Cyclin D1	Expressed in the nucleus during stage G1 of the cell cycle in some cell types but expression is not detected in normal lymphoid or haemopoietic cells; nuclear expression in mantle cell lymphoma and in about a fifth of cases of multiple myeloma

Antibody	Expression
MPO	Myeloperoxidase, a cytoplasmic antigen defining myeloid lineage; also expressed in MPAL
TdT	Terminal deoxynucleotidyl transferase: a nuclear antigen expressed by early T- and B-lineage cells; expressed in the majority of cases of B-lineage and T-lineage ALL and in a minority of cases of AML, particularly those with little maturation

Abbreviations: ALL, acute lymphoblastic leukaemia; AML, acute myeloid leukaemia; ATLL, adult T-cell leukaemia/lymphoma; CLL, chronic lymphocytic leukaemia; CMML, chronic myelomonocytic leukaemia; GPI, glycosylphosphatidylinositol; LGLL, large granular lymphocyte leukaemia; MPAL, mixed phenotype acute leukaemia; NHL, non-Hodgkin lymphoma; PNH, paroxysmal nocturnal haemoglobinuria; SMZL, splenic marginal zone lymphoma.

Molecular Terminology

Abbreviation	Gene	Location
ABL1	Abelson oncogene	9q34
AFF1	AF4/FMR2 family member 1	4q21
ALK	Anaplastic lymphoma kinase	2p23
BCL2	B cell lymphoma 2	18q21
BCL6	B cell lymphoma 6	3q27
BCR	Breakpoint cluster region	22q11
CALR	Calreticulin	19p13
CCND1	Cyclin D1	11q13
CDKN2A	Cyclin-dependent kinase inhibitor 2A	9p21
CDKN2B	Cyclin-dependent kinase inhibitor 2B	9p21
DKC1	Dyskeratosis congenita 1, dyskerin	Xq28
FANCA	Fanconi anaemia complementation group A	16q24
EVI1	Ecotropic virus integration site 1	3q26
ETV6	ETS variant 6	5q31-33
EWSR1	Ewing sarcoma gene	22q12
FLT3	FMS like tyrosine kinase 3	13q12
FIP1L1	FIP1 like 1	4q12
FGFR1	Fibroblast growth factor receptor 1	8p11
FGFR3	Fibroblast growth factor receptor 3	4p16
FLI1	Fli-1 proto-oncogene	11q24
GP1BA	Glycoprotein 1b alpha	17p13
HOX11 (TLX1*)	Homeobox gene 11	10q24
HOX11L2 (TLX3*)	Homeobox gene 11 L2	5q35
IGH	Immunoglobulin heavy chain locus	14q32
IGK	Immunoglobulin light chainkappa locus	2p12
IGL	Immunoglobulin light chainlambda locus	22q11
JAK2	Janus kinase 2	9p24
KIT	Stem cell factor receptor, CD117	4q12
MKL1	Megakaryocyte leukaemia 1	22q13

Abbreviation	Gene	Location
MLL(KMT2A*)	Mixed lineage leukaemia	11q23
MLLT10	Mixed lineage leukaemia translocated to 10	10p12
MLLT3	Mixed lineage leukaemia translocated to 3	9p22
MPL	Myeloproliferative leukaemia virus oncogene	1p34
MYC	Myc oncogene	8q24
NPM1	Nucleophosmin 1	5q35
NOTCH1	NOTCH1	9q34
PCM1	Pericentriolar material 1	8p22-p21.3
PDGRFA	Platelet-derived growth factor alpha	4q12
PDGRFB	Platelet-derived growth factor beta	12p12
PICALM	Phosphatidylinositol binding clathrin assembly protein	11q14
PML	Promyelocytic leukaemia	15q22
RARA	Retinoic acid receptor alpha	17q21
RBM15	RNA binding motif protein 15	1p13
RUNX1	Runt-related transcription factor	8q22
RUNX1T1	Runt-related transcription factor translocated to 1	21q22
STAT3	Signal transducer and activation of transcription 3	17q21
TAL1	T-cell acute lymphocytic leukaemia 1	1p32
TCRalpha (TRA*)	T-cell receptor alpha locus	14q11
TCRbeta (TRB*)	T-cell receptor beta locus	7q34
TCRdelta (TRD*)	T-cell receptor delta locus	14q11
TCRgamma (TRG*)	T-cell receptor gamma locus	7p15
TERC	Telomerase RNA component	3q26
TERT	Telomerase reverse transcriptase	5p15
WAS	Wiskott-Aldrich syndrome	Xp11.4-11.21

*Human Genome Project Nomenclature Committee approved name for gene or locus.

Classification of Cases According to Diagnosis

Myeloproliferative neoplasms

Cases 12, 25, 37, 64 and 78.

Myeloid and lymphoid neoplasms with eosinophilia and abnormalities of PDGRFA, PDGRFB or FGFR1

Cases 15 and 49.

Myelodysplastic/myeloproliferative neoplasms

Cases 9, 15 and 29.

Myelodysplastic syndromes

Cases 32, 67 and 80.

Acute myeloid leukaemia and related precursor neoplasms

Cases 3, 8, 12, 18, 22, 29, 32, 41, 47, 54, 57, 62, 64, 67, 72, 74, 76, 78, 85, 89, 91, 94 and 95.

Acute leukaemias of ambiguous lineage

Cases 61 and 82.

Precursorlymphoid neoplasms

Cases 36, 37, 45, 51, 70, 85, 87 and 97.

Mature B-cell neoplasms

Cases 2, 6, 10, 11, 14, 20, 23, 26, 28, 31, 33, 39, 40, 43, 46, 48, 53, 60, 77, 79, 81, 84, 90, 92, 96, 98, 99 and 100.

Plasma cell neoplasms

Cases 4, 19, 24, 52, 57, 65 and 69.

Mature T- and NK-cell neoplasms

Cases 1, 17, 34, 38, 55, 56, 58, 66, 68, 75 and 83.

Hodgkin lymphoma

Case 90.

Immunodeficiency-associated lymphoproliferative disorders

Cases 55 and 86.

Platelet disorders

Cases 7, 27 and 63.

Red cell disorders

Cases 16, 30, 59 and 71.

Marrow aplasia

Case 42.

Non-haemopoietic tumours

Cases 13, 35, 44, 73 and 93.

Reactive phenomena

Cases 5, 21, 30, 45, 50 and 88.

Index

Note: Please note that Page numbers in *italic* refers to figures.

acquired pure red cell aplasia
(PRCA), 194–5
acute EBV infection, *104*, 104–5, *105*
acute erythroid leukaemia
(erythroleukaemia), 189–92
acute erythrovirus infection, 59–61
acute kidney injury, hypercalcaemia with,
15–17
acute leukaemia (AL), 217
mixed phenotype, 300–5
acute lymphoblastic leukaemia (ALL), 116
CD20 expression in, 181
ETP ALL, 323
identification of, 181
immunophenotype, 181
isochromosome (9q), 181
Pro-B ALL, 128, 161
T-ALL, 307, 323
acute monoblastic leukaemia
CD14 detection, 13
CD14/CD64, *102, 103*
CD56, 103, *103*
dysplastic neutrophils, 100
with t(9:11)(p22;q23), *11–13*, 11–14
acute monocytic leukaemia, 27–30
acute myeloid leukaemia (AML), 65–7
accurate MRD assessment, 334–7
CD19 and CD7 expression, 260–5
lymphadenopathy and mediastinal mass,
260–5
with maturation (NK/myeloid type),
276–80
with myelodysplasia-related changes,
110–13, 284–8
myeloid sarcoma, 269–73
NPM1 and *FLT3* ITD mutations, 327–9,
351–4
with ring chromosome 18, 144–5
with t(3;3)(q21;q26.2), 129–31
with t(8;21), 227–31
therapy-related, 315–18
without maturation, 145, 327–9

acute promyelocytic leukaemia, 77–9
with CNS relapse, 166–7
acute undifferentiated leukaemia (AUL), 217
ADAMTS13 enzyme, 157, 158
aggressive systemic mastocytosis (ASM),
87–9
AL, *see* acute leukaemia (AL)
ALK, *see* anaplastic large cell lymphoma (ALK)
ALK-positive diffuse large B-cell lymphoma,
375–80
ALL, *see* acute lymphoblastic leukaemia (ALL)
all-*trans*-retinoic acid (ATRA), 166
AML, *see* acute myeloid leukaemia (AML)
amyloid, 234
anaplastic large cell lymphoma (ALK-positive)
CD2 staining for, 3, *4*
CD3 expression in, 2, *3*
CD30 staining for, 3, *5*
CD45 expression in, 2, *3*
CT imaging, 1, *1*
CXR, 1, *1*
FSC/SSC analysis, 2, *3*
H&E-stained core biopsy, 3
pleural fluid cell count, 1–3, *2–3*
t(2;5)(p23;q35) translocation, 4
angioimmunoblastic T-cell lymphoma,
119–21
anthracycline, 166
antibodies
flow cytometry, 386–8
immunohistochemistry studies, 381–5
aplastic anaemia, 146–50
Asian and Western sub-type lymphoma, 170,
340, 341

bacterial infections, 177–8
B-cell lymphoblastic leukaemia/lymphoma,
acute, 325–6
B-cell lymphoma
intravascular, 338–41
splenic B-cell lymphoma/leukaemia
unclassifiable (BCLU), 35–8, 136–9

B-cell lymphoproliferative disorder, 91
B-cell prolymphocytic leukaemia (B-PLL),
151–3
BCL2, 38
BCL6, 38
BCR-ABL1, 44
BEAM conditioning, 197
Bernard–Soulier syndrome (BSS),
24–6
platelet aggregation, 24, *25*
blastic NK-cell lymphoma, *see* blastic
plasmacytoid dendritic cell neoplasm
(BPDCN)
blastic plasmacytoid dendritic cell neoplasm
(BPDCN), 204–5
blastoid mantle cell lymphoma, 289–91
B/myeloid leukaemia, 300–5
bone marrow metastasis, 49, 158, 342–6
Burkitt lymphoma, 38, 114–16, 370–4

CD4+CD56+ haematodermic neoplasm, *see*
blastic plasmacytoid dendritic cell
neoplasm (BPDCN)
CD5-negative chronic lymphocytic leukaemia,
215
CD8 lymphocytosis, 20
CD236R, 190
chronic eosinophilic leukaemia, 172–6
chronic lymphocytic leukaemia (CLL), 41, 91,
183–5, 213–15
diffuse large B-cell lymphoma in, 281–3
Hodgkin lymphoma in, 330–3
with low CLL score, 310–14
trisomy 12 with atypical morphology,
310–14
chronic myeloid leukaemia (CML), 43–5
lymphoid blast phase, 292–6
chronic myelomonocytic leukaemia (CMML),
31–3, 31–4
with eosinophilia, 54–8
chronic obstructive pulmonary disease, 227
chylous pleural effusion, 9

Practical Flow Cytometry in Haematology: 100 Worked Examples, First Edition. Mike Leach,
Mark Drummond, Allyson Doig, Pam McKay, Bob Jackson and Barbara J. Bain.
© 2015 John Wiley & Sons, Ltd. Published 2015 by John Wiley & Sons, Ltd.

CLL, *see* chronic lymphocytic leukaemia (CLL)
Coombs-positive haemolytic anaemia, 338–41
cortical type T-cell lymphoblastic lymphoma, 359–64
cryoglobulins, 71
cutaneous T-cell lymphoma (CTCL), 236
cyclophosphamide/thalidomide/dexamethasone (CTD), 266–8
cytopenias, 23
cytospin, 266–8

de novo plasma cell leukaemia, 15–17
del(13q), 85
diffuse large B-cell lymphoma (DLBCL), 240
   activated B-cell subtype, 106–8
   ALK-positive, 375–80
   B-cell lymphoma, unclassifiable, 365–9
   CD10 CD10/HLA-DR, 7, *8*
   CD19+ B cells, 7, *8*
   chronic lymphocytic leukaemia, 281–3
   chylous pleural effusion, *9*
   CT scan, 6
   cytospin preparation, 6, *7*
   with germinal centre phenotype, 95–9
   intravascular large B-cell lymphoma, 168–71
   isolated lower spinal cord and intraconal CNS relapse, 297–9
   pleural fluid LDH, 6
   reactive pleural effusion, 80–1
disseminated intravascular coagulation (DIC), 79, 155
DLBCL, *see* diffuse large B-cell lymphoma (DLBCL)
double-hit lymphoma, 38
dual-energy X-ray absorptiometry (DEXA) scan, 230
dyskeratosis congenita (DKC), 148

EBV viraemia, 247
eosin-5-maleimide (EMA) binding studies, 210, 211
eosinophilia, chronic myelomonocytic leukaemia with, 54–8
eosinophilic leukaemia, 172–6
Epstein-Barr virus (EBV), 18–20, *18–20*
Epstein–Barr virus (EBV)
   HHV8 infection with, 108
erythrodermic mycosis fungoides, 236–9
erythrophagocytosis, 95
essential thrombocythaemia (ET), 218–22
EUTOS score, 45
EVI1, 130, 131
Ewing sarcoma, of tibia, 342–6
extracorporeal photopheresis, 236

FANCA gene, 148
Fanconi anaemia, 148
FIP1L1-PDGRFA, 57
FIP1L1-PDGRFA-associated chronic eosinophilic eukaemia, 172–6

FLT3-ITD mutation, 217
fludarabine therapy, chronic lymphocytic leukaemia, 330–33
follicular lymphoma (FL), 9
   in leukaemic phase, 163–5
   trephine biopsy, 98–9

Glanzmann thrombasthenia, 225–6
glycophorin C, 190
glycoprotein (Gp) expression, 224
GpIb-IX-V complex, 25

haematogones, 160–2
haemophagocytic syndrome, secondary, 244–8
haemophagocytosis, 198, *198*
   reactive, intravascular large B-cell lymphoma, 338–41
hairy cell leukaemia (HCL), 21–3, 139, 355–8
hereditary spherocytosis (HS), 105, 210, 212
Hodgkin lymphoma, chronic lymphocytic leukaemia with, 330–33
Howell–Jolly bodies, 104
human herpesvirus 8 (HHV8), 108
human immunodeficiency virus (HIV), 116
human T-cell lymphotropic virus 1 (HTLV-1), 274–5
hydroxycarbamide therapy, 218
hypercalcaemia, with acute kidney injury, 15–17
hypoplastic MDS, 148

IgA multiple myeloma, 183–5
IgG Donath–Landsteiner antibody, 60
IGH
   gene mutation, 153
   translocation, 85
IgM, 72
IgM paraprotein, 142
immunoglobulin G (IgG), 70, 73
indolent mantle cell leukaemia, 90–2
   CD5 expression, 91, *92*
   cyclin D1 expression, 91, *92*
infantile acute megakaryoblastic leukaemia, 347–50
intravascular large B-cell lymphoma (IVBCL), 168–71, 338–41
inv(14)(q11.2q32), 64
iron deficiency, 256–9

JAK2 mutation, 32, 33, 57, 221

large granular lymphocytes (LGLs), 132
leucoerythroblastic changes, 87, 154
leukaemia, *see Specific types*
lymphadenopathy, and mediastinal mass, AML, 260–5
lymphoid blast phase, chronic myeloid leukaemia, 292–6
lymphoplasmacytic lymphoma (LPL), 70–3, 72, 140–2

macrothrombocytopenia, 26
mantle cell lymphoma (MCL), 39–42
   meningeal relapse of blastoid, 289–91
marginal zone lymphoma (MZL), 41, 51–3, 91
   CD20 expression, 51, *52*
   CD21 expression, *53*
mast cell disease, 88
mastoiditis, 269–73
megakaryoblastic leukaemia, infantile acute, 347–50
meningeal and cutaneous relapse, of cortical-T lymphoblastic lymphoma, 253–5
meningeal relapse, of blastoid mantle cell lymphoma, 289–91
meningococcal septicaemia, 177–9
metastatic neuroblastoma, with bone marrow involvement, 122–5
microangiopathic haemolytic anaemia, 158
minimal residual disease (MRD) levels, 334–7
mixed lineage leukaemia *(MLL)* gene, 13
mixed phenotype acute leukaemia (MPAL), 217, 320–24
MLL gene, 13
molecular terminology, 389
monoblastic leukaemias, 12
monoclonal gammopathy of undetermined significance (MGUS), 68–9
monocytopenia, 23
monomorphic B-cell post-transplant lymphoproliferative disorder, 319–20
mucinous adenocarcinoma, 154–8
multiple myeloma (MM), 72, 266–8
   with blastoid morphology, 82–6
   CD20, 252
   CD38 expression, *85*
   CD45 expression, *84*
   CD56 expression, *86*
   CD138 expression, *85*
   IgM, 249–52
MYC rearrangement, 38, 85
   Burkitt lymphoma, 115, 116
mycosis fungoides (MF), 206, 208–9
   erythrodermic, 236–9
   with nodal involvement, 238
myelodysplastic syndromes (MDS)
   and associated monosomy 7, 319–20
   therapy-related, 240–3
myeloid hyperplasia, 202, *203*
myeloid sarcoma, 269–73

necrosis, focal, 196, *196*
necrotising lymphadenitis, 19
nephrotic syndrome, 233
neuroblastoma, metastatic, 125
neutropenia, 23
NK-cell leukaemia, 244–8
nodal marginal zone lymphoma, 50–3
non-haemopoietic tumour, 266–8
NPM1 and *FLT3* ITD mutation, 327–9
   acute myeloid leukaemia with, 351–4

p190 *BCR-ABL1*, 57
p210 *BCR-ABL1*, 57
panhypopituitarism, 130
paroxysmal nocturnal haemoglobinuria,
    256–9
parvovirus B19 infection, 59–61
PDGFRA, 57
peripheral T-cell lymphoma, 120
peripheral T-cell lymphoma, not otherwise
    specified (PTCL-NOS), 197, 199–200,
    200
    with nodal involvement, 306–9
PKC412, 89
plasma cell leukaemia, 15–17
    CD56 expression in, *16*
    proteinaceous staining, *16*
plasmacytoid dendritic cells (plasmacytoid
    monocytes), 204
platelet aggregation studies, 225
pleural effusion, diffuse large B-cell
    lymphoma, 80–1, 266–8
pleural metastasis, 266–8
PML-RARA, 78, 167
polychromasia, *154*
polyclonal B-cell lymphocytosis, 74–6
post-transplant lymphoproliferative disorder
    (PTLD), 194–5
    monomorphic, 319–20
pregnancy, 224
    Glanzmann thrombasthenia, 225–6
primary AL amyloidosis, 232–4
pro-B acute lymphoblastic leukaemia, 126–8
    prominent haematogones with, 162
programmed death 1 (PD-1), 119, *120*
prominent haematogones, 160–2
properdin deficiency, 179
pseudo-Chédiak-Higashi granules, 327

R-CHOP chemotherapy, 240
reactive T-cell lymphocytosis, and whooping
    cough, 325–6
relapsed follicular lymphoma, in leukaemic
    phase, 163–5
reticulin fibrosis, 23, *23*
Richter transformation/Richter syndrome,
    330–3
RUNX1, 130

secondary haemophagocytic syndrome,
    244–8
severe aplastic anaemia, 146–50
Sézary syndrome, 238–9
small cell carcinoma, 46–9
    CD45, 47
spherocytosis, 61, 105
spleen rupture, 18
splenectomy, for hereditary spherocytosis,
    105
splenic B-cell lymphoma/leukaemia
    unclassifiable, 136–9
splenic marginal zone lymphoma (SMZL),
    139, 186–8
STAT3 mutations, 135
superior vena cava (SVC) obstruction, 35
systemic mastocytosis (SM), CD25 expression,
    229
systemic mastocytosis with associated clonal
    haematological non-mast cell lineage
    disease (SM-AHNMD), 230–31

t(3;3)(q21;q26.2), 129–31
t(4;11)(q21;q23), 127, 128
t(4;14)(p16;q32), 84, 85
t(9;11)(p22;q23), 11
t(11;14)(q13;q32), 91

t(14;14)(q11.2;q32), 64
t(14;16)(q32;q23), 85
t(15;17)(q22;q12), 78
T lymphoblastic lymphoma, 253–5
tartrate-resistant alkaline phosphatase
    (TRAP), 138
T-cell large granular lymphocytic leukaemia,
    132–5
T-cell lymphoblastic lymphoma, 359–64
T-cell lymphoma
    HTLV-1 associated, 274–5
    peripheral, not otherwise specified, 306–9
T-cell receptor gamma, 132
TCR gene rearrangements, 135
therapy-related acute myeloid leukaemia
    (t-AML), 315–18
therapy-related myelodysplastic syndrome
    (t-MDS), 240–3
thrombocytosis, 34
thrombotic thrombocytopenic purpura
    (TTP), 154, 157
T-LGL leukaemia, with acquired pure red cell
    aplasia, 193–5
TP53, 153
T-prolymphocytic leukaemia (T-PLL), 62–4
tryptase IHC, 228
tyrosine kinase inhibitors (TKI), 43, 45

von Willebrand factor, 25

Waldenström macroglobulinaemia, 142
WAS gene mutation, 93–4
Whooping cough, and reactive T-cell
    lymphocytosis, 325–6
Wiskott–Aldrich syndrome (WAS), 94

X-linked thrombocytopenia, 93–4